Cytopathology of the Uterine Cervix

Alexander Meisels, MD, FRCPC
Professor of Pathology
Head, Department of Pathology and Cytology
Hôpital du Saint-Sacrement
Quebec City   Canada

Carol Morin, PhD
Clinical Professor of Pathology
Biologist, Department of Pathology
Hôpital du Saint-Sacrement
Quebec City   Canada

ASCP Press
American Society of Clinical Pathologists
Chicago

Acquisition & Development: Joshua Weikersheimer
Editor: Judy Hopping
Production Manager: Lisa Pollak
Production Coordinator: Michael Hudson

Technical Notes

All photomicrographs were taken using a Zeiss Photomicroscope on Kodak EPY film at a setting of 17 DIN. Magnifications (on the negatives) used for cytology were 63X, and for histology 10X and 20X. All cell preparations were stained with the Papanicolaou technique, as described in Chapter 14. Tissue sections were stained with hemalum-phloxine-saffron, as described in Chapter 15.

Electron microscopy was done with a Philips EM 300 and Hitachi H600-3 at a voltage of 80KV. Preparation of tissues and smears for EM examination was performed as described in Chapter 15. Staining and final magnification of EMs are indicated in the legend for each figure.

Chapter 15 also contains detailed information concerning the immunoperoxidase technique, in situ hybridization methods, and Southern and dot/blot techniques used herein.

Notice

Trade names and equipment and supplies described herein are included as suggestions only. In no way does their inclusion constitute an endorsement or preference by the American Society of Clinical Pathologists. The ASCP did not test the equipment, supplies, or procedures and, therefore, urges all readers to read and follow all manufacturers' instructions and package insert warnings concerning the proper and safe use of products.

Library of Congress Cataloging-in-Publication Data

Meisels, Alexander
    Cytopathology of the uterine cervix / by Alexander Meisels and Carol Morin; with the collaboration of Celine Bouchard . . . (et al)
    Includes bibliographical references.
    ISBN 0-89189-299-0
    1. Cervix uteri—Cytopathology. I. Morin, Carol. II. Title.
    [DNLM: 1. Cervix Uteri—pathology. WP 470 M515c]
RG310.M54   1990
681.1'4071—dc20
DNLM/DLC   90-309
for Library of Congress   CIP

Printed in Hong Kong by Everbest Printing Co Ltd.

95 94 93 92 91 5 4 3 2 1

⊚ Contents

▣ Tables

▣ Plates

Human Papillomavirus-Induced Changes

Squamous Intraepithelial Lesions

Invasive Squamous Carcinoma of the Cervix

Adenocarcinoma of the Cervix

The Gynecologic Smear

▣ Preface

This book was written with two readers in mind: 1. the student, either cytotechnologist or pathologist, who needs a complete source of information on one particular subject (ie, the cervix), and 2. the experienced pathologist or cytotechnologist who wants to look up a specific detail or wishes to read in more detail about some aspect of the cytopathology of the cervix. Because cytopathology deals with visual images and pattern recognition, illustrations are used generously throughout this volume, most of them in full color. It is, however, impossible to illustrate all the possible variations of cell patterns because their number is nearly infinite. The illustrations included here must therefore be considered as examples, as typical as possible, but by no means exhaustive, of the rich variety of visual patterns that can be appreciated through the microscope.

The only way to learn cytopathology is through experience. Cell patterns often seen before are registered in visual memory and recalled when a similar pattern is observed on a smear. This reliance on recalled patterns makes cytopathology a rather subjective science. The interpretation of cell patterns may vary from one observer to the other, and even the same observer may have a different interpretation at different times. This is true not only for cell spreads, but also for interpreting the subtle differences in certain histologic samples, for instance, in intraepithelial lesions of the cervix. Nevertheless, patient study of large collections of smears and tissue samples is essential, for it builds familiarity with established, recognised patterns. This book can only serve as a guide and a reference; it is no substitute for the microscope.

Cytopathology will detect significant lesions of the cervix if it is practised according to the state-of-the-art conditions outlined in this volume. However, it is only the first step in the process of diagnosis and treatment. The second step is often a tissue biopsy. We have therefore endeavored to illustrate the histologic presentation of many of the conditions that are detected on the smear.

The indispensable next step is treatment and adequate follow-up of all patients with significant cervical lesions. This is the responsibility of the gynecologist-colposcopist. In Chapter 11, two very experienced colposcopists, Céline Bouchard and Michel Fortier, from the Colposcopy Clinic of Hôpital du Saint-Sacrement Hospital, discuss the management of patients whose cervical lesions have been detected by cytopathology.

Techniques used in the cytology laboratory have evolved considerably from the time when all that was needed was the Papanicolaou staining method. At present, techniques such as electron microscopy, immunoperoxidase, molecular hybridization, and data processing are becoming ever more indispensable. We have therefore included two chapters with the practical details necessary to set up and use these modern techniques.

We were most fortunate to have the collaboration of two of the world's foremost experts in laboratory data processing. George Wied and Harvey Dytch, from the University of Chicago, who wrote Chapter 13: The Computerized Cytopathology Laboratory.

Nomenclature and reporting of cytologic findings has been a subject of much controversy. Chapter 2 is dedicated to this problem. We have adopted the *Bethesda System* throughout this volume.

This book was designed to be a practical guide to the complex domain of cervical cytopathology. We can only hope that the reader will find it useful.

◙ Acknowledgments

This work is based on the experience and knowledge of all members of the Department of Pathology and Cytology at Hôpital du Saint-Sacrement in Quebec City. Our thanks to all for their cooperation, patience, and support. Without our very competent staff of cyto-technologists and medical technologists, this book would not have been possible. Our special gratitude goes to Francine Parent, Louise Breton, and Michele Ward, who worked directly with us in various aspects of the preparation of the material included here.

CHAPTER ONE

The Normal Uterine Cervix

The cervix is the lower portion of the uterus, roughly cylindrical in shape and measuring about 3 cm in all directions. About half of its length protrudes into the vagina—the portio vaginalis (Figure 1.1). In general, the cervix points towards the posterior wall of the vagina, bending slightly just below its junction with the body of the uterus. However, there are many anatomic variations. Above the vagina, it is in close proximity with the ureters laterally, the bladder on its anterior aspect, and the rectum on its posterior side, where the peritoneum dips deeply to form the pouch (cul-de-sac) of Douglas.

The stroma of the cervix consists mainly of fibrous tissue and smooth muscle fibers, with branches of the uterine vessels penetrating into the deeper parts.

The cervix is perforated by the endocervical canal, which connects the endometrial cavity with the vagina. At the vaginal ending is the external os (orifice). The canal has a somewhat fusiform shape, with a slight enlargement in its midportion. The internal os is the point where the canal joins the endometrial cavity at the isthmus.

The vaginal aspect of the cervix (portio) is covered by a stratified squamous epithelium that turns back towards the vaginal wall, forming the fornices (Plate 1.1). The posterior fornix is deepest. The endocervical canal is lined by a mucosecreting monolayered columnar epithelium (Plate 1.2). The two epithelia meet at the squamocolumnar junction (Figures 1.1 and 1.2), which in the ideal cervix is situated at the external os. The squamocolumnar junction is not fixed, however, but wanders upwards or downwards at different times.

Histology

At birth and in infancy, the squamocolumnar junction is situated on the exocervix. At maturity it coincides approximately with the external os and after menopause, it recedes into the endocervical canal. At puberty, the columnar epithelium on the exocervix is gradually replaced by a squamous epithelium, by metaplasia. Squamous metaplasia is, therefore, a physiological process and needs not be mentioned as a diagnosis. The area of squamous metaplasia that covers pre-existing endocervical glands is called the transformation zone. Outside of the transformation zone is the "native" squamous epithelium of the exocervix; towards the canal, lies the columnar epithelium of the endocervix.

The squamous epithelium consists of several layers of cells; it is a true stratified epithelium (Plate 1.3). It rests on the basal membrane, which separates it from the stroma. The thickness and maturation of the epithelium depends on the hormonal stimulation: estrogen causes "maturation," that is, the complete expression of all layers of the epithelium. Progesterone, on the other hand, opposes complete maturation, while causing a thickening of the intermediate layers.

Although Fluhmann[1] divided the squamous epithelium into five layers (basal zone, parabasal zone, clear zone, condensation zone, and keratinized zone), Wied and Bibbo[2] more realistically recognized only three layers: a parabasal cell layer that consists of immature cells, an intermediate layer, and a superficial layer containing the most mature cells.

The basal or germinal cells lie directly on the basal membrane, to which they are fixed by half desmosomes. These small columnar-shaped cells actively divide by mitosis and produce all the overlying layers. Next come two or three layers of parabasal cells, which are rounded small cells with a vesicular nucleus occupying about half of the cell diameter (Plate 1.4). Then come the intermediate layers, in which cells are larger and contain a varying amount of glycogen (Plates 1.5 and 1.6; Figure 1.3). Finally, the superficial layers consist of large, polyhedral flat cells with pyknotic nuclei (Plate 1.7).

The columnar epithelium consists of a single layer of tall mucus-secreting cells (Plate 1.8). The nuclei are located near the basal membrane on which the columnar epithelium rests; they are vesicular and oval, and often contain a small nucleolus and the X-chromatin body affixed to the nuclear membrane, which is smooth and regular. The chromatin is finely reticular or granular. When irritated, the columnar cells may display cilia. Underneath the columnar cells are a few reserve cells, which are not easily observed on routine histologic sections. These reserve cells can multiply and differentiate to produce squamous metaplasia. The columnar epithelium invaginates deeply into the cervical stroma, producing clefts, crypts, and irregular spaces, which may become dilated by

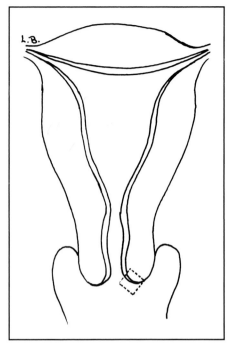

Figure 1.1 Schematic representation of the uterus. About half of the cervix protrudes into the vagina, forming the fornices. The transformation zone, ideally, is at the external os, and is illustrated in Figure 1.2

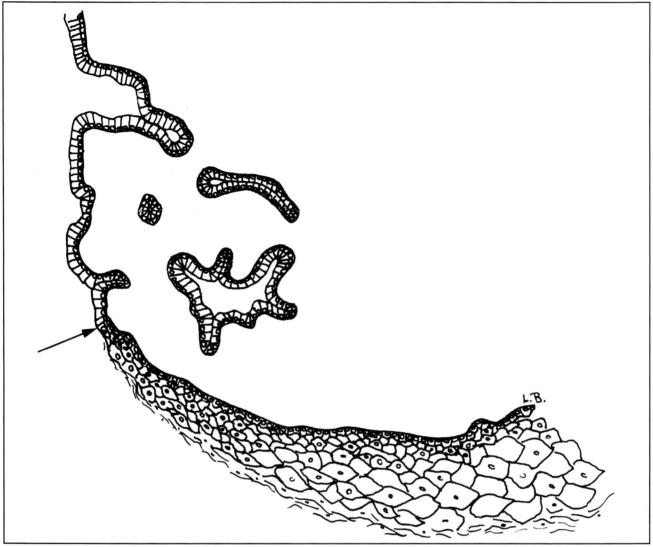

Figure 1.2 Schematic representation of the transformation zone. The arrow indicates the site where the exocervical squamous epithelium meets the endocervical columnar epithelium.

the accumulation of mucus when their outlets are obstructed (when visible to the naked eye, they are referred to as Naboth's eggs).

Cytology

In the absence of pathologic conditions, the smears contain mainly squamous and columnar cells. The squamous epithelium responds to ovarian hormonal production (see Chapter Three). Three types of squamous cells can be distinguished.[2] The _superficial cells_ (Plates 1.9 and 1.10; Figures 1.4 and 1.5) are large, flat, polygonal, and mostly eosinophilic. They contain a pyknotic nucleus, which is small (5 μm to 6 μm in diameter), dark, and featureless. The _intermediate cells_ (Plate 1.11) are somewhat smaller than the superficial cells, are usually flat and polygonal, and contain a vesicular nucleus

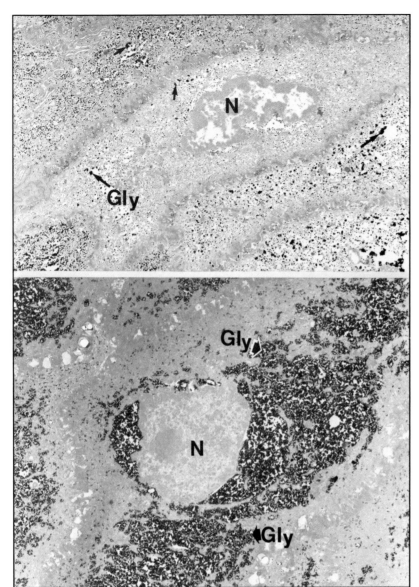

Figure 1.3 (Top) Electron microscopy illustration of cells from the superficial layers of the squamous epithelium of the uterine cervix. Very few dark glycogen granules (Gly) are visible in the cytoplasm. Periodic acid-thiocarbohydrazide-silver proteinate staining, 5,000×. (Bottom) Electron microscopy illustration of a cell of the intermediate layer of the squamous epithelium of the uterine cervix. A large area of glycogen (dark granules: Gly) is located in the cytoplasm surrounding the nucleus (N). Periodic acid-thiocarbohydrazide-silver proteinate staining, 5,000×.

with finely granular or reticular chromatin, a smooth nuclear membrane, and occasionally a small nucleolus and/or an X-chromatin body (a plano-convex dark structure, about 1 μm in diameter, firmly adherent to the inner aspect of the nuclear membrane). The cytoplasm is cyanophilic and may contain glycogen, which stains yellowish with the Papanicolaou technique. The *parabasal cells* (Plate 1.12) are small, rounded, and cyanophilic. They contain a large vesicular nucleus, similar to the nucleus of intermediate cells. Squa-

Superficial cell – less glycogen

glycogen – dark

glycogen – yellow = pap

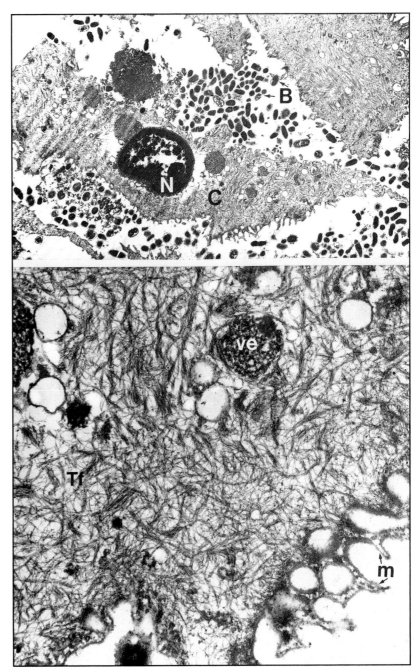

Figure 1.4 Electron microscopy illustration of a superficial cell reprocessed from a V–C–E smear. The nucleus (N) is dense and pyknotic. Numerous bacteria (B) are seen between cells. Individual tonofilaments (Tf) are scattered everywhere in the cytoplasm (C). Uranyl acetate and lead citrate staining; upper figure 3,000×; lower figure 17,500×.

mous cells are found singly or in small clumps, but show no tendency to form any special groupings.

Columnar endocervical cells are often shed in sheets or strips. They are elongated and cyanophilic, with a clear cytoplasm. The eccentric vesicular nucleus contains a finely distributed chromatin, a small nucleolus, and often an X—chromatin body (Plate 1.13).

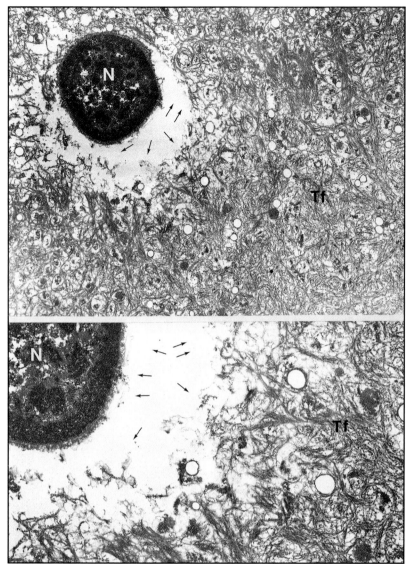

Figure 1.5 Electron microscopy illustration of a superficial cell reprocessed from a V–C–E smear. In this figure, the retraction of the nucleus (N) during the process of pyknosis has created a small halo (arrows). Uranyl acetate and lead citrate staining, upper figure 7,500×; lower figure 15,000×.

When present in sheets or strips, endocervical cells conserve their polarity, meaning that their orientation on a smear recalls their histologic structure. Endocervical cells may display a certain amount of anisokaryosis (variation in size and shape of the nuclei) (Plates 1.14 and 1.15).

Mucus can be found in abundance on smears obtained at midcycle. Within the mucus strands, endocervical cells tend to be devoid of cytoplasm. The naked nuclei may show budding protrusions at the time of ovulation and often have a very clear appearance, without much visible inner structure (Plate 1.16).

Endometrial glandular cells are observed normally during the first ten days of the cycle. They are smaller than endocervical cells, with scant, sometimes vacuolated, cyanophilic cytoplasm, and characteristically are grouped in tight three-dimensional clusters. The nuclei are vesicular and contain finely distributed chromatin, usually without visible nucleoli. From day 6 to day 10 of the cycle, endometrial glandular cells form tight balls surrounded by one or more layers of larger cells with pale cyanophilic cytoplasm, originating in the endometrial stroma (Plate 1.17). This typical formation has been called "exodus" by Papanicolaou.

Small histiocytes can be observed at the end of the menstrual cycle and during the first 10 days of the proliferative phase. They are thought to originate in the endometrial stroma. They are similar in size to parabasal cells, but their cyanophilic cytoplasm is foamy, their cellular outlines are indistinct, and their nucleus is often notched or kidney- or bean-shaped, with a prominent chromatin pattern (Plates 1.18 and 1.19). There may be two or more nuclei. When nuclei are numerous, histiocytes can become quite large, and are then designated as multinucleated giant cells (Plate 1.20). They may contain phagocytized material (hemosiderophages, for instance) (Plate 1.21), in which case they are called macrophages. In the absence of inflammation, macrophages are scavengers, removing debris and blood after menstruation.

Granulocytes (Plate 1.22) are commonly observed at the beginning and the end of the menstrual cycle and do not indicate the presence of infection or inflammation. Lymphocytes (Plate 1.23) and plasma cells (Plate 1.24) are rarely observed on normal smears. Psammomalike concretions are occasionally observed and probably represent inspissated mucus (Plate 1.25 and 1.26).

Plate 1.1

Cervical biopsy specimen illustrating normal squamous epithelium. Note the dense basal layer and the progressive maturation towards the surface. The lower layers contain small, rounded cells, which increase in size as they progress towards the surface, filling up with glycogen, and then, in the uppermost layers, becoming flattened, with small, pyknotic nuclei.

Plate 1.2

Cervical biopsy specimen illustrating normal endocervical columnar epithelium. A single layer of tall, mucosecreting cells lines the endocervical canal and the clefts and spaces around it.

Plate 1.3

Cervical biopsy specimen shows that the squamous epithelium is truly stratified. There are no blood vessels within the epithelium, but as illustrated here, a blood vessel carried by scanty stroma can invaginate within the epithelium and may reach the middle or even upper layers.

Plate 1.1

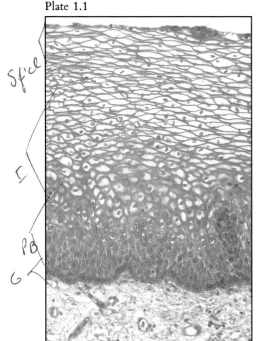

Plate 1.2

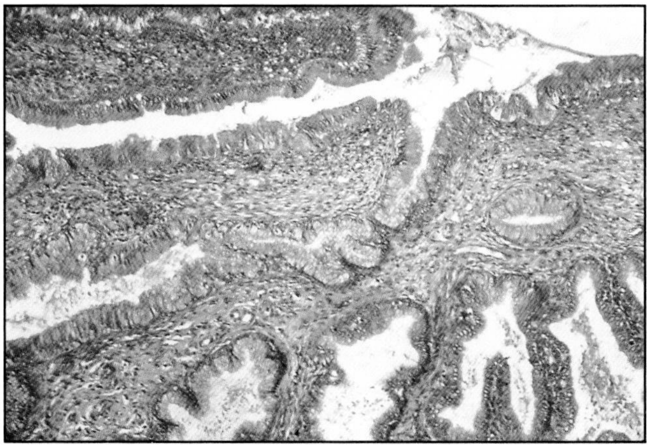

Plate 1.3

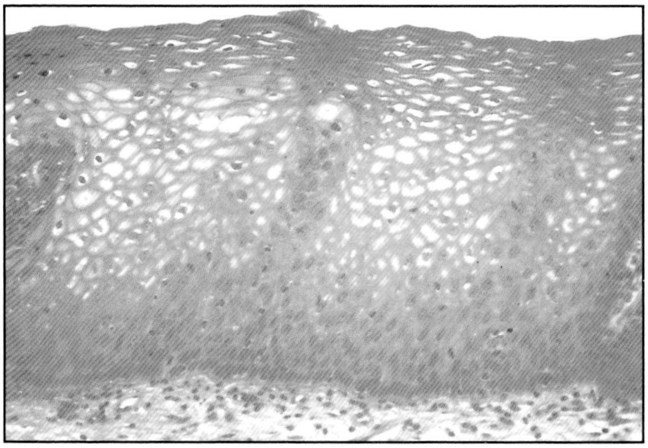

Plate 1.4

This higher magnification illustrates the lower levels of the cervical squamous epithelium. The cells are small and contain large, vesicular nuclei, often with prominent nucleoli, as shown here. Intercellular bridges (desmosomes) are clearly visible.

Plate 1.5

In the middle layers of the squamous epithelium of the cervix, the cells are larger and show empty-appearing spaces, which contain glycogen.

Plate 1.6

Demonstration of glycogen in normal epithelium of the uterine cervix. The intermediate layer has an intense red color indicating the presence of glycogen. PAS staining. 145×.

Plate 1.4

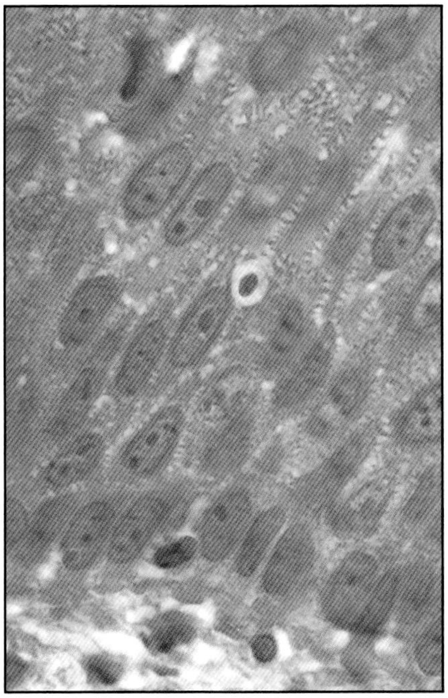

Plate 1.5

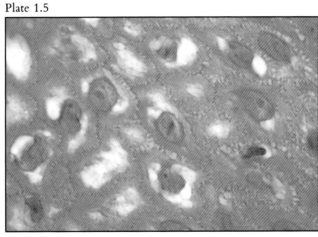

Int. cells

Plate 1.6

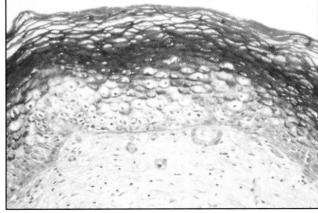

Plate 1.7

In the upper layers of the squamous epithelium the cells become flattened, and their nuclei are pyknotic, ie, uniformly dark and featureless.

Plate 1.8

Cervical biopsy specimen illustrating the endocervical columnar epithelium. The cells are tall and mucosecreting. When the clefts or spaces become obstructed, small cysts can form, as illustrated here.

Plate 1.9

Superficial squamous cells from a cellular sample of the cervix. These are entirely mature cells, showing a polyhedral shape, with abundant, flat, eosinophilic cytoplasm, and small, round, pyknotic nuclei.

Plate 1.7

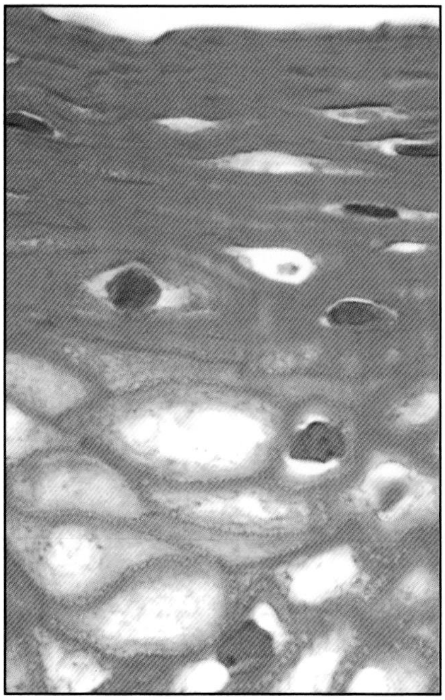

Plate 1.8

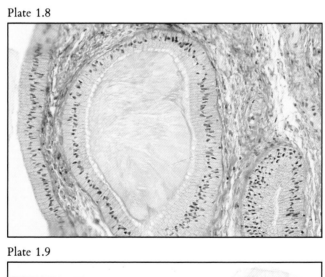

Plate 1.9

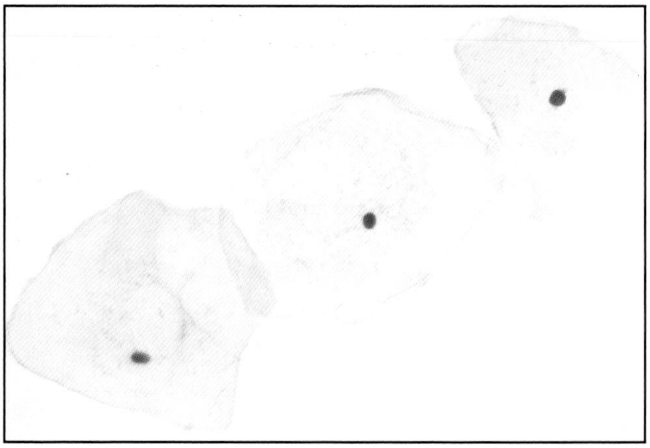

Plate 1.10
This mature squamous cell displays a commonly observed small clear perinuclear halo. Note also the dense eosinophilic cytoplasm.

Plate 1.11
Intermediate squamous cells from a cellular sample of the cervix. The shape is polyhedral, the cyanophilic cytoplasm is flat, and the nuclei are vesicular.

Plate 1.12
Parabasal cells from a cellular sample of the cervix. The cells are small and round, the cytoplasm is dense and sometimes vacuolated, and the nuclei are vesicular. These cells are usually observed in the absence of estrogenic stimulation (see Chapter 3). So are granulocytes.

Int cells, glans — around when estrogen is not.

Plate 1.13
Columnar endocervical cells from a cervical cell spread. These are tall columnar cells with large, vesicular nuclei. Many of the cells are ciliated. A sex chromatin body is clearly visible in the cell at the center. *— indicated by irritation*

Plate 1.10

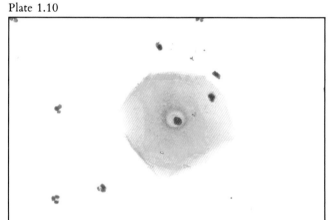

Plate 1.11

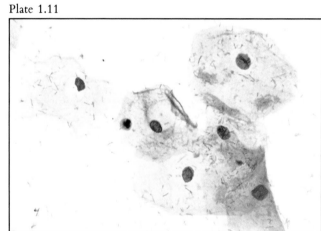

Plate 1.12

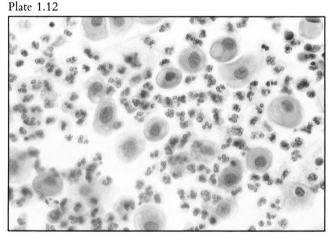

Plate 1.13

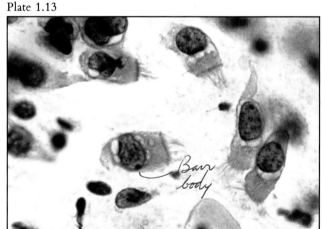

Barr body

Plate 1.14
A sheet of columnar endocervical cells. Some are mucosecreting and others are ciliated. The nuclei show a moderate variation in size and shape (anisokaryosis).

Plate 1.15
A tight grouping of mucosecreting endocervical cells, with a slight degree of anisokaryosis.

Plate 1.16
✳ Within a lightly stained strand of mucus, the columnar endocervical cells have lost their cytoplasm. There is some anisokaryosis. Some of the nuclei show partial clearing of their chromatin.

Plate 1.17
A tight cluster of endometrial glandular cells observed on the 7th day of a menstrual cycle. Small cells show much overlapping, and have scant cytoplasm and darkly stained nuclei.

Plate 1.14

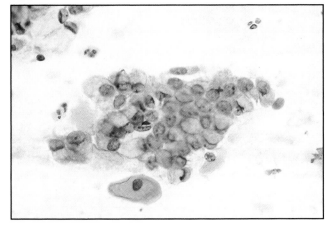

Plate 1.15

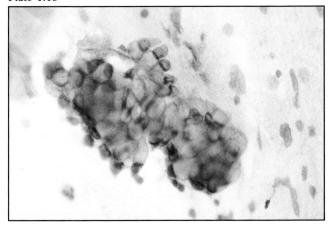

Plate 1.16

EC
cells
at
mid
cycle

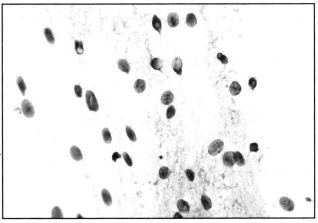

Plate 1.17

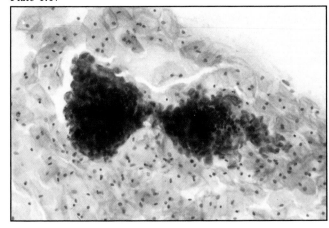

Plate 1.18

A loose group of small histiocytes observed on a cervical cell spread obtained on the 9th day of a menstrual cycle. Papanicolaou interpreted these cells as transformed endometrial stromal cells, which ⚹ function as scavengers after menstruation.

Plate 1.19

A small group of histiocytes from the same case as Plate 1.23. Note the vacuolated cytoplasm. The nuclei have a prominent, somewhat irregular, nuclear membrane. The chromatin structure is coarse, with several chromocenters and thickened chromatin bands.

Plate 1.20

A multinucleated giant histiocytic cell. The abundant, partly foamy cytoplasm contains a large number of nuclei, some of which display small nucleoli.

Plate 1.18

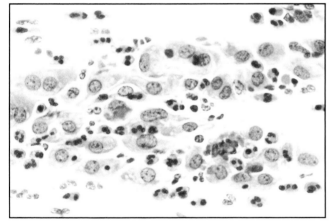

Plate 1.19

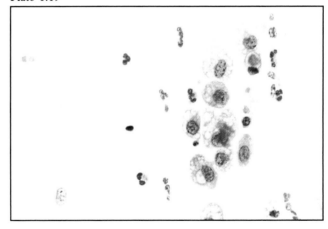

Plate 1.20

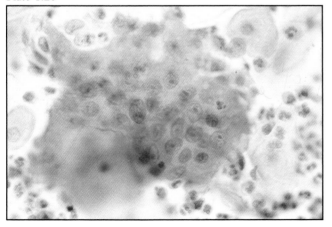

Plate 1.21
These histiocytes have ingested hemosiderin—they are hemosiderophages. Note the abundant hemosiderin within the cytoplasm. The smallest of these macrophages contains a kidney-shaped nucleus.

Plate 1.22
Granulocytes are commonly found just before and after menstruation. They contain three, or sometimes four, nuclear lobes.

Plate 1.23
Lymphocytes are rarely seen on normal smears. This is a case of lymphocytic cervicitis (see Chapter Five).

Plate 1.21

Plate 1.22

Grans—b4/after mens.

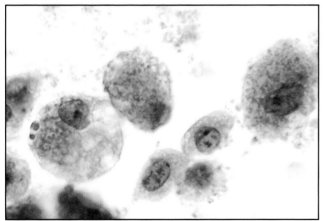

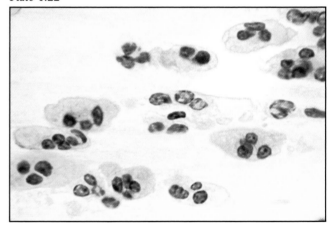

Plate 1.23

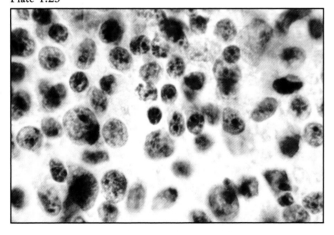

Lcytes —Rare

Plate 1.24
Plasma cells usually indicate the presence of a chronic inflammation. They are characterized by an eccentrically located nucleus, which displays the typical cartwheel chromatin distribution.

Plate 1.25
These psammomalike concretions can occasionally be found on cell spreads from the cervix. They are characterized by concentric circular markings, with a dense body in the center.

Plate 1.26
Psammomalike bodies in a cluster of glandular endocervical cells. They most probably are condensations of endocervical mucus.

Plate 1.24

Pl cells abn'l

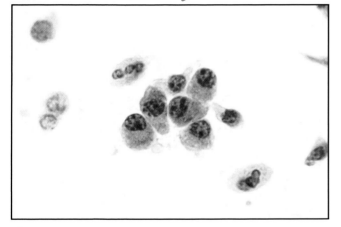

Plate 1.25

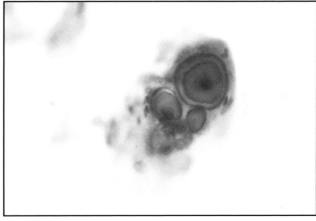

Plate 1.26

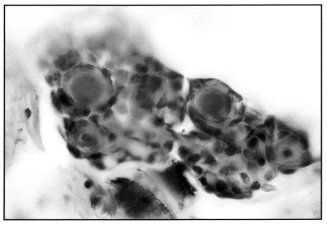

References

1. Fluhmann CF: The Cervix Uteri and its Diseases. WB Saunders, Philadelphia, 1961.
2. Wied GL, Bibbo M: Evaluation of endocrinologic condition by exfoliative cytology. In: Compendium on Diagnostic Cytology. Tutorials of Cytology, Chicago, 1988, pp33–42.

CHAPTER TWO

Nomenclature

Many schemes of nomenclature for intraepithelial changes of the squamous epithelium of the cervix have been advanced since Papanicolaou proposed his five classes. At that time, his system presented a good way of reporting his findings, because histologic correlations were not routinely obtained. Class I was "normal," and Class II indicated inflammation, repair, or other benign changes. Class III was used for those cases in which the diagnosis was debatable (another way of saying "I don't know"). Class IV was suspicious for malignancy, probably carcinoma in situ, and Class V was an invasive cancer. Papanicolaou's system provided a way for cytologists to be cautious in their diagnoses, but as diagnostic cytology became more sophisticated, this classification soon proved inadequate, and was replaced by various descriptive nomenclatures, which attempted to correlate the cytologic patterns with histology. Hence the terms *dysplasia* and *carcinoma in situ*.

In 1973 a WHO committee attempted without much luck to define the two terms above.[5] Time has shown that what seemed to be important differences between them had statistical significance only when applied to a large number of women, but for a given patient it was not possible to determine the true risk based on the morphology of the lesion. Furthermore, dysplasia means different things in different organs (eg, renal dysplasia, bone dysplasia, etc). And carcinoma in situ is not, by definition, real carcinoma, as it lacks two of the most important characteristics of malignant tumors: the ability to invade neighboring tissues, and to produce distant metastasis. For a time it became fashionable to split hairs, and to subdivide intraepithelial lesions of the cervix into a number of subcategories: mild, moderate, severe, metaplastic, keratinizing, etc.[3] One could attend serious meetings where interminable discussions centered on whether a particular slide showed "moderate metaplastic dysplasia" or "keratinizing severe dysplasia." The fact that there were no hard data to justify these subclassifications in the light of eventual outcome of the disease condemned this exercise to well-deserved oblivion. Furthermore, it is highly doubtful that the average cytotechnologist or cytopathologist can consistently classify cellular patterns, or even histologic sections, in these various subdivisions. It has been shown that there is a total lack of concordance among even experienced microscopists.[1] When the same smears and sections are reviewed after an interval of a few months the same individuals may disagree with their own previous diagnoses. Those who defend splitting should realize that it is a very subjective exercise.

Richart[4] introduced the term *cervical intraepithelial neoplasia* (CIN), which encompasses all noninvasive epithelial changes on the cervix, from condyloma to carcinoma in situ. At first he divided CIN into three grades: Grade 1 (CIN 1) was equivalent to mild dysplasia, Grade 2 (CIN 2) to moderate dysplasia, and Grade 3 (CIN 3) to severe dysplasia and carcinoma in situ. Later on he and others dropped the subclassfication of CIN, realizing that it had little if any predictive value. In our laboratory, CIN was used without subclassification for all lesions previously diagnosed as dysplasias or carcinoma in situ. This use is justified by the fact that management of the patient should not be influenced by the degree of severity of the intraepithelial change. Morphology in no way predicts the ultimate outcome of the disease for any particular woman. All patients must be referred to colposcopy, and biopsies must be obtained to confirm the diagnosis. The lesion can then be destroyed by laser or cryosurgery. Followup studies without treatment cannot ethically be justified in the light of our present knowledge.

The latest development is the proposed *Bethesda System of Nomenclature for Reporting Cervical/Vaginal Cytologic Diagnoses*[2] (Table 2.1), which represents the consensus of representatives of several American and international scientific societies who attended a special workshop organized by the American Cancer Institute in Bethesda, under the Chairmanship of Diane Solomon, in December of 1988. The Bethesda nomenclature is similar to Richart's in concept, but now includes HPV-related lesions of the cervix. As its name implies, it is a *complete system* for reporting gynecologic cytology—parts of it could also be used for reporting on the histology of cervical lesions. Several important features have been included: for instance, the *Bethesda System* requires *in every case* a statement concerning the adequacy of the sample received; limiting intraepithelial lesions to just two categories removes much of the subjectivity of previous systems. A second meeting of the Bethesda Workshop is scheduled for the spring of 1991 and it is to be expected that some modifications will be proposed, in response to suggestions received from various quarters. In effect, the *Bethesda System* is a flexible, reproducible system, that can be adapted to the needs of each laboratory, for instance by adding descriptive terms. Because of the importance of achieving a uniform system of reporting, and because the Bethesda System has found wide acceptance, it is hoped that it will soon be in general use.

Table 2.1
The Bethesda System

In the introduction, the participants to the Workshop agreed that:

The cytopathology report is a medical consultation.

The Papanicolaou classification for reporting consultations is not acceptable in the modern practice of diagnostic cytopathology.

The Bethesda System should serve as a guideline for cytopathology reports of cervical/vaginal specimens.

They further recommended that a cervical/vaginal cytopathology report address each of the following elements: 1) a Statement on Adequacy of the Specimen for diagnostic evaluation, 2) a General Categorization of the diagnosis, and 3) Descriptive Diagnosis.

Statement on Specimen Adequacy
  Satisfactory for interpretation,
  ~~Less than optimal~~ *Satisfactory, but limited by*
  Unsatisfactory

  Explanation for "less than optimal/unsatisfactory specimen:
    Scant cellularity
    Poor fixation or preservation
    Presence of foreign material (eg, lubricant)
    Partially or completely obscuring inflammation
    Partially or completely obscuring blood
    Excessive cytolysis or autolysis
    No endocervical component in a premenopausal woman who has a cervix
    Not representative of the anatomic site
    Other

General Categorization
  Within normal limits
  Other:
    See descriptive diagnosis
    Further action recommended

Descriptive Diagnosis
  Infection
    Fungal
      Fungal organisms morphologically consistent with *Candida* species
      Other
    Bacterial
      Microorganisms morphologically consistent with *Gardnerella* species
      Microorganisms morphologically consistent with *Actinomyces* species
      Cellular changes suggestive of *Chlamydia* infection, subject to confirmatory studies
      Other
    Protozoan
      Trichomonas vaginalis
      Other
    Viral
      Cellular changes associated with cytomegalovirus
      Cellular changes associated with herpesvirus simplex
      Other
      (Note: For human papillomavirus (HPV) refer to "Epithelial Cell Abnormalities, Squamous cell")
    Other

(Continued.)

Reactive and Reparative Changes
  Inflammation
    Associated cellular changes
    Follicular cervicitis
  Miscellaneous (as related to patient history)
    Effects of therapy
    Ionizing radiation
    Chemotherapy
    Effects of mechanical devices (eg, intrauterine contraceptive device)
    Effects of nonsteroidal estrogen exposure (eg, diethylstilbestrol)
    Other
Epithelial Cell Abnormalities
  Squamous cell
    Atypical squamous cells of undetermined significance (recommended follow-up and/or type of further investigation: specify)
    Squamous intraepithelial lesion (SIL) (comment on presence of cellular changes associated with HPV, if applicable)
      Low-grade squamous intraepithelial lesion, encompassing:
        Cellular changes associated with HPV
        Mild (slight) dysplasia/cervical intraepithelial neoplasia grade I (CIN 1)
      High-grade squamous intraepithelial lesion, encompassing:
        Moderate dysplasia/CIN 2
        Severe dysplasia/CIN 3
        Carcinoma in situ/CIN 3
    Squamous cell carcinoma
  Glandular cell
    Presence of endometrial cells in one of the following circumstances:
      Out of phase in a menstruating woman
      In a postmenopausal woman
      No menstrual history available
    Atypical glandular cells of undetermined significance (recommended followup and/or type of further investigation; specify)
      Endometrial
      Endocervical
      Not otherwise specified
    Adenocarcinoma
      Specify probable site of origin: endocervical, endometrial, extrauterine
      Not otherwise specified
    Other epithelial malignant neoplasm: specify
  Nonepithelial Malignant Neoplasm: Specify
✗ Hormonal Evaluation (Applies to Vaginal Smears Only)
  ✓ Hormonal pattern compatible with age and history
  ✓ Hormonal pattern incompatible with age and history: specify
  ✓ Hormonal evaluation not possible
    Cervical specimen /
    Inflammation
    Insufficient patient history
  Other

Explanatory Notes on the Bethesda System

Statement on Specimen Adequacy

Three possible responses are listed under the first element of the recommended report format.

(a) "Satisfactory" indicates the specimen is an adequate sample that can be interpreted without qualification based on sampling or preparation.

(b) "Less than optimal" indicates the specimen may provide useful diagnostic information but is less than optimal (for example, because of *partially* obscuring inflammation). Use of the category *Less than Optimal* is optional.

(c) "Unsatisfactory" indicates the specimen is not acceptable for diagnostic evaluation and repeat sampling may be warranted.

An explanation should be provided for any specimen designated either "Less than Optimal" or "Unsatisfactory." The Bethesda System includes the entry "No endocervical component in a premenopausal woman who has a uterine cervix" to indicate that none of the following elements are present: (a) endocervical cells, (b) endocervical mucus, or (c) squamous metaplastic cells. The cytopathologist should recommend a repeat smear when reporting an unsatisfactory specimen. For less than optimal specimens, the cytopathologist may choose to recommend a repeat smear or other followup.

General Categorization

The second element of the report format sorts reports (except those classified as "Unsatisfactory") to either "Within normal limits" or "Other." If "Other" is selected the report may include an additional notation if further action is recommended. The general categorization is not a substitute for specific descriptive diagnoses, which should be included elsewhere in the report. Rather, it is to assist the referring physician and support personnel to sort the cases that need review and, possibly, further action.

Descriptive Diagnosis

The final element of the report format is the descriptive diagnosis, which is largely self-explanatory as outlined. The terms with the exception of two new ones are in general use. However, a few points are clarified below.

Infection
Under this heading belong those infectious agents associated with cervical/vaginal disease whose presence can be suggested by cytologic examination. However, definitive diagnosis of some of these agents may require confirmatory studies. The qualifying phrases accompanying the identification of certain pathogens (such as "fungal organisms morphologically consistent with *Candida*") reflect the level of diagnostic certainty achieved by routine light microscopy alone. These phrases can be modified to suit the individual cytopathologist.

Epithelial Cell Abnormalities
Use of the term "atypical cells" is limited to those cases in which the cytologic findings are of undetermined significance. Atypia

should *not* be used as a diagnosis for otherwise defined inflammatory, preneoplastic, or neoplastic cellular changes.

To assist the referring physician, a report in which cells are described as "atypical" should include a recommendation for further evaluation that may help to determine the significance of the atypical cells.

The only new diagnostic terms are "Low-grade squamous intraepithelial lesion (LGSIL)" and "High-grade squamous intraepithelial lesion (HGSIL)." They encompass the spectrum of terms currently used for squamous cell precursors to invasive squamous cell carcinoma, including the grades of cervical intraepithelial neoplasia (CIN) and the degrees of dysplasia and carcinoma in situ (CIS). "Grade," as used with SIL, does *not* connote invasive carcinoma.

While "Low-grade SIL" and "High-grade SIL" are the preferred terms, their use does not preclude the addition of degree of dysplasia or grade of CIN for cytopathologists who wish to retain these designations. Examples are "low-grade squamous intraepithelial lesion: cellular changes associated with HPV, "low-grade squamous intraepithelial lesion: mild dysplasia and cellular changes associated with HPV or "high-grade squamous intraepithelial lesion: cervical intraepithelial neoplasia, Grade 3 (CIN 3)."

The statement "cellular changes associated with HPV" should be added to the report of either Low-grade SIL or High-grade SIL when appropriate. The same statement (if the changes show no features of dysplasia or CIN) may be listed separately, although it is preferably placed under the designation of LGSIL. Terms such as "koilocytic atypia," "keratinizing atypia," and "dyskaryosis" are not included in the Bethesda System lexicon.

As with every change in nomenclature and reporting systems, the Bethesda System has met its share of criticism and opposition. In particular, it has been said that the term "grade" is usually employed in relation to invasive cancer and thus may cause some confusion. Of course, CIN also uses grades, so the term is not really new. Not only does the Bethesda System offer a systematic format for reporting cervical/vaginal smears, which can be followed (and adapted) by all cytopathologists, but it also reduces the subdivisions of preneoplastic lesions of the cervix to only two, leaving much less room for subjectivity in the interpretation of cellular changes. In view of the currently held opinion that HPV is a necessary component in the process of cervical carcinogenesis, and that all women with morphologic signs of either HPV infection, low-grade SIL, or high-grade SIL should be referred to colposcopy and confirmatory biopsy, it would have been conceivable to encompass all these lesions in a single category of SIL, without grades or divisions. The Bethesda System was elaborated by a large committee including representatives from all groups and associations interested in the problem of prevention of cervical cancer, and it was necessary to reach a consensus; compromises had to be worked out amongst the "splitters" and the "lumpers." The fact that a consensus could be reached is an indication that this system might find general acceptance.

References

1. Meisels A, Alonso de Ruiz P: Human papillomavirus-related changes in the genital tract. In: Human Papillomavirus and Cervical Cancer. Muñoz N, Bosch FX, Jensen OM, eds. IARC Scientific Publication No. 94, International Agency for Research on Cancer, Lyon, 1989, pp 67–85.

2. National Cancer Institute Workshop. The 1988 Bethesda system for reporting cervical/vaginal cytological diagnoses. *JAMA* 262:931–934, 1989.

3. Patten SF: Morphologic subclassification of preinvasive cervical neoplasia. In: Compendium on Diagnostic Cytology, Wied GL, Keebler CM, Koss LG, Reagan JW (editors), The Tutorials of Cytology, Chicago, 1988, pp 105–113.

4. Richart RM: Cervical intraepithelial neoplasia: A review. In: Pathology Annual, Vol. 8, Sommers SC, ed. Appleton-Century-Crofts, Norwalk, 1973, p 301.

5. Riotton G, Christopherson WM, Lunt R: Cytology of the Female Genital Tract. Geneva, World Health Organization, 1973.

CHAPTER THREE

Hormonal Cytology

When a hormonal evaluation is requested, it is necessary to obtain a special smear, which should be taken with a wooden or metallic spatula at the junction of the upper and middle thirds of the lateral vaginal wall. That area is chosen because it is usually free of detritus, bacteria, and other contaminants, so that the smear is generally clean and the cellular patterns can easily be recognized. Smears from the posterior fornix may give an indication of extremes of hormonal action, or lack of it, but do not usually permit a precise assessment of gonadal activity. The exocervical smear is useless for hormonal evaluation.

Assessment of Hormonal Activity

The vaginal epithelium is quite sensitive to the action of gonadal hormones. It matures under the effect of estrogen and thickens when acted upon by progestrone. Under the effect of unopposed estrogen, smears contain a predominance of superficial squamous cells. Progesterone impedes the complete maturation of the squamous epithelium, resulting in a predominance of intermediate cells on the smear. When the gonads are quiescent, the epithelium becomes thin and immature and smears contain mostly parabasal cells.

One must remember that the smear samples the surface of the epithelium. All cells on the smear are therefore superficial in the sense that they are lying on top. Estrogen ensures that the uppermost layers of the epithelium are mature, that is, consisting of large polygonal flat eosinophilic cells, each with a pyknotic nucleus. Pyknosis in this sense is defined as a featureless darkly stained nucleus, with a diameter not exceeding 5 μm to 6 μm. Only estrogen can produce complete maturation. The finding of mature superficial cells on the smear, therefore, is definite proof that estrogen is present.

Cytology

The general pattern of cervical smears depends on the level of gonadal hormones, on the vaginal microbiology, and on other local factors. It varies considerably with age.

At Birth

Gonadal hormones are produced in large amounts during pregnancy and pass readily through the placenta into the fetal circulation. The squamous epithelium of the cervix and of the vagina of the newborn girl responds to this strong hormonal stimulation with a marked maturation. A vaginal smear can be obtained with a thin cotton applicator. It will contain a clear predominance of superficial cells, with a general pattern very similar to that of a mature woman at midcycle[2,22] (Plate 3.1). At this time, also, the baby's breasts may sometimes be slightly increased in volume with a few drops of "witches' milk."

In Childhood

Within a few days to 1 week after birth, the maternal hormones are eliminated and the genital crisis sets in; the more mature layers of the squamous epithelium are desquamated and the smears will contain mostly parabasal cells (Plate 3.2). This atrophic pattern persists until the onset of puberty.

At Puberty

Even before the first menstrual period occurs, the vaginal smear begins to change; intermediate cells replace the parabasal cells of childhood and a few scattered superficial cells reflect the onset of estrogen secretion (Plate 3.3). This pattern may appear several months before clinical menarche.

During the Reproductive Years

Day 1 of the cycle is the first day of menstruation. The first 5 days are characterized by a smear containing blood, cellular debris, inflammatory cells, and endometrial glandular and stromal cells. Endometrial glandular cells are often found in compact groups, with little nuclear detail (Plate 3.4). Endometrial stromal cells which resemble small histiocytes are shed as clusters or discrete cells. There are many superficial cells, but there is often a false eosinophilia, ie, the cytoplasm of intermediate cells stains pink.

From day 5 to day 10, the smear usually contains a predominance of intermediate squamous cells, which may display a slightly wrinkled cytoplasm. The cells may occur in clusters but are mostly isolated. Endometrial glandular and stromal cells are found in tight groupings, which Papanicolaou called "exodus" (Plate 3.5). The stromal cells form the inner part of the cluster; they are tightly grouped and somewhat hyperchromatic. The glandular cells have more cytoplasm than the stromal cells, and form the periphery of the clump. The smear cleans up and by day 10 there are few if any inflammatory cells and no more blood is seen (Plate 3.6).

Days 11 to 15 comprise the ovulatory phase, characterized by very clean smears with many superficial squamous cells, mostly isolated and quite flat (Plate 3.7). Just before, or at the time of ovulation, the endocervical mucus is very abundant and can be stretched outside of the vagina when grabbed with a forceps; this is called *Spinnbarkeit.* When this mucus is spread on a glass slide and allowed to air-dry without fixation or staining, it will reveal a special fern-like crystallization under the microscope (Plate 3.8).

The secretory phase begins around day 16 of the cycle. During the first few days the cells tend to group together and to lose some of their flatness. Eventually the cellular membrane becomes crinkled and the cells form dense aggregates in which the cellular outlines are indistinct (Plate 3.9). The predominant cell during the secretory phase is the intermediate cell, which contains large amounts of glycogen.

At the end of the cycle leukocytes and histiocytes in varying numbers may be seen. With the degeneration of the corpus luteum, progesterone secretion ceases, but estrogen levels are maintained by the developing follicles, so that the predominant cells are of the intermediate type, with a few scattered superficial cells.[6,10,13,15,23]

Anovulatory cycles can be detected by the absence of signs of progesterone activity during the second half of the cycle. For this purpose, a smear taken on days 22 to 24 of a 28-day cycle is particularly useful[9,10] (Plate 3.10). Contraceptive pills mostly contain estrogenlike substances associated with progesteronelike chemicals, which causes smears to resemble those observed during the secretory phase[3,18] (Plates 3.11 and 3.12).

In amenorrheas, the cytohormonal smear may reveal whether the ovaries are functional. If the smear shows atrophy, then there is no hormonal production. This finding is of prognostic significance, particularly in primary amenorrheas.[1]

During Pregnancy

During the first trimester of pregnancy the hormonal support is supplied by the corpus luteum, which produces increasing amounts of estrogens and progesterone. At the end of the 14th week, the placenta takes over the function of the corpus luteum, which degenerates and ceases to function. The fetal adrenal glands supply the building blocks for the synthesis of placental hormones. This transition sometimes is not smooth and progesterone production may diminish. After the 15th week, with increasing size of the fetus and the placenta, the synthesis of estrogens and progesterone increases considerably, reaching levels up to 100 times higher towards the end of pregnancy than those existing during the menstrual cycle. Shortly before labor begins, the production of placental hormones sometimes diminishes.

Vaginal smears reflect the balance of hormones during pregnancy. Generally, the high levels of progesterone do not allow complete maturation of the squamous epithelium. Therefore, superficial cells are rare after the first trimester. Even exogenous estrogens in high doses will fail to produce superficial cells.

During the first trimester, the cellular pattern often resembles that of the secretory phase. Around the 14th week, superficial cells may appear in small numbers. The pregnancy smear has two characteristic features: (1) the presence of numerous "navicular" cells (Plate 3.13), so called by Papanicolaou because of their shape; these small intermediate cells contain a large amount of glycogen, which pushes the cytoplasm out to the periphery where it becomes dense and cyanophilic; the nucleus is eccentrically located; and (2) a marked cytolysis (Plate 3.14) related to the abundance of lactobacilli, which thrive in the glycogen-rich environment.

Cellular patterns can reveal hormonal imbalances occurring during pregnancy. In any situation where there is fetal suffering (for instance, in imminent miscarriage) fetal adrenal activity diminishes, resulting in a lower level of progestrone production in the placenta. Consequently, estrogen can again manifest itself by the presence of superficial cells on the hormonal smear (Plate 3.15). The presence of numerous superficial cells during pregnancy can therefore be used as an alarm signal.[8,11,12,14]

If the fetus dies inside the uterus, all hormone production ceases.[4] Since the ovary is not functioning during the later trimesters of pregnancy, atrophy sets in[20] (Plate 3.16). In such cases, even small doses of estrogens will produce a prompt response and superficial cells will appear on the smear (Plate 3.17). This is the estrogen test[5] that has been used to confirm fetal death in utero.

After delivery of the placenta, the levels of estrogen and progesterone rapidly decrease, and the smear soon becomes atrophic[7,19] (Plate 3.18). This situation lasts until the ovaries begin their normal cycles, which may take from a few weeks to a few months. Breast feeding may prolong this atrophic period for 1 year, or longer.

After Menopause

Menopause is generally defined as the cessation of menses. Unless the ovaries are surgically removed or otherwise rendered inactive (by ionizing radiation, for example), estrogen production may continue for prolonged periods of time. The cellular pattern after the menopause depends on the amount of residual estrogen secreted by the ovarian stroma and the adrenal cortex. Superficial cells may persist on the smear for many years.[21] Eventually the cellular pattern becomes atrophic, when and if estrogen production effectively ceases. The smear then consists mostly of parabasal cells (Plate 3.19).[17]

Interpretation of the Hormonal Patterns

The response of the squamous epithelia of the vagina and the cervix to the various hormonal stimuli can show great variations from patient to patient. The only two absolute cell patterns are: a predominance of superficial cells—large polygonal flat cells containing a pyknotic nucleus that indicates the presence of estrogen (Plate 3.20), and a predominance of parabasal cells—small round cyanophilic cells containing a round or oval vesicular nucleus that indicates absence of estrogenic stimulation (Plate 3.21). Therefore, it is possible to judge the presence or absence of estrogen from the smear. Various indices have been proposed to report hormonal patterns: the maturation index, the maturation value,[16] the karyopyknotic index, the eosinophilic index, the folded cell index, etc.[23] These indices have no value whatsoever because there is no continuity in the epithelial response to the gonadal hormones. Intermediate cells occur in a great variety of circumstances and have little diagnostic value. With the Bethesda System the information transmitted to the clinician is limited to a statement indicating that the hormonal pattern is consistent with the age and anamnesis, or if that is not the case, a simple specification of the abnormality observed.

Plate 3.1
Vaginal smear of a 1-day-old girl. The smear contains superficial and intermediate cells, reflecting the effect of maternal hormones absorbed through the placenta.

Plate 3.2
Vaginal smear of a 3-month-old girl. The cell spread contains only parabasal cells, reflecting the absence of gonadal hormones. This pattern subsists until puberty.

Plate 3.3
At puberty, the smear contains mature cells, mostly intermediate, with a few superficial cells, indicating the beginning of estrogen production in the ovaries.

Plate 3.4
Day 3 of a menstrual cycle. The smear has a "dirty" appearance and contains tight clumps of endometrial cells.

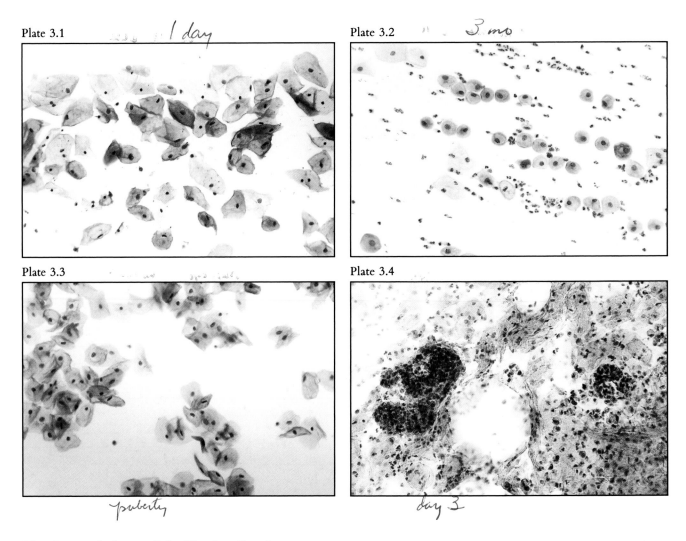

Plate 3.1

Plate 3.2

Plate 3.3

Plate 3.4

Plate 3.5

Day 7 of a menstrual cycle. This pattern was described by Papanicolaou under the name of "exodus." There are two cell-types: a denser inner core, made up of endometrial stromal cells, and an outer layer of endometrial glandular cells. Exodus is commonly observed between days 6 and 10 of the cycle.

Plate 3.6

Day 11 of a menstrual cycle. The smear is now "clean" and contains a mixture of flat intermediate and superficial cells, showing distinct cell boundaries.

Plate 3.7

Day 14 of a menstrual cycle. Estrogen effect is at its highest point. Superficial flat cells predominate on the smear.

Plate 3.8

At midcycle the endocervical mucus shows the characteristic fern-like crystallization when left to dry on a glass slide without fixation or staining.

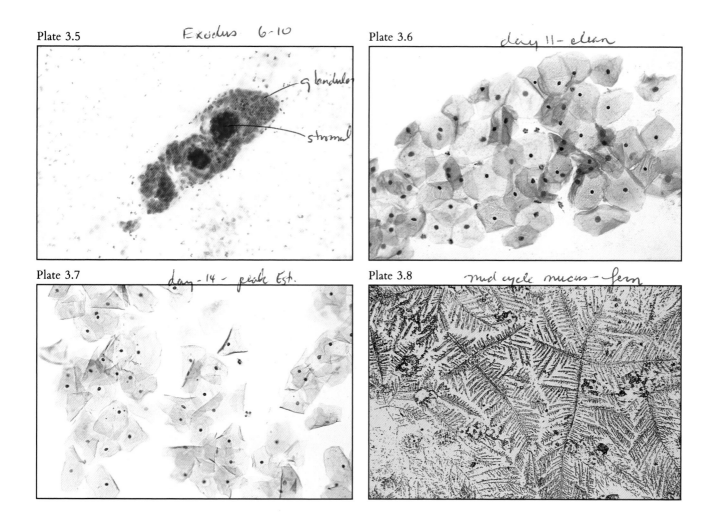

Plate 3.5   Exodus 6-10   glandular   stromal

Plate 3.6   day 11 - clean

Plate 3.7   day 14 - peak Est.

Plate 3.8   mid cycle mucus - fern

Plate 3.9

Day 21 of a menstrual cycle. Progesterone secretion from the corpus luteum produces clumping of the squamous cells, with loss of distinct cell boundaries and wrinkled cell membranes. Intermediate cells predominate.

Plate 3.10

Day 23 of a menstrual cycle. There is no progesterone effect here. The smear contains flat intermediate and superficial cells, indicating that ovulation has not taken place.

Plate 3.11

Day 12 of a menstrual cycle. The patient is taking contraceptive medication. The smear contains mostly glycogen-filled intermediate cells in dense groupings.

Plate 3.12

Effect of contraceptive medication. The smear—taken at any time before day 24 of the cycle—shows a pattern reminiscent of the secretory phase.

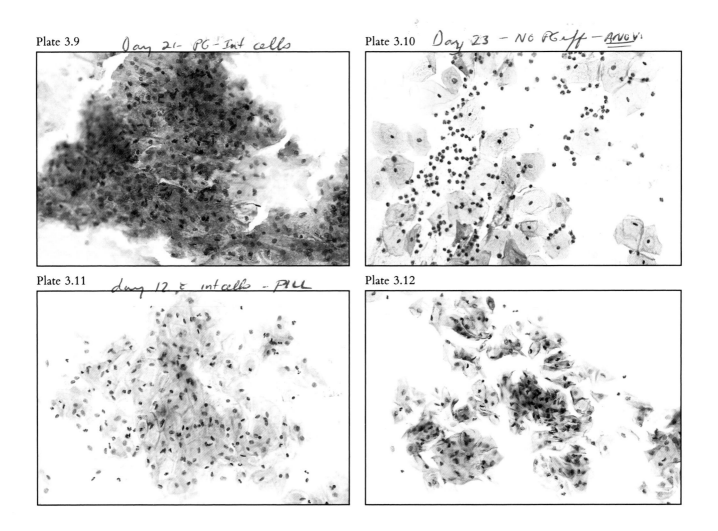

Plate 3.9   *Day 21 - PG - Int cells*

Plate 3.10   *Day 23 - No PG eff - ANOV*

Plate 3.11   *day 12, c int cells - PILL*

Plate 3.12

Plate 3.13
Smear obtained during the 16th week of pregnancy, illustrating the "navicular" pattern. In this pattern, intermediate cells predominate, usually containing a droplet of glycogen, which pushes the nucleus into an eccentric position.

Plate 3.14
The cytolytic pattern of pregnancy. The smear contains abundant Döderlein bacilli. The intermediate cells have lost their cytoplasm (cytolysis). Only the nuclei remain. This pattern is normal and does not require treatment.

Plate 3.15
Smear obtained during the 14th week of pregnancy. No progesterone effect is visible. This pattern indicates a possible threatened abortion.

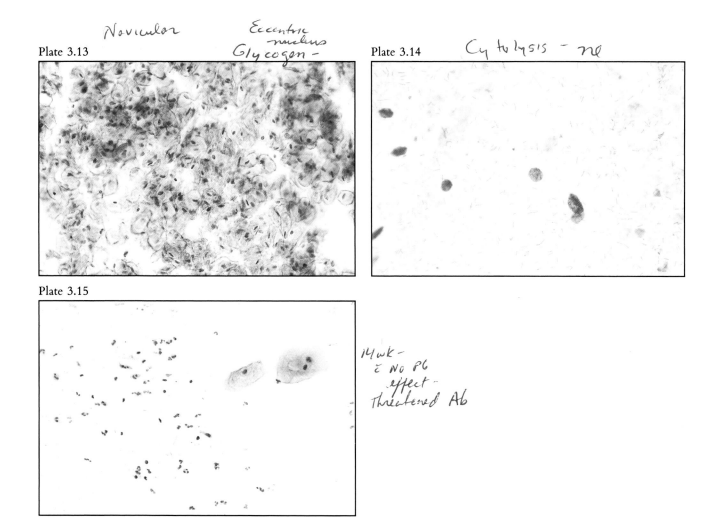

Plate 3.13   Navicular   Eccentric nucleus   Glycogen -

Plate 3.14   Cytolysis - ne

Plate 3.15   14 wk - č No PG effect - Threatened Ab

Plate 3.16
Smear obtained during the 14th week of pregnancy. The pattern is atrophic, indicating loss of hormonal support. The possibility of fetal death in utero must be considered.

Plate 3.17
Smear obtained from the same patient as Plate 3.16 after oral administration of estrogen. The smear now contains mostly superficial cells, confirming the diagnosis of fetal death in utero. Estrogen administration does not produce maturation when the pregnancy is normal.

Plate 3.18
Smear obtained 4 weeks after delivery. The ovaries have not resumed their function; the cell pattern is atrophic.

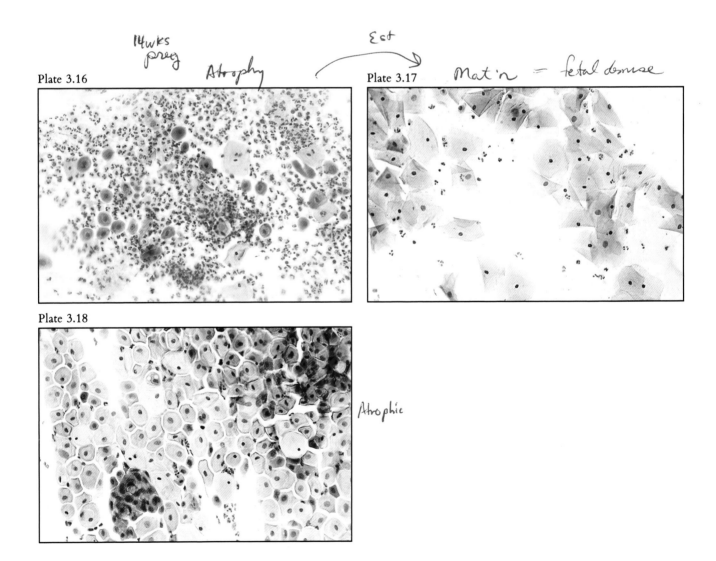

Plate 3.16

Plate 3.17

Plate 3.18

Plate 3.19

Smear obtained from a 64-year-old woman. No hormonal medication had been given. The smear is atrophic.

Plate 3.20

The effect of estrogen is reflected on the vaginal smear by the presence of superficial squamous cells.

Plate 3.21

A predominance of normal parabasal cells on a vaginal smear (excluding immature squamous metaplasia) indicates absence of gonadal hormone effect.

Plate 3.19

Plate 3.20

Plate 3.21

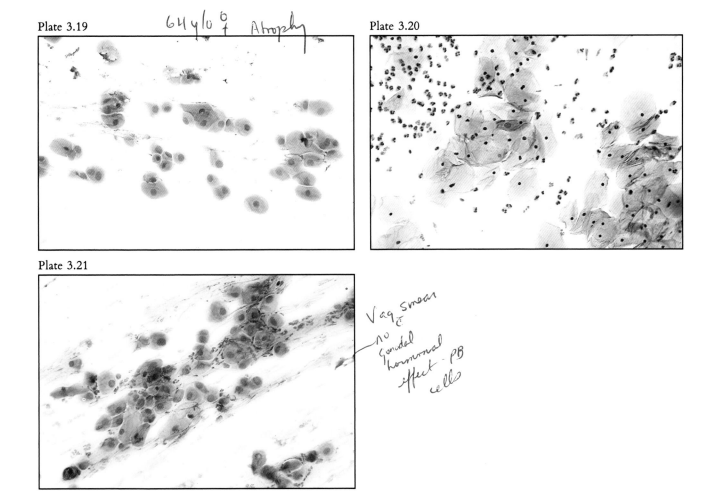

References

1. Batrinos ML, Eustratriades MG: Vaginal cytology in primary amenorrhea. *Acta Cytol* 16:376–380, 1972.

2. Butler EB, Taylor DS: The postnatal smear. *Acta Cytol* 17:237–240, 1973.

3. Heber KR: The effect of progestogens on vaginal cytology. *Acta Cytol* 19:103–109, 1975.

4. Holmquist ND, Danos M: The cytology of early abortion. *Acta Cytol* 11:262–266, 1967.

5. Keebler CM, Wied GL: The estrogen test: an aid in differential diagnosis. *Acta Cytol* 18:482–493, 1974.

6. Kobilkova J: Cytologic study of the level of estrogen during the reproductive age. *Acta Cytol* 11:497–500, 1967.

7. McLennan MT, McLennan CE: Hormonal patterns in vaginal smears from puerperal women. *Acta Cytol* 19:431–433, 1975.

8. Meisels A, Dubreuil-Charrois M: Hormonal cytology during pregnancy. *Acta Cytol* 10:376–382, 1966.

9. Meisels A, Schneider V: Hormonal cytology. *Clini Perinatol* 1:53–63, 1974.

10. Meisels A: Computed cytohormonal findings in 3307 healthy women. *Acta Cytol* 9:328–333, 1965.

11. Meisels A: Cytologic diagnosis of pregnancy. *Acta Cytol* 11:252, 1967.

12. Meisels A: El diagnóstico hormonal durante el embarazo. *Prensa Med Mex* 30:85–91, 1965.

13. Meisels A: Hormonal cytology. In: *Compendium on Diagnostic Cytology*, Wied GL, Keebler CM, Koss LG, Reagan JW (editors), The Tutorials of Cytology, Chicago, 1988, pp 43–48.

14. Meisels A: Le cytodiagnostic hormonal durant la grossesse. *Laval Med* 34:551–560, 1963.

15. Meisels A: Letter to the editor: Cytohormonal findings and high estrogen levels. *JAMA* 200:262, 1967.

16. Meisels A: The maturation value. *Acta Cytol* 11:249, 1967.

17. Meisels A: The menopause. A cytohormonal study. *Acta Cytol* 10:49–55, 1966.

18. Reyniak JV, Sedlis A, Stone D, Connell E: Cytohormonal findings in patients using various forms of contraception. *Acta Cytol* 13:315–322, 1969.

19. Soloway HB: Vaginal and cervical cytology of the early puerperium. *Acta Cytol* 13:136–138, 1969.

20. Soszka S, Wisniewski L: Cytologic evaluation of fetal death and an attempt to determine the time of its occurrence. *Acta Cytol* 11:403–409, 1967.

21. Stone DF, Sedlis A, Stone M, Turkel WV: Estrogen-like effects in the vaginal smears of postmenopausal women. *Acta Cytol* 11:349–352, 1967.

22. Uyanwah PO: Influence of maternal factors on the postnatal smear. *Acta Cytol* 29:800–804, 1985.

23. Wied GL, Boschann HW, Férin J, Frost JK, Luksch F, Meisels A, Montalvo-Ruiz L, Terzano G, Teter J, Wachtel E: Symposium on hormonal cytology. *Acta Cytol* 12:87–127, 1968.

CHAPTER FOUR

Microbiology

It is essential for the cytologist to recognize the microorganisms that occur on routine smears. The microbiologic diagnosis is a valued side benefit of screening programs. Volumes have been written on this subject and no attempt is made here to review the literature, but only to describe the more common microorganisms that have clinical importance and can be readily identified on the smears.

Bacteria

Although the lactobacillus of *Döderlein* (Plate 4.1) has been considered to represent the "normal" flora, it is found in only about 20% of patients screened.[2] It is a rod of variable length, usually associated with cytolysis. Cytolysis occurs when, in the presence of lactobacilli, the cytoplasm disappears, resulting in the presence of "naked" nuclei. The *Döderlein* bacillus feeds on glycogen, which is found in intermediate cells and is more abundant during the second half of the menstrual cycle and during pregnancy. The naked nuclei represent the remains of intermediate cells. Cytolysis occurs with a "clean" background (Plate 4.2), as opposed to autolysis, which is the destruction of the cytoplasm by the action of other agents, and which is accompanied by numerous inflammatory cells.

In about 35% of women screened,[2] the smears display either mixed (Plate 4.3) or coccoid bacteria[5,6] (Plate 4.4). These microorganisms can not be identified with certainty by cytology. "Mixed" flora consist of cocci and rods, and may be found in the absence of any sign of inflammation. Coccoid bacteria appear on the smear in the form of a cloudy whitish background. Lactobacilli and mixed and coccoid bacteria can be grouped together in the category of non-pathogenic flora and can be reported as such.

(handwritten margin note: LB mixed, coccoid } non pathogenic)

Cytology can identify, with more or less certainty, a number of pathogenic microorganisms. *Gardnerella vaginalis* (previously *Haemophilus vaginalis* or *Corynebacterium vaginalis*) adhere to the surface of squamous cells, forming a uniform grainy cyanophilic cover known as "clue cells" (Plates 4.5 and 4.6). *G vaginalis* can be cultured in the vast majority of cases when clue cells are present. Other bacteria may adhere to squamous cells, but they are usually longer and their distribution is irregular (compare Plate 4.7—a "true" clue cell with Plate 4.8—a "false" clue cell). About one fifth of women screened harbor *G vaginalis*, often with signs of mild to moderate inflammation. Recognition of the gonococcus (*Neisseria gonorrhoeae*)[15] is more debatable. The presence of diplococci within the cytoplasm of leukocytes is suggestive and should elicit further microbiologic investigation.

(handwritten margin note: 20% – clue cells = G. vaginalis)

Chlamydia trachomatis is an extremely small intracellular microorganism responsible for trachoma and inclusion conjunctivitis, lymphogranuloma venereum, and sexually transmitted infections of the genital tract that may cause pelvic inflammatory disease and infertility. Previously thought to be a virus, *Chlamydia* went under various names: TRIC agent, *Bedsonia*, and *Miyagawanella*. It was finally decided that it is a bacterium and a special genus, *Chlamydia*, was created for it. This genus comprises two species, *C trachomatis* and *C psittaci*, the latter being responsible for psittacosis, a disease transmitted by parrots.

Chlamydial infection of the cervix is diagnosed by culture, monoclonal antibodies, and enzyme-linked immunoassays.[6,11] The Papanicolaou smear is unreliable.[1] The cellular changes that have been described[3,7,13,16,18,28] consist of small eosinophilic coccoid bodies found within the cytoplasm. Later, fine vacuoles appear with larger cyanophilic inclusions. The vacuoles are of uniform size and have distinct outlines. They are grouped around the nucleus and tend to mold to each other (Plate 4.13). The life-cycle of the organism takes about 35 hours. Cellular abnormalities are sometimes found associated with chlamydial infections.[7] These changes are subtle, *(handwritten: Key)* difficult to differentiate from degenerative vacuoles (Plate 4.14), and show little correlation with the results of the other tests mentioned above. The systematic search for *C trachomatis* on routine smears is a futile and time-consuming exercise.

Protozoa

Trichomonas vaginalis appears on smears as a pale, greyish pear-shaped body, which resembles partially lysed cytoplasm. It often contains a small, dense, eccentric nucleus. The cytoplasm displays small, round, eosinophilic granulations[10,17,29] (Plate 4.9). Rarely, it is possible to observe the flagellae (Plate 4.10). Trichomonads may occur without signs of inflammation, but frequently produce a marked reaction, trichomoniasis, with abundant inflammatory exudate. Mature squamous cells often display perinuclear halos in the presence of trichomoniasis, and the smear is poorly stained, most cells being faintly eosinophilic (Plate 4.11). Because trichomoniasis is easily detected on smears, and because its treatment is effective and simple, this infestation has decreased in frequency: in the 1960s our laboratory reported finding *T vaginalis* in about 13% of the women screened;[22] in the 1970s the rate was down to 6%[21] and presently it is of the order of 2% to 3%. This rate varies widely from one area to another (at the University of Chicago Clinics in 1987 it was still 15%).[5]

A thin, elongated bacterium known as *Leptothrix* is often found associated with trichomonads and can be easily recognized on smears (Plate 4.12). It varies in length and does not seem to have much clinical significance when present without other pathogens.

Leptothrix — no sig.

Fungi

Actinomycetes are occasionally found on smears in patients wearing an intrauterine contraceptive device.[12] They are recognized by their characteristic "dust-ball" appearance: small, round, poorly delineated formations of microorganisms from which thin filaments radiate in all directions (Plates 4.15 and 4.16).

Among the fungal diseases that can be recognized on the smears, most are due to *Torulopsis glabrata*, which produces small yeast cells without elongated forms[27] surrounded by a thin clear halo (Plate 4.17). *Candida* are larger yeast cells with elongated segmented forms. They are identified by their budding and pseudomycelia (Plates 4.18 and 4.19).[10,14,29] *Geotricum* produces mycelia and spores (Plates 4.20 and 4.21). Squamous cells on the smear are often poorly stained, with a pale, sometimes eosinophilic vacuolate cytoplasm (Plate 4.22). The presence of fungi on smears should be reported, but it is difficult to be specific because these microorganisms closely resemble each other. It is best to signal the presence of fungi and remain descriptive.

Viruses

The most common viral infection of the genital tract is produced by human papillomavirus (see Chapter Six). Cellular manifestations of herpesvirus II (HSV) infection are not seen frequently, probably because the acute stage lasts only for 2 or 3 weeks, and it is a matter of chance to receive a routine smear obtained during that short period of time. When present, the cytologic findings are characteristic:[4,9,24-26,29,30] the chromatin degenerates and the nuclei take a ground-glass appearance, with the remnants of chromatin forming a thin irregular rim beneath the nuclear membrane. Multinucleation is frequent and the nuclei tend to cluster close to each other and to become molded (Plates 4.23 and 4.24). Eventually the degenerative phenomenon also involves the cytoplasm, which becomes amphophilic and takes the same color as the nucleus. The end stage is karyorrhexis and karyolysis. Another characteristic of HSV-infected nuclei is the presence of a large, irregular, eosinophilic nuclear inclusion, surrounded by a clear halo. The chromatin is relegated to the periphery of the nucleus. Inclusion-bearing cells may also form syncytia (Plates 4.25–4.29).

Other viral infections can occur on the cervix.[20] Cytomegalovirus produces intranuclear inclusions difficult—if not impossible—to differentiate from those produced by HSV.[19,23,24]

In tropical countries the smear may contain various other microorganisms and parasites: *Entamoeba histolytica* (Plate 4.30), *Ascaris lumbricoides, Enterobius vermicularis* (Plate 4.31), *Trichiuris trichiuria,* etc, discussion of which goes beyond the scope of this volume.

Plate 4.1

Lactobacillus Döderlein. These rod-like organisms thrive on the glycogen contained within the cytoplasm of intermediate cells and produce cytolysis: only the nuclei of the squamous cells persist. Döderlein bacilli live in an acid environment.

Plate 4.2

Higher magnification of the smear depicted in Plate 4.1. Cytoplasmic debris are seen in the background.

Plate 4.3

Mixed flora. The smear contains small rods of varying sizes and some coccoid organisms.

Plate 4.4

Pure coccoid flora. The microorganisms form a cloudy background on the smear.

Non pathogenic flora

Plate 4.1

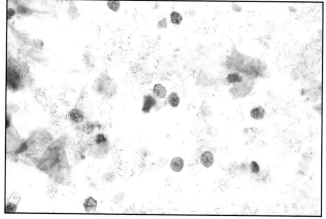

Plate 4.2

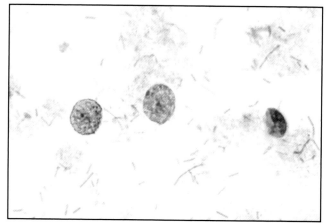

Plate 4.3

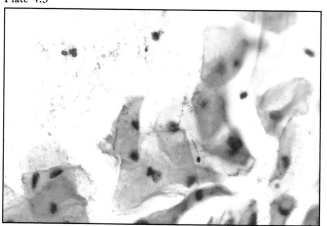

Plate 4.4

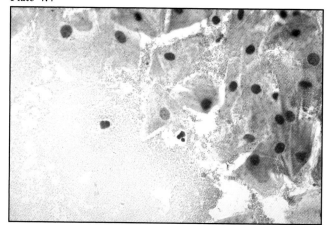

Plate 4.5
Gardnerella vaginalis. The clue cells can be recognized even at low magnification by their characteristic purple color.

Plate 4.6
Higher magnification of a clue cell. *G vaginalis* is a tiny rod-like organism that clings to the cellular membrane. The background is clean.

Plate 4.7
Clue cell. In spite of the pinkish staining, the microorganisms are firmly attached to the cell membrane without spilling over into the background. Compare with Plate 4.8.

Plate 4.8
This is a false clue cell. The staining is cyanophilic and the microorganisms spread out into the background. Compare with Plate 4.7.

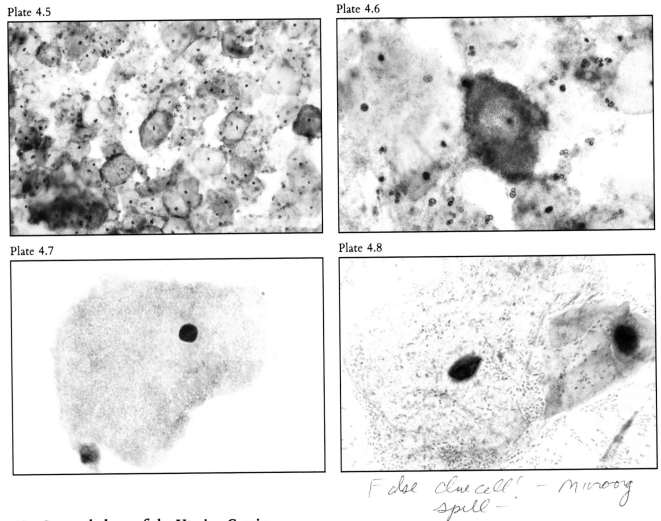

Plate 4.5

Plate 4.6

Plate 4.7

Plate 4.8

False clue cell! — microorg spill —

Plate 4.9

Trichomonas vaginalis. These are flagellate parasites with a small eccentric nucleus and characteristic pink granules in the cytoplasm.

Plate 4.10

Trichomonas vaginalis (arrows). The pink granules are clearly visible.

Plate 4.11

Halo formation in trichomoniasis. The squamous cells tend to lose their cytoplasmic staining affinity. These intermediate cells all stain pink instead of blue-green.

Plate 4.12

Leptothrix, often associated with trichomonads. The very long hair-like organisms can be seen with trichomonads, which appear here like cytoplasmic blobs.

Plate 4.9

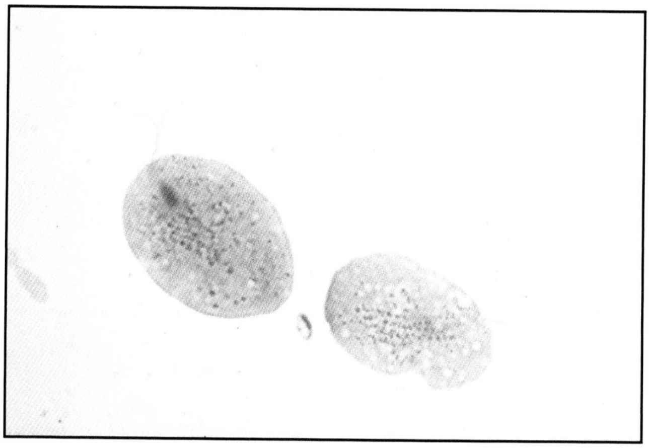

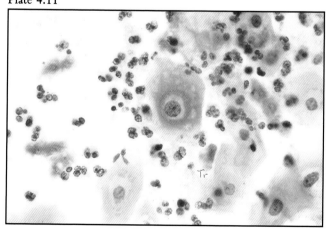

Plate 4.10

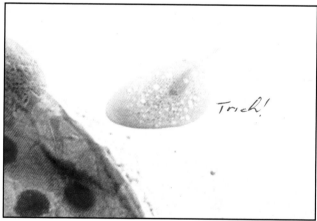

Plate 4.11

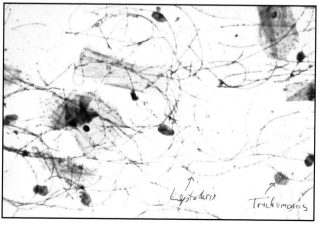

Plate 4.12

Plate 4.13
This cell shows the morphologic changes that have been described in cases of *Chlamydia trachomatis* infection. The cytoplasm contains a number of sharply demarcated vacuoles that contain pinkish material.

Plate 4.14
Parabasal cell containing degenerative vacuoles in the cytoplasm.

Plate 4.15
Actinomycetes in characteristic dust-ball formation.

Plate 4.16
At higher magnification, the actinomycetes can be seen to project rod-like structures outwards from the tight ball formation. Actinomycetes are sometimes observed in women wearing intrauterine contraceptive devices (IUDs).

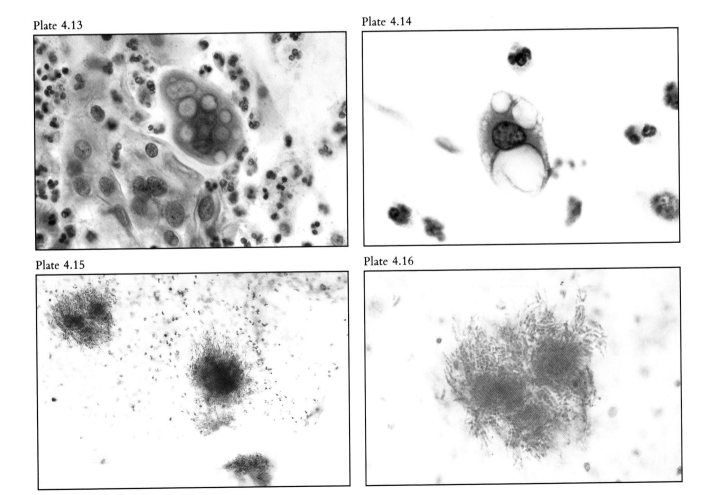

Plate 4.13

Plate 4.14

Plate 4.15

Plate 4.16

Plate 4.17
Tiny spores identified as *Torulopsis glabrata*.

Plate 4.18
Candida is identified by its pseudomycelia (protoplasm is not continuous between the main stem and the various branches) and the buds emerging from the stems.

Plate 4.19
Candida alters the cytoplasmic staining affinity of squamous cells, much as *Trichomonas vaginalis* does. The cells tend towards eosinophilia.

Plate 4.20
Geotricum produces true mycelia with characteristic branching.

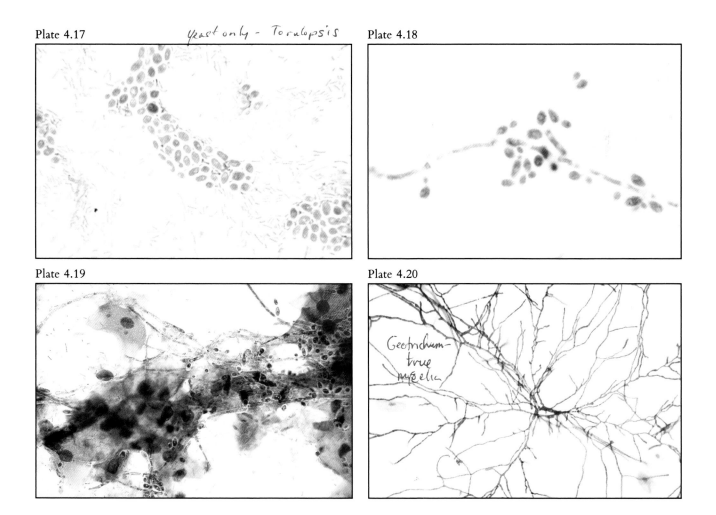

Plate 4.17   *yeast only - Torulopsis*   Plate 4.18

Plate 4.19   Plate 4.20   *Geotrichum - true mycelia*

Plate 4.21

Geotricum. Note that the protoplasm is continuous between the branches and the stems.

Plate 4.22

Cellular pattern of fungal infections. Notice the poor staining reaction of the cytoplasm of the squamous cells.

Plate 4.23

Characteristic cellular changes of herpesvirus infection. The nuclei take a "ground-glass" texture and tend to agglutinate and mold to each other.

Plate 4.24

Herpesvirus II infection. Very bizarre cells with agglutinated ground-glass type nuclei.

Plate 4.21

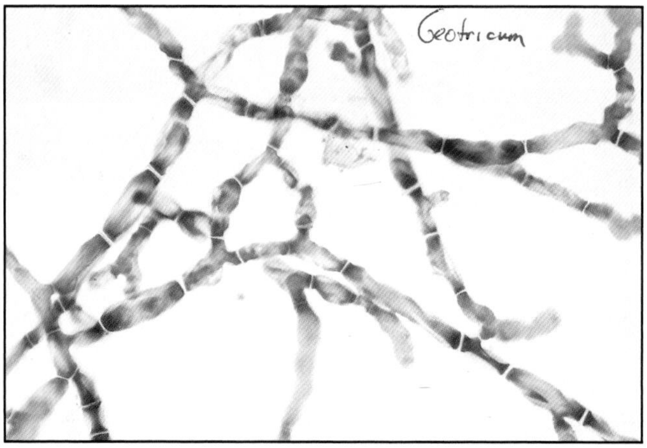

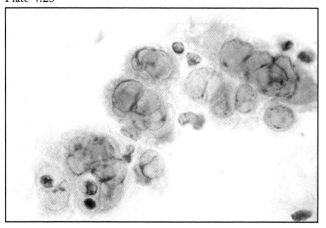

Plate 4.22

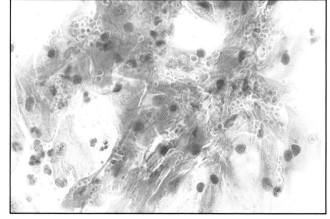

Plate 4.23

Plate 4.24

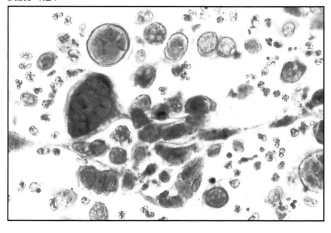

Plate 4.25

Herpesvirus II infection. This tadpole-shaped cell contains several molded nuclei, each of which is centered by a large, darkly stained, irregular inclusion, surrounded by a clear halo.

Plate 4.26

A multinucleated cell from a herpesvirus II infection. Note the large intranuclear inclusions surrounded by a clear space. The remaining chromatin can be seen at the inner aspect of the nuclear membrane.

Plate 4.27

In this group of cells displaying characteristic changes of herpesvirus II infection, both ground-glass nuclei and nuclei with large inclusions can be observed.

Plate 4.28

Section from a biopsy of a herpetic lesion of the cervix. The epithelial cells show multinucleation with intranuclear inclusions. Note the marked inflammatory infiltrate.

Plate 4.25

Plate 4.26

Plate 4.27

Plate 4.28

Plate 4.29

Higher magnification of the tissue specimen illustrated in Plate 4.28. Ground-glass type nuclei can be seen alongside others containing large viral inclusions.

Plate 4.30

Entamoeba histolytica found in a case of cervical amebiasis. Note the erythrocytes within the cytoplasm of the parasite.

Plate 4.31

Enterobius vermicularis found on a V–C–E smear, probably a fecal contaminant.

Plate 4.29

Plate 4.30

E histolytica

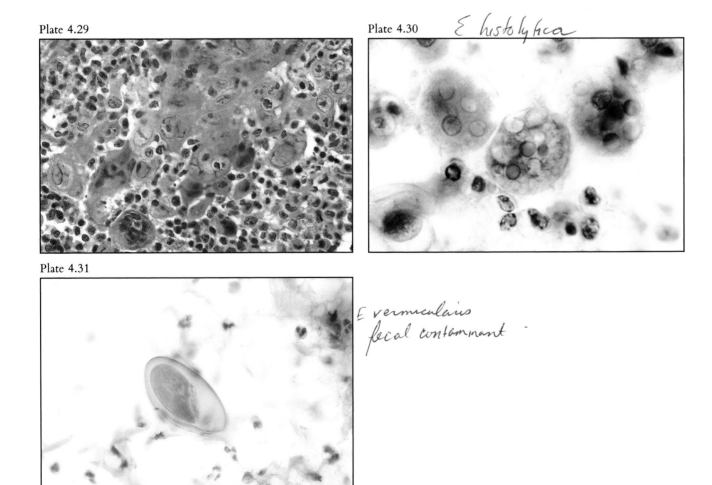

Plate 4.31

E vermicularis
fecal contaminant

References

1. Arroyo G, Linnemann C, Wesseler T: Role of the Papanicolaou smear in diagnosis of chlamydial infections. *Sex Tr Dis* 16:11–14, 1989.

2. Bartlett JG, Moon NE, Goldstein PR, Goren B, Onderdonk AB, Polk BF: Cervical and vaginal bacterial flora: Ecologic niches in the female lower genital tract. *Am J Obstet Gynecol* 130:658–661, 1978.

3. Bartlett JG, Onderdonk AB, Drude E, Goldstein C, Anderka M, Alpert S, McCormack WM: Quantitative bacteriology of the vaginal flora. *J. Infect Dis* 136:271–277, 1977.

4. Beilby JOW, Cameron CH, Catterall RD, Davidson D: Herpesvirus hominis infection of the cervix associated with gonorrhoea. *Lancet* 1:1065–1066, 1968.

5. Bibbo M, Wied GL: Microbiology and inflammation of the female genital tract. In: Compendium on Diagnostic Cytology, Wied GL, Keebler CM, Koss LG, Reagan JW (editors), The Tutorials of Cytology, Chicago, 1988, pp 54–62.

6. Burns DCM, Darougar S, Thin RT, Lothian L, Nicol CS: Isolation of *chlamydia* from women attending a clinic for sexually transmitted disease. *Br J Venereal Dis* 51:314–318, 1975.

7. Carr MC, Hanna L, Jawetz E: *Chlamydiae*, cervicitis, and abnormal Papanicolaou smears. *Obstet Gynecol* 53:27–30, 1979.

8. Catterall RD: Trichomonal infections of the genital tract. *Med Clin North Am* 56:1203–1209, 1972.

9. Chang TW: Genital herpes and type 1 herpesvirus hominis. *JAMA* 238:155, 1977.

10. Eriksson G, Wanger L: Frequency of *N. gonorrhoeae, T. vaginalis,* and *C. albicans* in female venereological patients. A one year study. *Brit J Vener Dis* 51:192–197, 1975.

11. Ghadirian FD, Robson HG: *Chlamydia trachomatis* genital infections. *Brit J Vener Dis* 55:415–418, 1979.

12. Gupta PK, Hollander DH, Frost JK: Actinomycetes in cervico-vaginal smears: An association with IUD usage. *Acta Cytol* 20:295–297, 1976.

13. Gupta PK, Lee EF, Erozan YS, Frost JK, Geddes ST, Donovan PA: Cytologic investigation in *Chlamydia* infection. *Acta Cytol* 23:315–320, 1979.

14. Heller CJ, Hoyt V: Squamous cell changes associated with the presence of *Candida* sp. in cervical Papanicolaou smears. *Acta Cytol* 15:379–384, 1971.

15. Heller CJ: *Neisseria gonorrhoeae* in Papanicolaou smears. *Acta Cytol* 18:338–340, 1974.

16. Hilton AL, Richmond SJ, Milne JD, Hinley F, Clarke SKR: *Chlamydia* A in the female genital tract. *Brit J Vener Dis* 50:1–10, 1974.

17. Jirovec O, Petru M: *Trichomonas vaginalis* and *Trichomoniasis. Adv Parasitol* 6:117–188, 1968.

18. Johanisson G, Löwhagen GB, Lycke E: Genital *Chlamydia trachomatis* infection in women. *Obstet Gynecol* 56:671–675, 1980.

19. Jordan MC, Rousseau WE, Noble GR, Steart JA, Chin TDY: Association of cervical cytomegaloviruses with venereal disease. *N Engl J Med* 288:932–934, 1973.

20. Laverty CR, Russell P, Black J, Kappagoda N, Benn RAV, Booth N: Adenovirus infection of the cervix. *Acta Cytol* 21:114–117, 1977.

21. Meisels A, Gagné O: Microbiology of the female genital tract. V. Changing patterns within one decade in a French Canadian population. *J Reprod Med* 18:66–68, 1977.

22. Meisels A: Microbiology of the female reproductive tract as determined in the cytologic specimen. I. Influence of gonadal hormones. *J Reprod Med* 1:603–612, 1968.

23. Montgomery R, Youngblood L, Medearis DM: Recovery of cytomegalovirus from the cervix in pregnancy. *Pediatrics* 49:524–531, 1972.

24. Morse AR, Coleman DV, Gardner SD: An evaluation of cytology in the diagnosis of herpes simplex virus infection and cytomegalovirus infection of the cervix uteri. *J Obstet Gynaecol Br Commonwealth* 81:393–398, 1974.

25. Naib ZM, Nahmias AJ, Josey WE: Cytology and histopathology of cervical herpes simplex infection. *Cancer* 19:1026–1032, 1966.

26. Naib ZM: Exfoliative cytology of viral cervico-vaginitis. *Acta Cytol* 10:126–129, 1966.

27. Omer EFE, Gummaa SA, El-Naeen HA, Hagali M: *Torulopsis glabrata* and *Candida albicans* in female infections in the Sudan. *Br J Vener Dis* 57:165–166, 1981.

28. Oriel JD, Powis PA, Reeve P, Miller A, Nicol CS: Chlamydial infections of the cervix. *Br J Vener Dis* 50:11–16, 1974.

29. Thin RNT, Atia W, Parker JDJ, Nicol CS: Value of Papanicolaou-stained smears in the diagnosis of trichomoniasis, candidiasis, and cervical herpes simplex virus infection in women. *Br J Vener Dis* 51:116–118, 1975.

30. Vesterinen E, Purola E, Saksela E, Leinikki P: Clinical and virological findings in patients with cytologically diagnosed gynecological herpes simplex infections. *Acta Cytol* 21:199–205, 1977.

CHAPTER FIVE

Benign Morphologic Changes

Squamous Metaplasia

When the squamocolumnar junction is located distal to the external os, on the exocervix, the mature endocervical columnar epithelium is progressively replaced by a more or less mature squamous epithelium, beginning around puberty. This normal development results in an area on the cervix in which squamous epithelium overlays glandular spaces: the transformation zone (Plate 5.1). Although squamous metaplasia as such has no diagnostic significance, its presence indicates that an adequate smear has been obtained from the transformation zone.

If the squamous metaplasia has matured completely, it cannot be recognized on cellular samples; the cells are identical to the mature squamous cells of the cervix. Only cells from an incompletely mature or immature metaplasia can be identified with certainty. Such cells are parabasal cells with a normal nuclear/cytoplasmic (N/C) ratio and one round or oval nucleus containing finely granular or reticular chromatin; the nuclear membrane is smooth and thin, small nucleoli may be present. The cytoplasm is dense and cyanophilic. Metaplastic cells show great uniformity of size and shape. They may occur singly or in small groups or chains, rarely in loose sheets[11] (Plates 5.2–5.7). Often they will be found within streaks of mucus.

Keratinization and Epidermization

The squamous epithelium of the cervix does not normally keratinize. The uppermost layers are flattened and display pyknotic nuclei. The cells may contain keratin precursors (hyalokeratin), but no real keratin. In some circumstances the surface layers may become keratinized and are then made up of anucleated squames (Plate 5.8). In epidermization there is, in addition, a granular layer in the epithelium (Plate 5.9). Underneath the keratin layer, the epithelium may appear normal, or it may show any of the changes due to HPV, intraepithelial squamous lesions, or even squamous carcinoma. Since it is the surface which is scraped, the smear obtained from areas of keratinization or epidermization usually contains anucleated squames, with no indication of underlying abnormalities (Plate 5.10). The presence of anucleated squames on a smear may also indicate that the sample was obtained from the lower third of the vagina or the vulva. Anucleated squames are not diagnostic, and the only mention that can be made of them, if there is evidence that the smear was obtained from the cervix, is the fact that there is an area of keratinization.

Inflammation

Inflammatory changes are characterized by the presence of an abundant exudate consisting mainly of granulocytes intermingled with a few histiocytes in a dirty background containing cellular debris and a serous/mucoid exudate (Plate 5.11). Epithelial cells show signs of degeneration: nuclei are pyknotic or karyorrhectic, and the cytoplasm is pale and amphophilic or eosinophilic (Plate 5.12). In the presence of *Trichomonas vaginalis* there often is perinuclear halo formation (Plate 5.13). Metaplastic cells may become vacuolated in the presence of *Chlamydia trachomatis* (Plate 5.14). With *Candida* the smear sometimes has a normal appearance; more often the squamous cells are pale and eosinophilic (Plate 5.15). With experience, the presence of *T vaginalis* or *Candida* can be inferred by the overall cellular changes on the smear (Plate 5.16).

Follicular or lymphocytic cervicitis is seen in postmenopausal women, rarely in younger age groups. Lymphoid follicles lodge under the epithelium, which may become eroded (Plate 5.17). Lymphocytic cervicitis is characterized by the presence on the smear of loose aggregates of lymphoid cells, mainly mature and immature lymphocytes (Plate 5.18), with a few plasma cells and macrophages containing "tingible bodies" (Plate 5.19). The latter are useful for identifying the pattern because they are not found in lymphomas, which are generally monomorphic.

If the inflammatory changes are very marked and the exudate is covering most of the smear, then the sample must be considered *unsatisfactory* and a repeat smear should be submitted after appropriate local treatment.

Repair and Therapy Effects

The squamous epithelium of the cervix will regenerate when it has been destroyed by inflammation (ulceration), injury, biopsy, or local destruction by cautery, freezing, or laser vaporization. During active repair cellular samples display sheets of elongated, large, immature cells, containing enlarged nuclei with pale chromatin and a prominent macronucleolus. The cytoplasm is abundant and cyanophilic. The sheets are arranged in a regular fashion, with conserved polarity (the cells lay parallel to each other in an orderly manner), and generally no overlapping (there is a single layer of cells) (Plates 5.20 and 5.21). Mitotic figures may be found (Plate 5.22); cells in the tissue actively proliferate. Single cells are rare in repair.[1,4] Repair must be differentiated from invasive large cell squamous carcinoma (see Chapter Nine). In the latter there are isolated malignant cells in addition to clusters in which the cells overlap considerably; the N/C ratio is elevated, the chromatin is irregular, the nucleoli are smaller, and the nuclear membrane is more prominent.

Various types of treatment may leave their mark on the squamous epithelium of the cervix. The cellular changes observed in these cases are difficult or impossible to interpret in the absence of pertinent clinical information.

Ionizing Radiation

The effect of irradiation on cells depends directly on the dose administered and inversely on the differentiation of the cells. The most radiosensitive cells are those that reproduce most frequently, since radiation has its greatest effect during mitosis. Since cancer cells retain the capacity for reproduction, they are the prime target of radiation effect. However, their mitotic rhythm may be slow, and for this reason repeated applications of radiotherapy are necessary to reach the largest possible number of cells, as they enter mitosis at various intervals. The basal (germinal) layer of the squamous epithelium is the site of most radiation-induced changes in benign tissues of the cervix. Irradiation may kill the cell, or it may cause genotypic changes with phenotypic consequences, which can be observed on smears. These modified cells reside in the basal layers and form clones which may persist for months or many years.

The effect of irradiation on benign cells can be classified into two main groups: the acute stage and the chronic stage. In the acute stage, occurring during the first month after therapy, an exudate contains leukocytes and debris resulting from local necrosis. Mononucleated and multinucleated histiocytes are often present. Signs of repair (see preceding section) are also observed. Squamous cells show the classical signs of irradiation: vacuolization (Plates 5.23 and 5.24), macrocytosis (Plates 5.25 and 5.26), nuclear enlargement (Plate 5.27), binucleation and multinucleation (Plates 5.28 and 5.29), bizarre shapes, and altered cytoplasmic staining reaction. The vacuoles are irregularly distributed in the cytoplasm and vary in size. The cells are enlarged and contain an enlarged nucleus, without increase in the N/C ratio. The chromatin remains bland and regular, and the nuclear membrane is uniformly thin, sometimes with an irregular outline. The cells often show bizarre shapes with irregular cytoplasmic extensions. The cytoplasm may take various hues with the Papanicolaou stain; often it is amphophilic or eosinophilic.[13]

During the chronic stage, the inflammatory changes disappear, repair ceases, and the smear becomes atrophic. Since irradiation produces clonal changes in the squamous basal cells, some of the changes described above can persist for many months or years. Often the only residue will be the atrophy and the presence of a small number of enlarged cells. In other cases, more profound cellular changes appear, which Patten has called "postradiation dysplasia"[12] (Plate 5.30). These changes are essentially identical to those observed in cases of high-grade squamous intraepithelial neoplasia, but the N/C ratio is not usually much increased. The significance of postradiation dysplasia is not clear: according to Patten it may indicate a probability for local recurrence or may indicate the presence of metastasis, while von Haam[13] stated that these dysplastic cells showed a generally decreased viability and generally could either disappear within days, or remain for the rest of the patient's life, without other evidence of malignant disease. Cells from postradiation dysplasia should not be confused with persistent or recurrent malignant cells.

Malignant cells disappear from the smears during or shortly after irradiation therapy. While still present, they display changes similar to those in benign cells: macrocytosis, swelling of the nucleus, clumping of the chromatin with tendency towards pyknosis, and vacuolization. The degenerative changes in malignant cells are more pronounced than in their benign counterparts (Plate 5.31). Malignant cells without radiation effect indicate persistent or recurrent tumor. Morphologically, they are identical with the cells from the original neoplasia, before treatment. Their presence signifies a poor prognosis.

Chemotherapy

Several chemotherapeutic agents used in the treatment of malignant tumors, particularly lymphomas, cause cellular changes similar to the effects (described above) that routinely occur after irradiation. Benign cells show marked degenerative changes, with cytoplasmic vacuolization (Plate 5.32), enlargement of the cytoplasmic volume and also of the nuclei (Plate 5.33), disruption of the chromatin structure, pyknosis, and karyorrhexis[8] (Plate 5.34). Since chemotherapy is mostly administered systemically, these changes can be seen in extra-genital areas: for example, in urine and bladder washings, sputum, etc. Adequate information concerning chemotherapy must be given by the clinician. When this information is not available, the correct interpretation of the smears may be extremely difficult, and errors are likely.

Electrocoagulation, Cryosurgery, Laser Vaporization

Local destruction of the mucous lining of the cervix produces acute and protracted changes. During the acute phase, the smear contains necrotic material and inflammatory cells with an abundant serous and bloody exudate. No cytologic interpretation is possible. Obtaining Pap smears within the first three months following treatment by electrocoagulation, cryosurgery, or laser vaporization is not recommended. Later there will be cytologic evidence of repair and regeneration. Inflammatory changes diminish and eventually the smear returns to a normal appearance, if the lesions have been completely destroyed.[2,6]

Hormone Therapy

Synthetic or organic gonadal-type hormones have a direct effect on the squamous epithelia of the cervix and vagina. Estrogens cause maturation, with exfoliation of mature squamous cells (Plate 5.35). Progesteroids cause a proliferation of the intermediate layers of the epithelium, without complete maturation. The smear will show a predominance of intermediate cells (Plate 5.36). Androgens impede maturation and result in smears containing many large, round, parabasal cells, sometimes containing glycogen (Plate 5.37). In most cases, these hormones are not administered singly, so a combined effect can be observed.

During pregnancy there is occasionally a decidual reaction on the cervix (Plate 5.38). Smears may contain large, pale, cyanophilic or eosinophilic cells, with one or two large vesicular nuclei containing a prominent nucleolus (Plates 5.39 and 5.40). When they form clusters, the cellular borders remain discrete. Decidual cells should not be misinterpreted as originating from a squamous carcinoma. Rarely one sees similar cells in patients taking oral contraceptive hormones (a morphologic appearance know as pseudo-decidualization of the cervix).

Trophoblasts may appear on gynecologic smears during pregnancy or in the weeks following delivery. Cytotrophoblasts have one, or rarely two, nuclei with finely distributed, regular chromatin and a prominent nucleolus, and a cyanophilic, sometimes vacuolated cytoplasm (Plate 5.41). They occur singly, or more frequently, in clusters in which the cellular boundaries are indistinct. Syncytiotrophoblasts form clumps of varying size and shape. The cytoplasm is dense, cyanophilic, and contains a variable number of darkly stained nuclei with coarse chromatin and small nucleoli (Plates 5.42 and 5.43).

Trophoblasts are rarely found on routine Pap smears from nonpregnant women. When they are numerous, or if they present morphologic abnormalities, the possibility of a trophoblastic tumor (ie, hydatidiform mole, invasive mole, or choriocarcinoma) should be taken into consideration.

Intrauterine Contraceptive Devices

Cellular changes due to an intrauterine contraceptive device (IUD) can be confusing if pertinent information is not provided by the clinician. More commonly, the smear displays clusters of glandular cells on a clean background. Cytoplasmic vacuolization is not infrequent and granulocytes may be seen within the vacuoles (Plate 5.44). Since many IUDs are provided with a string extending through the endocervical canal, both irritated endometrial and endocervical glandular cells can be observed.[3,5,7,9] Endometrial glandular cells are smaller and their nuclei are more darkly stained (Plate 5.45), than their endocervical counterparts (Plates 5.46 and 5.47). *Actinomycetes* organisms have been reported on smears from patients wearing IUDs of different types; they are rarely pathogenic.[10] They form small ball-like structures from which thin filaments radiate in all directions (see Plate 4.15, page 44).

Without information concerning the presence of an IUD, the endometrial cell changes should be interpreted as either "presence of endometrial cells out of phase in a menstruating woman or atypical endometrial glandular cells of undetermined significance" (Bethesda System). In our experience these changes have only rarely justified the removal of the IUD followed by further investigation (direct endometrial sample).

Patterns of Atrophy

In atrophy, the squamous epithelial lining of the cervix becomes very thin (Plate 5.48). Atrophic smears consist predominantly, or exclusively, of parabasal cells. In simple atrophy, the background is clean with few if any leukocytes. The most common difficulty arises in the presence of atrophic vaginitis or cervicitis. In those cases the background contains necrotic debris, the inflammatory exudate is abundant, and the parabasal cells show a range of degenerative changes (Plates 5.49 and 5.50). Many of the cells are very small, sometimes with an eosinophilic cytoplasm and a pyknotic nucleus. Other cells contain larger hyperchromatic or karyorrhectic nuclei. Occasionally, so-called blue blobs are observed (Plates 5.51 and 5.52). At first sight, they look like much enlarged hyperchromatic nuclei, sometimes with a prominent nucleolus. Closer examination reveals, however, that they are degenerated parabasal cells stained with hematoxylin; what looks like a nucleolus is actually the shrunken nucleus. Sheets of small cells with very scanty cytoplasm are sometimes seen; they form a single layer with well-preserved polarity.

Although atrophic vaginitis or cervicitis may display a few enlarged hyperchromatic nuclei, it is generally not necessary to administer estrogens in order to clean up the smear (Plate 5.53).

Plate 5.1
Tissue section illustrating an area of squamous metaplasia surrounding a glandular opening.

Plate 5.2
Cytologic presentation of squamous metaplasia. The cells are of the parabasal type. They form coherent sheets with a mosaiclike arrangement of the cells.

Plate 5.3
Squamous metaplasia. Parabasal cells in a small strip.

Plate 5.4
Higher magnification of a group of cells from squamous metaplasia. The cytoplasm may contain degenerative vacuoles. The nuclei are sometimes slightly irregular.

Plate 5.1

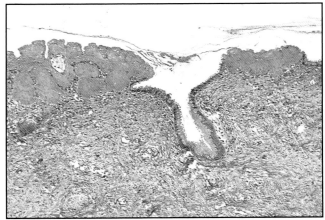

Plate 5.2

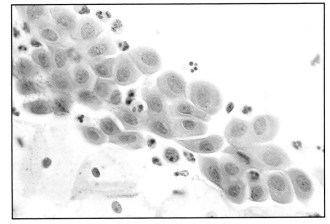

Plate 5.3

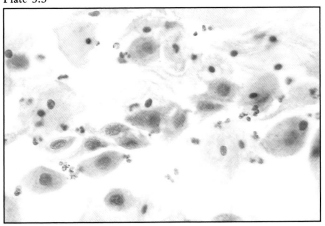

Plate 5.4

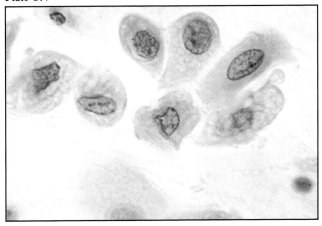

Plate 5.5
Cells from squamous metaplasia often form small "Indian files," with molding of the cell borders.

Plate 5.6
Tissue section demonstrating the histogenesis of squamous metaplasia. The reserve (subcolumnar) cells multiply and start a squamous differentiation, beneath the columnar epithelium. Eventually, the columnar cells are shed and the area is then seen as an immature squamous metaplasia (see Plate 5.1), which later may become mature (see Plate 5.7).

Plate 5.7
Mature squamous metaplasia can be seen on this tissue section surrounding a glandular opening.

Plate 5.8
Tissue section illustrating keratinization of the squamous epithelium of the cervix. The surface of the epithelium is covered by a layer of keratin.

Plate 5.5

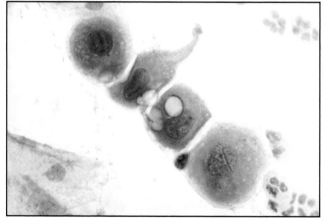

Plate 5.6

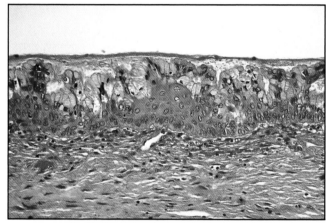

Plate 5.7

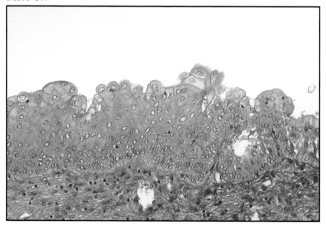

Plate 5.8

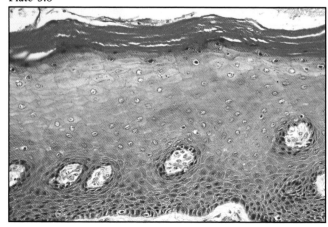

Plate 5.9

Epidermization is characterized histologically by the presence of a granular layer. The surface is keratinized.

Plate 5.10

On smears, keratinization of the squamous epithelium results in the presence of anucleated squames stained a brilliant orange with the Papanicolaou technique.

Plate 5.11

Inflammatory changes. The cells are poorly stained, there are numerous granulocytes, and sometimes a mucoid exudate can be seen in the background.

Plate 5.12

Inflammatory changes. The cytoplasm become eosinophilic even in the intermediate cells (these have vesicular nuclei). Nuclei tend to be swollen, without distinct chromatin detail.

Plate 5.9

Plate 5.10

Plate 5.11

Plate 5.12

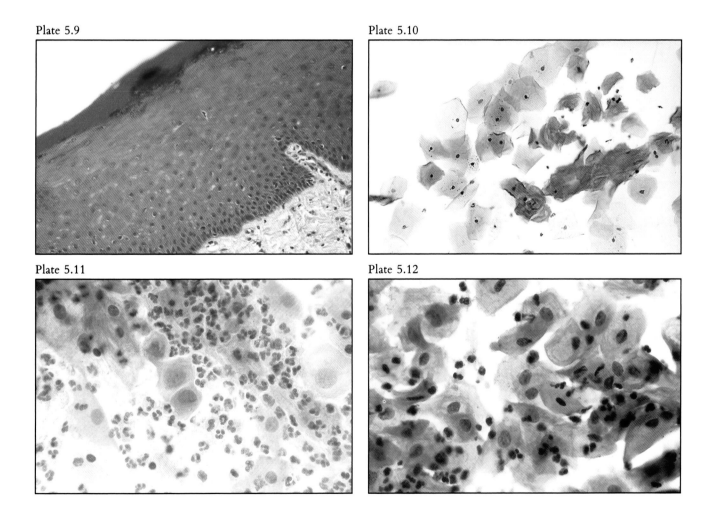

Plate 5.13

Inflammatory changes. Perinuclear halos and eosinophilia in a case of trichomoniasis.

Plate 5.14

Inflammatory changes. Cytoplasmic vacuolization in metaplastic cells. In this case, the vacuoles have sharp limits and contain an eosinophilic material, suggesting the presence of *Chlamydia* organisms.

Plate 5.15

Inflammatory changes. Cytoplasmic eosinophilia in the presence of *Candida* species.

Plate 5.16

Inflammatory changes. The smear has a dirty background and the cytoplasmic staining is irregular. Nuclei have a smudged appearance. Trichomonads and *Candida* species can be seen here.

Plate 5.13

Plate 5.14

Plate 5.15

Plate 5.16

Plate 5.17
Tissue section illustrating a case of lymphocytic (follicular) cervicitis.

Plate 5.18
Cell spread of a case of lymphocytic cervicitis. Lymphoid cells are grouped in discrete areas of the smear and usually comprise small lymphocytes and larger centrocytes.

Plate 5.19
Lymphocytic cervicitis. In the center, a characteristic macrophage containing tingible bodies.

Plate 5.17

Plate 5.18

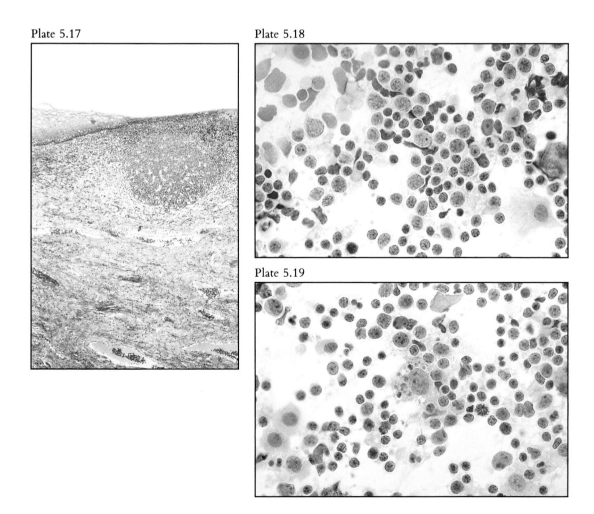

Plate 5.19

Plate 5.20
Cellular pattern of repair. The cells are large with cyanophilic or amphophilic cytoplasm, and contain large nuclei with smooth membranes and finely granular or reticular chromatin. A mitotic figure can be seen near the center of this illustration.

Plate 5.21
Cellular pattern of repair. The cells are arranged in sheets with little or no overlapping. Nucleoli are common. A mitotic figure can be seen near the center of this illustration.

Plate 5.22
Tissue section of an area of active repair following a recent biopsy. Nests of large cells are appearing in the damaged area and tend to grow towards each other. Nucleoli can be appreciated even at this low magnification.

Plate 5.23
Effect of ionizing radiation. There is considerable cytoplasmic vacuolization, with granulocytic inclusions.

Plate 5.20

Plate 5.21

Plate 5.22

Plate 5.23

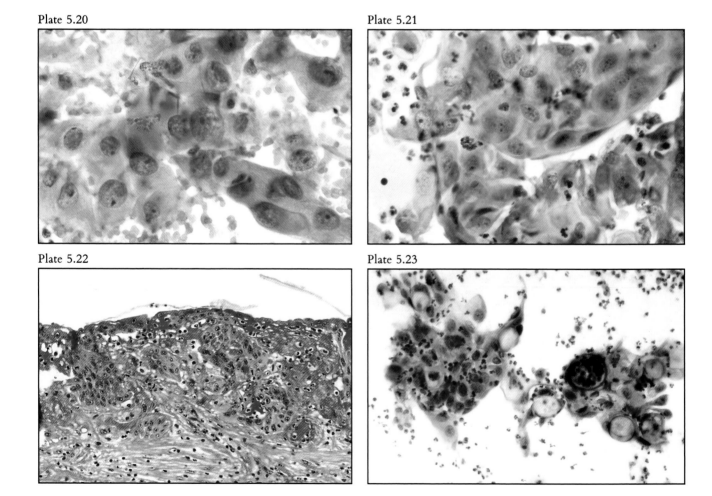

Plate 5.24

Higher magnification of Plate 5.23. The nuclei are within normal limits. The cytoplasm is abundant and vacuolated. One of the vacuoles contains numerous granulocytes.

Plate 5.25

Effect of ionizing radiation. Macrocytosis without significant nuclear changes. This pattern is often seen years after radiation therapy.

Plate 5.26

Effect of ionizing radiation. Here macrocytosis is associated with nuclear enlargement. The chromatin structure and the nuclear membrane remain within normal limits.

Plate 5.27

Effect of ionizing radiation. There is considerable nuclear enlargement. One nucleus contains a macronucleolus.

Plate 5.24

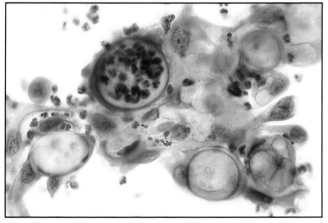

Plate 5.25

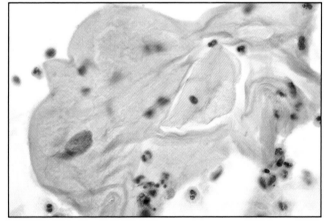

Plate 5.26

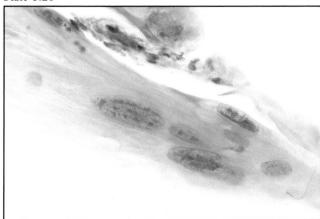

Plate 5.27

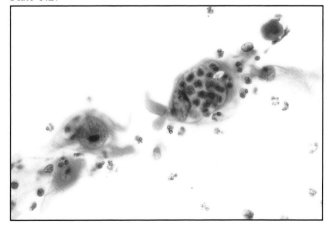

Plate 5.28

Effect of ionizing radiation. Multinucleation is often seen in these cases.

Plate 5.29

Effect of ionizing radiation. A multinucleated benign cell.

Plate 5.30

Pattern of postradiation dysplasia. The N/C ratio is increased, the nuclear membrane is slightly irregular, and the chromatin is coarsely granular.

Plate 5.31

Effect of ionizing radiation on a malignant cell. Note the degenerative vacuoles within this very large, darkly stained nucleus.

Plate 5.28

Plate 5.29

Plate 5.30

Plate 5.31

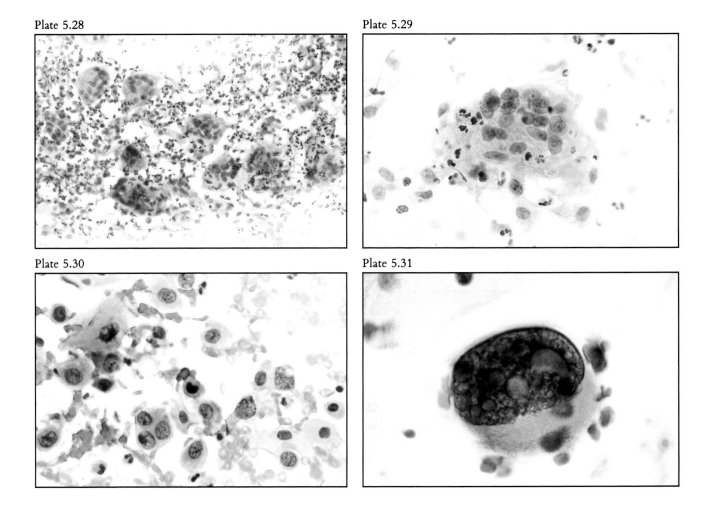

Plate 5.32
Effect of chemotherapy. The cells display marked cytoplasmic vacuolization.

Plate 5.33
Effect of chemotherapy. Macrocytosis, perinuclear halo formation, and slight enlargement of the nucleus.

Plate 5.34
Effect of chemotherapy. The cytoplasm is eosinophilic, the nucleus is pyknotic, and karyorrhexis has begun.

Plate 5.35
Effect of estrogen administration. Predominance of superficial squamous cells on a very clean background. The cells are isolated from each other and quite flat.

Plate 5.32

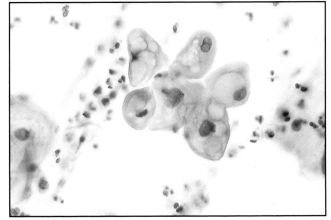

Plate 5.33

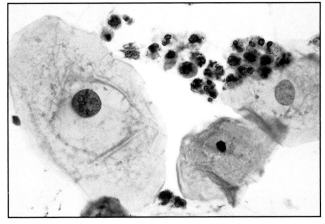

Plate 5.34

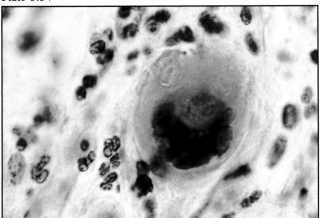

Plate 5.35

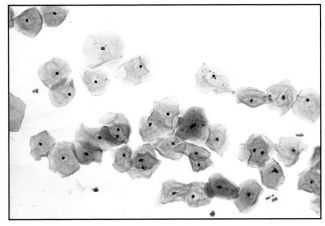

Plate 5.36

Effect of progesteroid administration. Predominance of intermediate squamous cells, which tend to cluster together and show some wrinkling of their membranes.

Plate 5.37

Effect of androgen administration. Predominance of small intermediate and parabasal squamous cells. The yellowish substance in the cytoplasm is glycogen.

Plate 5.38

Tissue section from a pregnant patient showing marked decidualization of the cervical stroma.

Plate 5.39

Cell spread from a patient in the 7th week of pregnancy. The cell at the center has a dense cytoplasm and three nuclei with coarsely granular chromatin. This cell originated in an area of decidualization of the cervix.

Plate 5.36

Plate 5.37

Plate 5.38

Plate 5.39

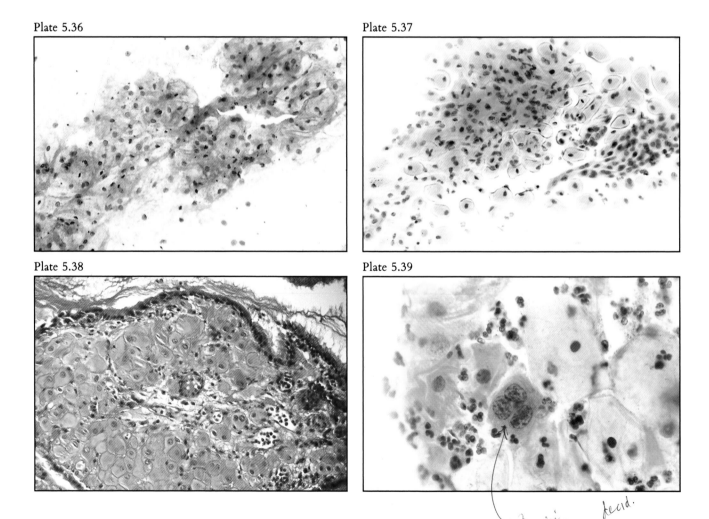

3 nuclei   decid.

Plate 5.40
A decidual cell from the smear illustrated in Plate 5.39

Plate 5.41
Cytotrophoblasts found on a V–C–E smear obtained shortly before delivery.

Plate 5.42
The multinucleated cells depicted here are syncytiotrophoblasts. Note the very large number of nuclei, filling almost all space within the cell.

Plate 5.43
A syncytiotrophoblast found on a V–C–E smear.

Plate 5.40

Plate 5.41

Plate 5.42

Plate 5.43

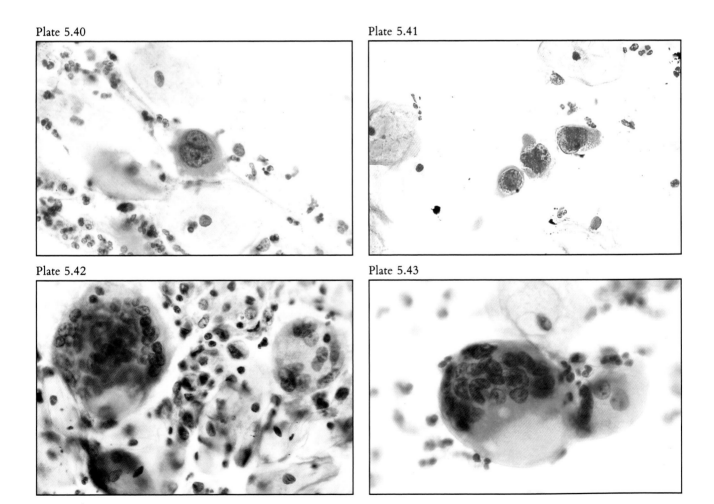

Plate 5.44
Effect of intrauterine contraceptive device (IUD). A tight, three-dimensional grouping of vacuolated glandular cells, often containing granulocytes within the cytoplasm.

Plate 5.45
Effect of IUD. Desquamation of vacuolated endometrial glandular cells on a clean background.

Plate 5.46
Effect of IUD. A group of vacuolated endocervical cells.

Plate 5.47
Effect of IUD. The endocervical cells are vacuolated and contain granulocytes within some of the vacuoles.

Plate 5.44

Plate 5.45

Plate 5.46

Plate 5.47

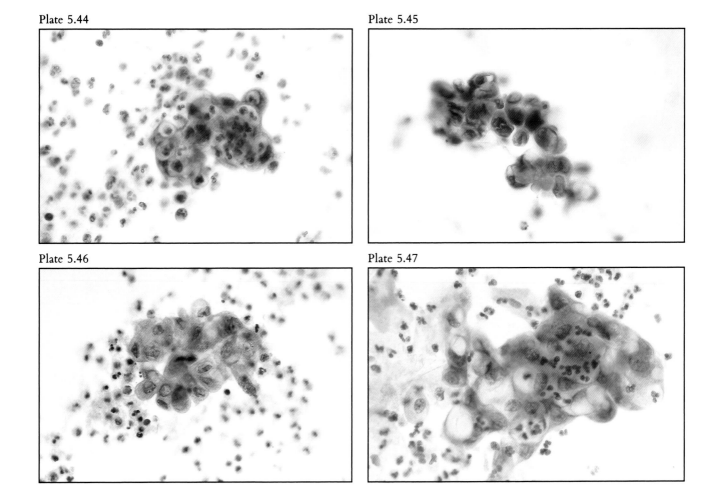

Plate 5.48
Tissue section of an atrophic squamous epithelium of the cervix.

Plate 5.49
Cell pattern of atrophy. Predominance of parabasal squamous cells with an exudate containing many granulocytes.

Plate 5.50
Cell pattern of atrophy. Marked inflammatory reaction with poor staining of the cytoplasm of the parabasal squamous cells.

Plate 5.48

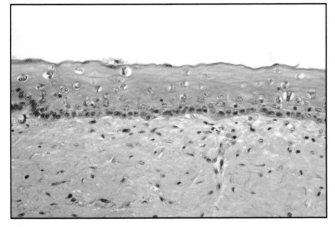

Plate 5.49

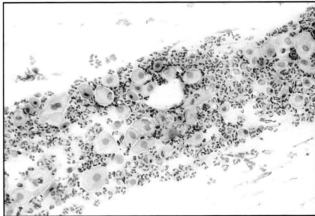

Plate 5.50

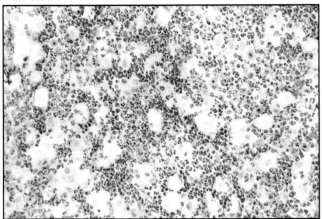

Plate 5.51

Cell pattern of atrophy. A blue blob is seen at the center of this illustration. It is a degenerated parabasal cell. The cytoplasm has taken the hematoxylin stain.

Plate 5.52

Cell pattern of atrophy. A field of blue blobs.

Plate 5.53

Cell pattern after local administration of estrogen to a patient whose previous smear is illustrated in Plate 5.52. There is now a predominance of intermediate squamous cells. The background is clean, and the blue blobs have disappeared.

Plate 5.51

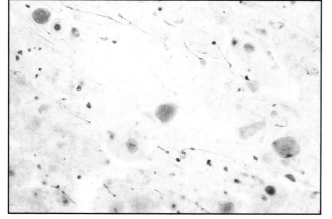

Plate 5.52

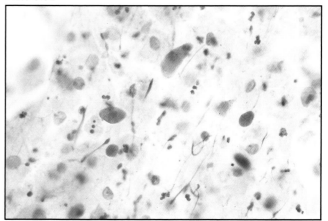

Plate 5.53

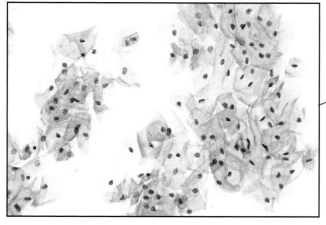

INT cells — ↑ est. in atrophy (5.51-2)

References

1. Bibbo M, Keebler CM, Wied GL: Tissue repair. In: Compendium on Diagnostic Cytology, Wied GL, Keebler CM, Koss LG, Reagan JW (Editors), Tutorials of Cytology, Chicago, IL, 1988, pp. 69–70.

2. Bukovsky A, Zidovsky J: Cytologic phenomena accompanying uterine cervix coagulation. *Acta Cytol* 29:353–362, 1985.

3. Engineer AD, Misra JS, Tandon P: Long-term cytologic studies of copper-IUD users. *Acta Cytol* 25:550–556, 1981.

4. Geirssom G, Woodworth FE, Patten SF Jr, Bonfiglio TA: Epithelial repair and regeneration in the uterine cervix: an analysis of the cells. *Acta Cytol* 21:371–378, 1977.

5. Gupta PK: Intrauterine contraceptive devices. Vaginal cytology, pathologic changes and clinical implications. *Acta Cytol* 26:571–613, 1982.

6. Holmquist, ND, Bellina JH, Danos ML: Vaginal and cervical cytologic changes following laser treatment. *Acta Cytol* 20:290–294, 1976.

7. Kobayashi TK, Fugimoto T, Okamoto H, Harami K, Yuasa M: The cells from intrauterine contraceptive devices. *Acta Cytol* 26:614–617, 1982.

8. Kraus H, Schuhmann R, Ganal M, Geier G: Cytologic findings in vaginal smears from patients under treatment with cyclophosphamide. *Acta Cytol* 21:726–730, 1978.

9. Luthra UK, Mitra AB, Prabhakar AK, Agarwal SS, Bhatnagar P: Cytologic monitoring of women using copper-containing intrauterine devices. *Acta Cytol* 26:619–622, 1982.

10. Nayar M, Chandra M, Chitraratha K, Kumari Das S, Chowdhary GR: Incidence of actinomycetes infection in women using intrauterine contraceptive devices. *Acta Cytol* 29:111–116, 1985.

11. Patten SF: Benign proliferative reactions of the uterine cervix. In: Compendium on Diagnostic Cytology, Wied GL, Keebler CM, Koss LG, Reagan JW (Editors), Tutorials of Cytology, Chicago, IL, 1988, pp. 83–87.

12. Patten SF: Postradiation dysplasia of the uterine cervix: cytopathology and clinical significance. In: Compendium on Diagnostic Cytology, Wied GL, Keebler CM, Koss LG, Reagan JW (Editors), Tutorials of Cytology, Chicago, IL, 1988, pp. 267–270.

13. von Haam E: Radiation cell changes. In: Compendium on Diagnostic Cytology, Wied GL, Keebler CM, Koss LG, Reagan JW (Editors), Tutorials of Cytology, Chicago, IL, 1988, pp. 239–253.

CHAPTER SIX

Human Papillomavirus-Induced Changes

Human papillomavirus (HPV) infection manifests itself by characteristic changes of the squamous epithelium. The lesions detectable on tissue sections have in common the presence of vacuolated cells (koilocytes)[41] in the intermediate and superficial layers of the epithelium, with a tendency towards monocellular keratinization, surface dyskeratosis, papillomatosis, elongation of the rete pegs, and increased thickness of the epithelium.[9,30,40,53,55,56,89] The following main types can be distinguished:

The most frequently encountered type of lesion is the *flat lesion*[51,53,56] in which the basal layer and the epithelial surface are parallel to each other (Plate 6.1). The upper layers contain numerous koilocytes, which can be distinguished from glycogen-laden cells by their shrunken, hyperchromatic nucleus (Plate 6.2). Periodic acid–Schiff (PAS) staining will demonstrate that these cells contain no glycogen, or very small amounts (Plates 6.3 and 6.4), in contrast to the middle layers of normal squamous epithelium (see Plate 1.6, page 9). Electron microscopy confirms the scarcity of glycogen in tissue koilocytes (Figures 6.1 and 6.2). On the surface, there may be a few layers of keratinized flattened cells with elongated dark small nuclei (Plates 6.5–6.7).

The flat lesion sometimes shows small outward projections or spicules, which are formed by thin strands of stroma (generally surrounding a small blood vessel) that protrude through the epithelium.[56] Such a lesion is called a *spiked* lesion (Plates 6.8 and 6.9).

The *papillary*, or *exophytic lesion*, has thin fingerlike projections on the surface, each containing a blood vessel (Plates 6.10–6.14).

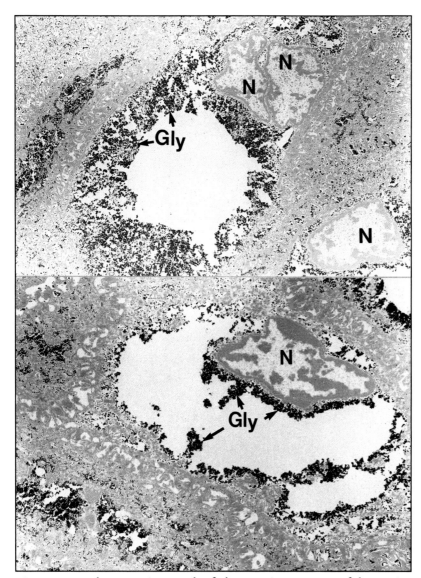

Figure 6.1 Electron micrograph of glycogen in an LGSIL of the uterine cervix. The koilocytotic cavity reveals a large clear area devoid of glycogen granules. Binucleation is seen in the upper part of this figure. Periodic acid–thiocarbohydrazide–silver proteinate staining; upper figure 4,500×; lower figure 5,000×.

When the papillary form reaches a large volume, it becomes the *condyloma acuminatum*, whose counterparts on the vulva and penis are well known.

The *inverted lesion* grows into the glandular clefts and spaces, replacing the columnar epithelium (Plates 6.15 and 6.16). It differs from simple squamous metaplasia by the cellular changes characteristic of HPV infection (koilocytosis, dyskeratosis). The inverted lesion is rare on the cervix.

Cytology

HPV infection produces characteristic changes in squamous cells, two of which are pathognomonic: koilocytosis and dyskeratosis.

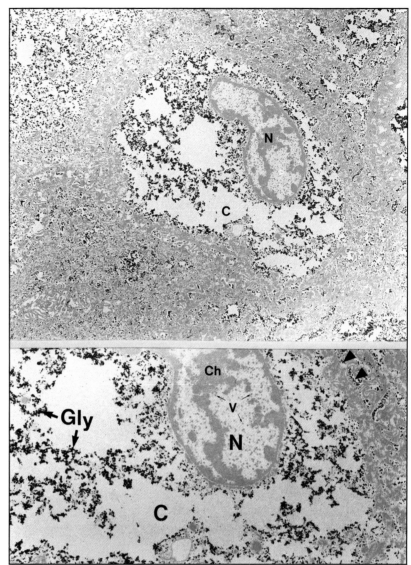

Figure 6.2 Electron micrograph of glycogen in an LGSIL of the uterine cervix. Little glycogen granules (Gly) are visible in the cytoplasm (C). A few virus particles are faintly visible in the nucleus. Periodic acid–thiocarbohydrazide–silver proteinate staining; upper figure 4,500×; lower figure 8,500×.

Koilocytosis

It is interesting to review briefly the history of this particular cell pattern, because it has given rise to some controversy. The first description of the cells and their tissue counterpart was published by Ayre in 1949.[1] His detailed characterization and illustrations are still valid today. He already suspected that this morphological change was in some way related to cancer of the cervix, and he called the cells "balloon cells" and later coined the term "nearocarcinoma."[2] This somewhat awkward appellation did not survive, however, and Koss, in 1956, introduced the expression (koilocytotic atypia,"[41] whence the present term "koilocytes" is derived.

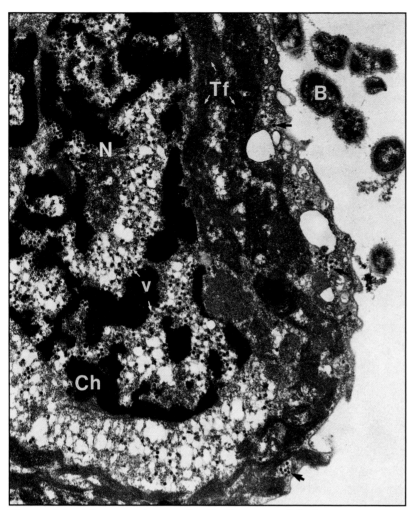

Figure 6.3 Electron micrograph of a degenerated dyskeratocyte. Tonofilaments (Tf) appear as homogeneous keratinized bundles. Karyorrhexis and cytoplasmic vacuolization are present. Virus particles (v, arrows) are visible in the cytoplasm. Nucleus (N); chromatin (Ch); bacteria (B). Uranyl acetate and lead citrate, 6,500×.

Koss did not then suspect the relationship of this change with a virus infection, but rather stated that patients with koilocytosis should be followed, as it was not then clear what the outcome would eventually be. In a later publication, he wrote that koilocytotic atypia should "best be interpreted as a warning that cancer may be present elsewhere in the cervical epithelium." It "should not be considered as either cancerous or precancerous in nature." A relatively large body of literature concerning koilocytotic atypia followed these early publications, without ever hinting at the etiologic role of papillomaviruses. For a more complete review of the literature of this fascinating subject, see Reference 49. It was not until 1976 that Meisels and Fortin[52] were able to establish the etiology of the koilocyte, demonstrate that many so-called dysplasias were in reality manifestations of HPV infection, and confirm zur Hausen's suspicion of the role of HPV in the etiology of cancer of the cervix.[90,91]

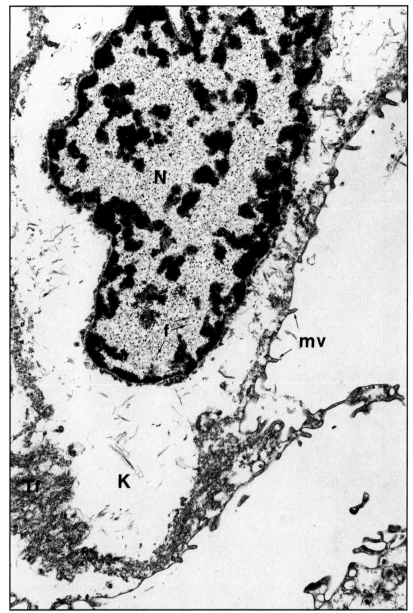

Figure 6.4 Electron micrograph of a koilocyte. A large cavity (K) surrounds the nucleus (N). Tonofilaments (Tf) are located at the inner cytoplasmic periphery. A few microvillosities (mv) are visible. Uranyl acetate and lead citrate, 10,500×.

Koilocytes are mature squamous cells (intermediate or superficial) characterized by a large perinuclear cavity (Plates 6.17 and 6.18). This cavity has sharply cut borders and appears very lightly stained, usually cyanophilic (Plates 6.19 and 6.20). Peripheral to this cavity, the cytoplasm is very dense, and may stain intensely eosinophilic or cyanophilic. When eosinophilic, it sometimes appears as dense as hyalin (Plate 6.21). The nucleus of koilocytes displays various degrees of degeneration, depending on the stage of HPV infection; sometimes the chromatin may appear almost normal (Plate 6.23). More often, however, it is smudged, without any clear

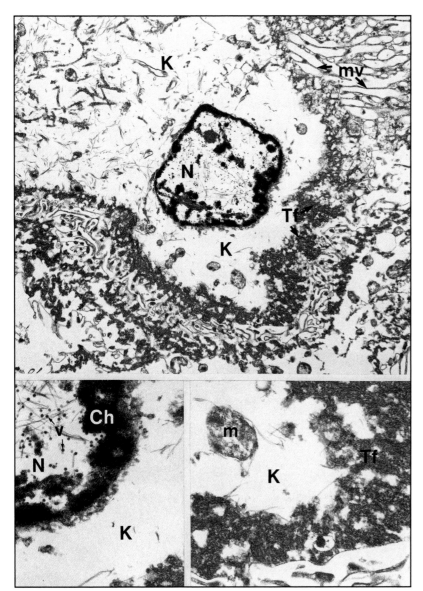

Figure 6.5 Electron micrograph of a koilocyte reprocessed from a V–C–E smear. The koilocytotic cavity (K) contains a few degenerated organelles (m). Tonofilaments (Tf) are mostly keratinized in the outer part of the cytoplasm which reveals microvillosities (mv). Dense chromatin (Ch) is visible at the inner periphery of the nucleus (N). Intranuclear virus particles (v) are present. Uranyl acetate and lead citrate; upper figure 7,500×; lower left 27,000×; lower right 27,000×.

detail (Plate 6.24). The nuclear membrane is usually not apparent. There are neither nucleoli nor inclusion bodies. Binucleation is frequent (Plate 6.22) and multinucleation can be observed, but without molding of the nuclei, as occurs in herpesvirus infections. The final stage of degeneration is karyorrhexis (Plate 6.25). Koilocytes occur singly, or more frequently, in clusters, which may be thick, obscuring the cellular features. Koilocytes are pathognomonic; their presence is definite proof of HPV infection. However, the Papanicolaou stain must be of excellent quality, so that the finer char-

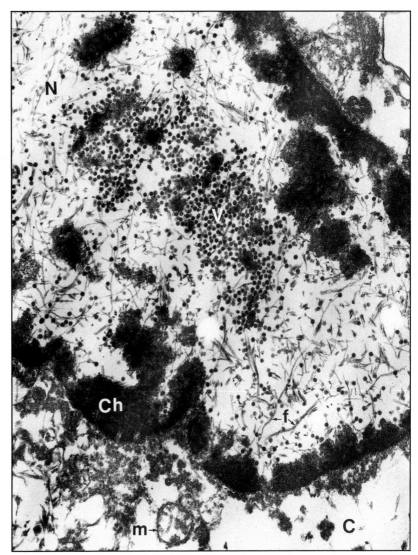

Figure 6.6 Electron micrograph of a nucleus (N) containing many virus particles (v), filaments (f), and dense chromatin (Ch). A degenerated mitochondrion (m) can be seen in the cytoplasm (C). Uranyl acetate and lead citrate, 40,000×.

acteristics of cytoplasmic amphophilia may be discerned.[6,7,11–13, 17,24,43,44,64,65,67–69,71,76]

Dyskeratosis

This cellular pattern[52,65] has been reported to be as important a sign for HPV infection as koilocytosis. Unfortunately some investigators have ignored this change, with the result that many cases of HPV infection, in which there is no koilocytosis, go undiagnosed, or are labelled "keratinizing dysplasia."[63,66]

Dyskeratocytes are keratinized squamous cells, staining a brilliant orange with the OG-6 of the Papanicolaou technique. They occur mostly in thick, three-dimensional clusters, characterized by

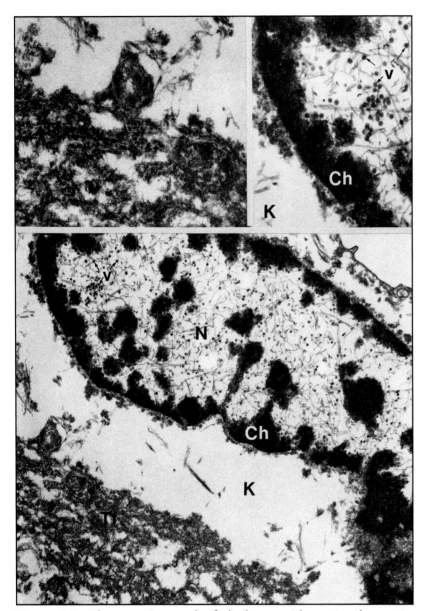

Figure 6.7 Electron micrograph of a koilocyte with a perinuclear cavity (K), tonofilaments (Tf), and a nucleus (N) with dense chromatin (Ch) distributed at the periphery, and scarce virus particles (v). Uranyl acetate and lead citrate; upper left 42,000×; upper right 40,000×; lower figure 21,500×.

the presence of vesicular nuclei with indistinct chromatin detail, identical to the nuclei of koilocytes (Plates 6.26–6.31). When of small size, dyskeratocytes have been called "miniature squamous cells"[63] (Plate 6.32). Other authors use the terms "parakeratosis" or "pseudo-parakeratosis" for the cellular pattern.[63] However, the latter terminology refers to the epidermis, when nuclei persist in superficial squames (ie, in psoriasis). Since the squamous lining of the cervix does not keratinize under normal circumstances, the expression dyskeratosis, meaning abnormal keratinization, seems more appropriate.

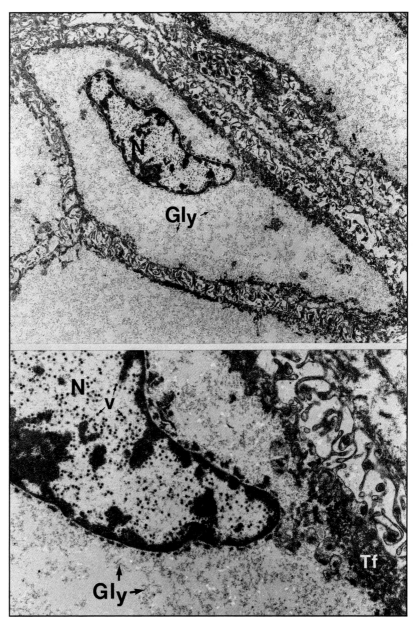

Figure 6.8 Electron micrograph of a biopsy of a low-grade intraepithelial lesion showing a koilocyte. The nucleus (N) is surrounded by a clear area containing dispersed glycogen granules (Gly). Tonofilaments (Tf) are located against the cytoplasmic membrane surrounding the koilocytotic cavity. Virus particles (v) are visible in the nucleus. Uranyl acetate and lead citrate; upper 5,000×; lower 22,000×.

Dyskeratocytes may occur in the absence of HPV infection; in those cases they form small keratinized pearls (Plates 6.33 and 6.34) or small aggregates of elongated keratinized cells in parallel arrangement, with mostly pyknotic nuclei (Plates 6.35–6.37). In contrast, HPV-related dyskeratocytes occur singly or in thick clusters without any discernible polarity. These features are also pathognomonic for HPV infection. In many cases, dyskeratosis is the only signal of the presence of HPV, and the diagnosis should be made even in the total absence of koilocytes.

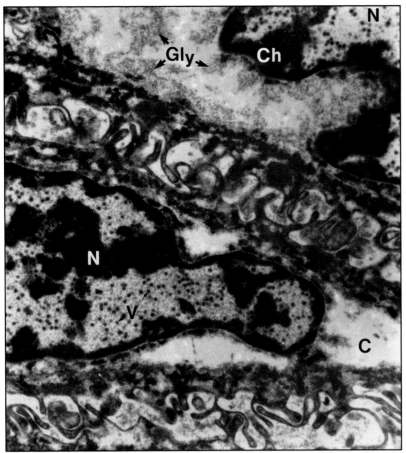

Figure 6.9 Electron micrograph of a biopsy of a low-grade intraepithelial lesion. Virus particles (v) and chromatin (Ch) are visible in the nucleus (N). Cytoplasmic granules corresponding to remnants of glycogen (Gly) are still visible in the cytoplasm (C). Uranyl acetate and lead citrate, 24,000×.

It is incorrect to describe the features of HPV infection as koilocytosis, since this is only one of the earmarks of the infection. Ignoring the dyskeratotic changes is tantamount to deliberately missing the correct diagnosis in a large number of cases.

Although in our hands, a definite diagnosis of HPV infection is made in about 4% of the 150,000 cases screened each year, the real incidence is probably near 30%, according to de Villiers,[23] who screened a large population of asymptomatic women in the Heidelberg area of West Germany by means of membrane filter hybridization. The patients whose smear does not display clear-cut evidence of HPV infection, but whose infection is demonstrated by hybridization, may be entirely negative at colposcopy and biopsy. Revision of the smears may show very minute changes that can be retrospectively ascribed to HPV infection.[86] These changes consist of binucleation, amphophilia (Plate 6.38), presence of miniature keratinized squamous cells (Plate 6.39), etc. They are not sufficiently diagnostic, however, to warrant a prima facie conclusion of HPV infection. One must remember that we are dealing here with a sexually transmitted disease and that such a diagnosis can have se-

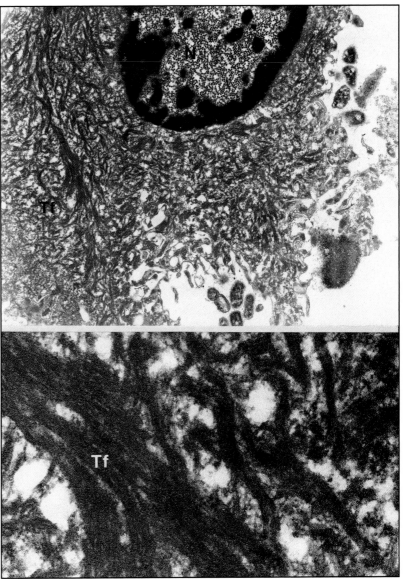

Figure 6.10 Electron micrograph of a dyskeratocyte reprocessed from a V–C–E smear. The cytoplasm is completely filled with keratinized tonofilaments (Tf) forming large bundles as seen in the lower part of this micrograph. The nucleus contains numerous virus particles. Uranyl acetate and lead citrate; upper figure 9,000×; lower figure 36,000×.

rious social and medical implications. It is, therefore, prudent to offer such a diagnosis only when the morphologic evidence is irrefutable. It must be realized, however, that cytology severely underestimates the true incidence of HPV infection. In a recent review of the literature,[50] we found the estimated sensitivity of cytology (and histology) to be only between 15% and 36%.

If a patient is proven by molecular hybridization to harbor HPV, but all other tests are negative, it can be surmised that she is in immunologic equilibrium with the virus and that, as in the vast majority of such cases, the virus will eventually disappear. It is also doubtful that she can transmit the virus to her sexual partner(s) at this stage: the epithelial cells are not producing virus particles, be-

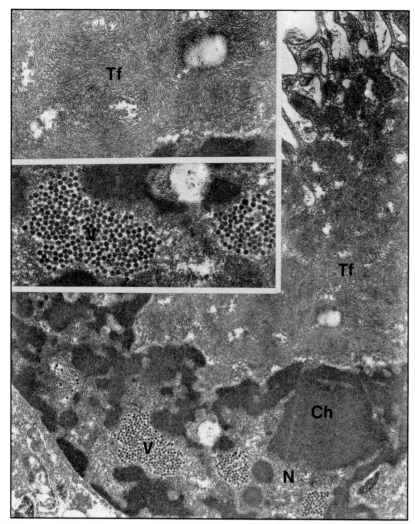

Figure 6.11 Electron micrograph of a dyskeratocyte reprocessed from a V–C–E smear. Tonofilaments (Tf) are homogeneously distributed in the cytoplasm. Virus particles (v) are visible in the nucleus. Uranyl acetate and lead citrate; upper and center figures 44,000×; lower figure 24,000×.

cause when they do, they must show morphologically recognizable changes. It will be necessary to establish long-term followup protocols for this large group of women in order to learn more about the eventual outcome of the infection.

On the other hand, when morphologic signs of HPV infection are present, one can demonstrate complete infective viral particles by immunoperoxidase or electron microscopy in about 50% of the cases.[28,58,59,77–79, 83,87] These are infective and represent the prime target for preventive therapy. It is, therefore, justified to recommend a colposcopic examination, with biopsies and local eradication of all visible lesions in all these patients.

Associated Lesions

In about 10% to 15% of patients with morphologic evidence of HPV infection, the cellular pattern proves to be extremely bizarre:

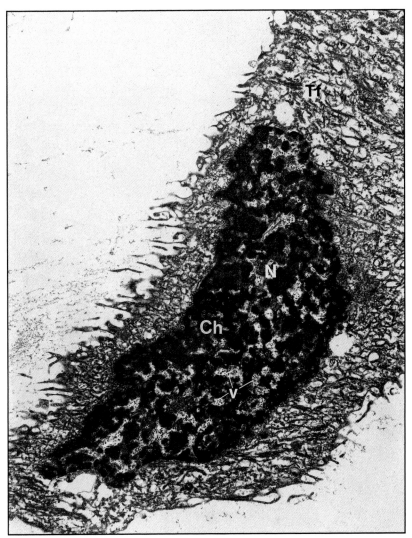

Figure 6.12 Electron micrograph of a cell reprocessed from a V–C–E smear, consistent with a high-grade intraepithelial lesion. The nucleus (N) is enlarged and irregular. It contains virus particles (v) located between large areas of dense chromatin (Ch). Bundles of tonofilaments (Tf) are filling the cytoplasm. Uranyl acetate and lead citrate, 10,000×.

the smear will contain thick aggregates of large dyskeratotic cells with enlarged, irregular, hyperchromatic nuclei. These cells show no good chromatin detail, no nucleoli, no apparent nuclear membrane, but considerable anisokaryosis (Plates 6.40–6.47). These changes may be important enough to give rise to suspicion of invasive keratinizing squamous carcinoma. Previous to our 1981 publication on the subject,[57] (we then called this pattern the "atypical condyloma") many cases were erroneously diagnosed as cancer.

On tissue sections koilocytes are found in the intermediate and superficial layers (Plate 6.48). They contain enlarged, irregular, hyperchromatic nuclei (Plate 6.49). Even the deeper layers of the epithelium are affected (Plate 6.50). The nuclei are increased in size and darkly stained, often with smudged chromatin and indistinct nuclear membrane (Plate 6.51). Anisokaryosis can be marked (Plate 6.52). This histologic presentation is quite different from that of

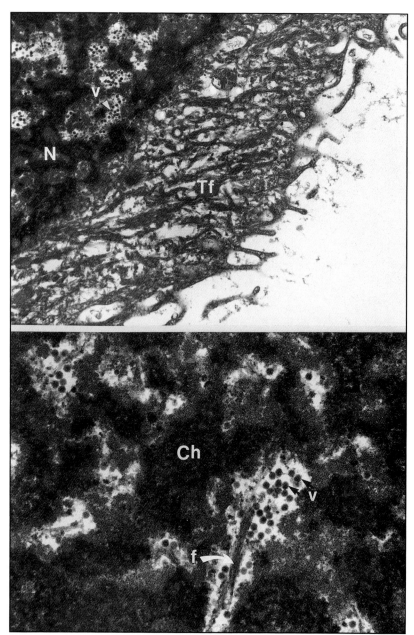

Figure 6.13 Higher magnification of Figure 6.12. Nucleus (N); tonof-ilaments (Tf); chromatin (Ch); filaments (f, arrow). Uranyl acetate and lead citrate; upper figure 22,500×; lower figure 44,000×.

high-grade squamous intraepithelial lesions, in which there is little or no differentiation, and the cells show only slight variation in size and shape throughout the epithelial lining.

The differential diagnosis is sometimes very difficult to establish. HGSIL is a more aggressive lesion: we found HPV-16 DNA in the vast majority of the cases studied (unpublished data) and our fol-lowup studies have shown that these lesions progress to pure HGSIL at a rate about double that of ordinary flat condylomas and in about half the time.[54,57] This lesion should be classified within the group of lesions known as HGSIL, most of which contain HPV-16 DNA, except that afflicted patients do produce infective viral particles and

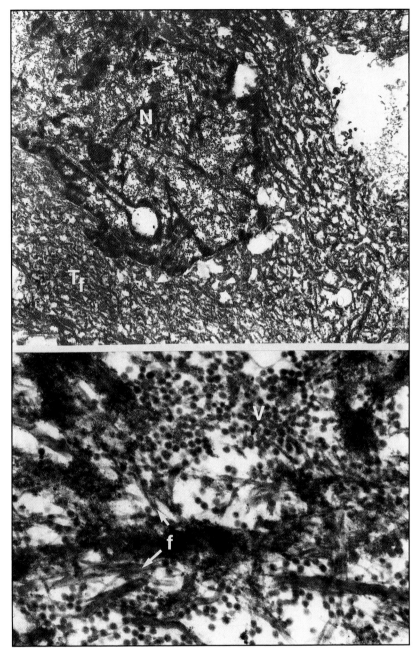

Figure 6.14 Electron micrograph of a cell reprocessed from a V–C–E smear, consistent with a high-grade intraepithelial lesion. In the upper part, an enlarged nucleus (N) is surrounded by numerous bundles of tonofilaments (Tf). The lower part shows intranuclear virus particles (v) and filaments (f). Uranyl acetate and lead citrate; upper 10,000×; lower 52,000×.

can therefore transmit the virus to their sexual partner(s). It represents what I call the mixed type of association, in which the same cell manifests morphologic changes due to HPV infection and to HGSIL. It is important, from the standpoint of prevention, to alert the clinician to this situation, so that both the patient and her partner(s) can be treated simultaneously. It is best to report this particular change as "HGSIL with evidence of HPV infection," to

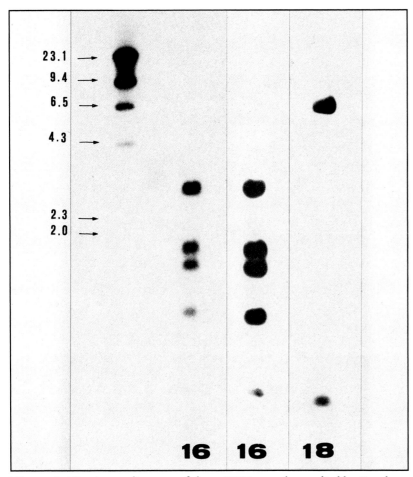

Figure 6.15 Autoradiogram of three DNA samples studied by Southern blot. On the left, a size marker (λ-Hind III) ranging from 2.0 to 23.1 kilobases is indicated. Three DNAs extracted from HGSIL are also illustrated: two of them were proved to contain HPV–16 and the other HPV–18 as revealed by their Pst I pattern and high–stringency conditions of hybridization.

make sure there is no misunderstanding the ominous nature of this lesion.

There are two other forms of association between an HPV infection and HGSIL. I have termed them the *vertical* and the *horizontal* associations. In the latter, the cervix shows evidence of HPV infection and of HGSIL either adjacent to each other, or at different sites (Plates 6.53–6.57). It is also possible that the HGSIL is limited to the cervix, while the HPV infection is found in the vagina. In those cases, the smear will contain cells typical of HPV infection, often of the mixed type described above, and cells characteristic of pure HGSIL (Plate 6.58).

In the vertical association there is an area of HGSIL on the cervix, in which the uppermost layers show changes due to HPV, while the rest of the epithelium is typical HGSIL (Plates 6.59–6.64). In those cases, the smear may only show the HPV changes, since the scraping instrument can not gather deeper cells. This is one reason why some cases are underdiagnosed by cytology.

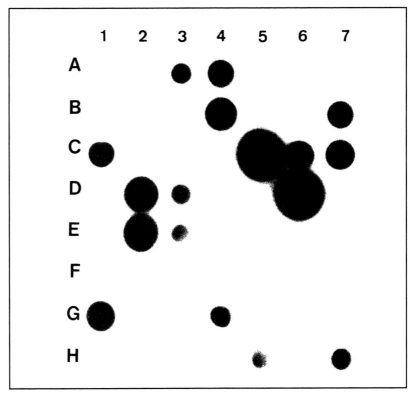

Figure 6.16 Autoradiogram of a dot blot. A total of 56 DNA samples extracted from LGSIL and HGSIL were dot-blotted and hybridized with HPV–16 under stringent conditions. Dark spots indicate the presence of corresponding HPV type.

HPV Infection

At the beginning of 1990, 62 types of HPV had been identified. In order to be considered a distinct type, an HPV must have less than 50% homology, meaning that of the 7,900 base pairs that constitute its circular DNA molecule, no more than 50% should match completely. This means that each of the over 60 types is quite different from all others. No simple mutation can transform one type of HPV into another. More than twenty types have been found in genital lesions. Types 6, 11, and 42[4,21,31,32] are mostly associated with condylomata acuminata and have not been seen in invasive carcinomas. Types 16, 18, and 31[8,25,45] have been found in about 90% of invasive cancers, as well as in SIL and in flat condylomas. Some other types (HPV 33, 35, 39)[3,5,46] occur in isolated instances of carcinomas or SIL (for details, see Table 6.1).

Differentiated keratinocytes are necessary for HPV particle production and such differentiation has not as yet been achieved in culture. Thus, HPVs have not been propagated in vitro as yet. However, the DNA of various types has been entirely characterized, ie, the complete sequence of bases is known.[15,16] The various genes have been identified and the genes responsible for in vitro transformation (E6 and E7)[82] can be cloned and studied separately from the rest of the virus DNA. The techniques of molecular virology

Table 6.1
Human papillomavirus types, location, and associated lesions

Location	Disease	HPV types
Skin	Various types of warts	1–4,7,10,57,26–29,49,60
Skin	Keratoacanthoma	37
Skin	Malignant melanoma	38
Skin	Squamous cell carcinoma	48
Skin	Epidermodysplasia verruciformis (benign)	5,8,9,12,14,15,17,19, 20–25,36,46,47,50
Skin	EV (malignant)	5,8,14,17,20
Skin & mucosa	Laryngeal carcinoma	30
	Focal epithelial hyperplasia	13
	Oral papilloma	32,57
	Cutaneous squamous cell carcinoma	41
	Bowenoid papulosis	55
Genital mucosa	Condyloma acuminatum	6,11,42,54
Genital mucosa	Normal mucosa	53
Genital mucosa	Intraepithelial squamous lesion	6,11,16,18,30,31,35, 39,40,42–45, 51,52,58,59
Genital mucosa	Cervical carcinoma	16,18,31,33,35,39,45,51, 52,56

De Villiers EM: Heterogeneity of human papillomavirus group. *J Virol* 63: 4898–4903, 1989.

have allowed for rapid advances in the intimate knowledge of these agents.

Several techniques are available to demonstrate HPV within a cell or tissue: Electron microscopy (EM)[20,28,36–39,44,57,59,73,80,84] (Figures 6.3–6.14), immunocytochemistry (IC)[19,26–28,35,37,58,60,74,77,78,83,84,88] (Plates 6.65 and 6.66) or molecular hybridization (MH)[5,8,10,18,22,29,33,34,42,61,62,70,75,81,86,87] (Figures 6.15 and 6.16; Plates 6.67 and 6.68). With EM or IC, HPV is only demonstrated when its protein envelope is present, that is, when the virus exists as a complete virion. Virions are only produced by mature squamous cells, the so-called "permissive" cells. Not all mature squamous cells are permissive. For unknown reasons, in about half of all cases of HPV infections there are no permissive cells. It is clear, therefore, that EM and IC are only useful when positive. A negative finding does not rule out HPV infection.

Molecular hybridization directly demonstrates the presence of viral DNA within cells or tissues. Specific probes must be obtained for the various HPV types to be investigated. These probes are then marked either with radioactive phosphorus or an avidin-biotin complex and then put in contact with the cellular DNA. This can be done in situ on smears or sections, or after homogenization of a tissue sample on a membrane, or by the Southern technique. Molecular hybridization is the only method to determine which particular HPV type is present in a given lesion.

½ cases
no permissive
cells - no complete
virions

HPV infection may be entirely asymptomatic.[23,47,85,87] Even the cytologic sample may fail to reveal the characteristic changes. Zur Hausen and his group from the Krebsforschungsinstitut in Heidelberg found that about 10% of asymptomatic women harbored HPV.[23] In pregnant women this percentage was 30%.[72] Yet in a mass screening program like ours in Quebec City, smears show evidence of HPV infection in only about 4% of women. It may well be that subtle cytologic changes occur, which have not as yet been identified as manifestations of HPV infection. However, when all the morphologic signs of HPV infection—signs revealed through cytology, histology, and colposcopy—are missing, and yet there is HPV DNA demonstrable in the cells, one may surmise that there are only a few virus copies present, possibly as naked DNA. The patient would not be able to infect her sexual partner. Whether she will ever develop symptoms and signs of her infection is not known at present. Screening for HPV DNA would therefore seem somewhat of an overkill. Only when lesions (those demonstrable by morphologic studies) appear is treatment available. Only at that time can the virus be transmitted.

Morphology does not generally identify the precise HPV type. Identification can only be made by MH. From the standpoint of patient care, it is therefore preferable to consider all cases of HPV infection as potentially dangerous and recommend colposcopy with multiple biopsies in order to confirm the diagnosis. All lesions should then be eradicated by laser, cryosurgery, or diathermy, since the removal of the lesions decreases the critical biomass of the virus significantly, so that the patient's immunological defense can overcome the remaining HPV. Sexual partners should also be examined and treated.

In condyloma and HGSIL associated with HPV infection, HPV is present as a complete virion and can therefore be transmitted to the sexual partner(s). In HGSIL without morphologic evidence of HPV infection and in invasive cancer, the HPV DNA is either integrated into the host's DNA or it exists as an episome,[14,48] without any protein coat. It can not be transmitted in those cases.

Plate 6.1
Colposcopically directed biopsy illustrating the flat low-grade squamous intraepithelial lesion (LGSIL), or flat condyloma. The basal membrane is parallel to the surface. Koilocytes are visible in the middle and upper layers, with a few keratinized cells on the surface.

Plate 6.2
Flat LGSIL. There is a mild degree of papillomatosis. Blood vessels surge towards the surface. Koilocytes contain small, shrunken nuclei, with an empty-appearing perinuclear area.

Plate 6.3
A flat LGSIL stained with PAS to demonstrate the lack of glycogen in the perinuclear clear areas of the koilocytes.

Plate 6.4
PAS staining of a flat LGSIL. Glycogen is present in very small amounts, surrounding the perinuclear area of the koilocytes. Notice also the dyskeratotic layers on the surface.

Plate 6.1

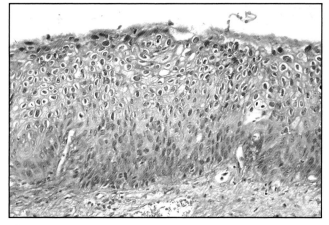

Plate 6.2

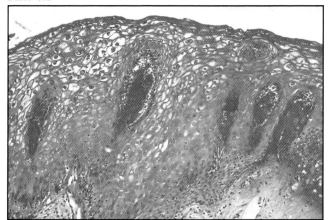

Plate 6.3

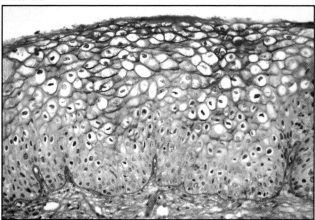

Plate 6.4

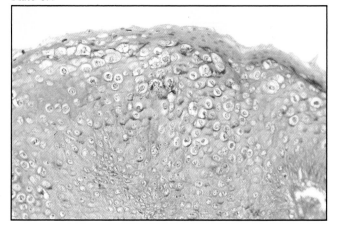

Plate 6.5
Flat LGSIL illustrating the dyskeratotic cells on the surface. A smear obtained by scraping such a lesion may contain only dyskeratotic cell clusters, and no koilocytes.

Plate 6.6
Demonstration of keratin in a flat LGSIL of the uterine cervix. All layers of the epithelium are stained with a brownish color at the cytoplasmic location of keratin. Peroxidase antiperoxidase technique.

Plate 6.7
Higher magnification of the previous lesion. Note that keratin is mainly located in the ectoplasm of superficial koilocytes as revealed by the distribution of the brown staining. Peroxidase antiperoxidase technique.

Plate 6.8
Flat LGSIL illustrating the formation of a spike. A blood vessel, surrounded by a small amount of stroma, ascends through the epithelium and seems to push the upper layers outwards.

Plate 6.5

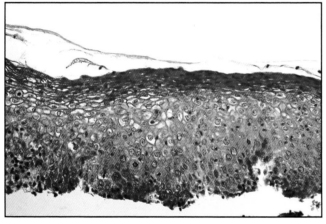

Plate 6.6

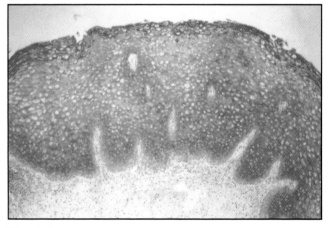

Plate 6.7

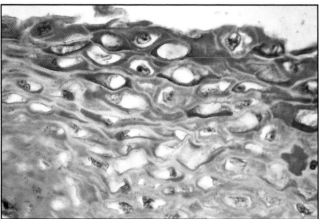

Plate 6.8

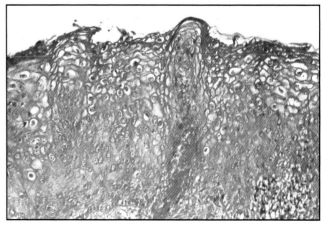

Plate 6.9

A spiked LGSIL. Note the blood vessel within the spike. The uppermost layers on the spike are keratinized and may show up on a smear as a clump of dyskeratotic cells.

Plate 6.10

The papillary type of LGSIL shows papillomatosis and acanthosis. Koilocytes are visible in the middle layers.

Plate 6.9

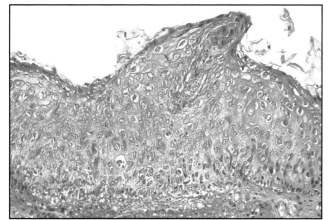

Plate 6.10

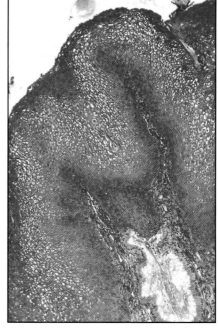

Plate 6.11
PAS staining of a papillary LGSIL. Little glycogen material is visible ⟨⟩
in some area of the intermediate layers.

Plate 6.12
Histologic section of a papillary LGSIL of the uterine cervix with
koilocytosis and superficial dyskeratosis.

Plate 6.11

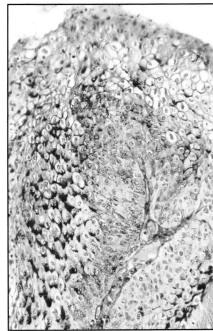

Plate 6.12

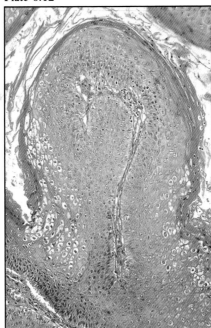

Plate 6.13

PAS staining of a papillary projection of the previous LGSIL. Small amounts of glycogen (red) are visible. A layer of dyskeratotic cells (yellow) is covering the papillary projection.

Plate 6.14

PAS staining of an LGSIL with papillomatosis. Small amounts of glycogen (red) are visible in the intermediate layers. A layer of dyskeratocytes is undulating at the surface of this lesion.

Plate 6.15

This section illustrates the inverted LGSIL. The lesion grows into the glandular clefts and spaces of the cervix, mimicking stromal invasion.

Plate 6.13

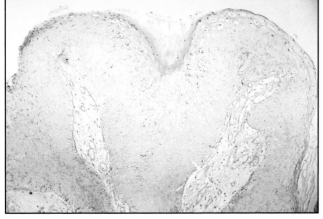

Plate 6.14

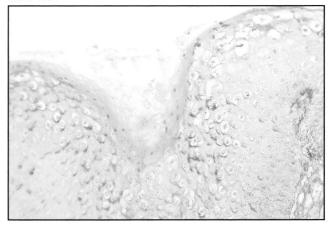

Plate 6.15

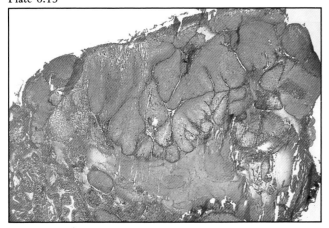

Plate 6.16

A higher magnification of the inverted LGSIL shown in the previous illustration. The glandular spaces are entirely occupied by the abnormal epithelium, but there is no stromal invasion.

Plate 6.17

Smear obtained from an LGSIL illustrating koilocytes, pathognomonic for HPV infection. These are mature (intermediate or superficial) cells with a large perinuclear cavity.

Plate 6.18

Koilocytes with a very large perinuclear cavity. The remaining cytoplasm is pushed out to the periphery of the cell.

Plate 6.16

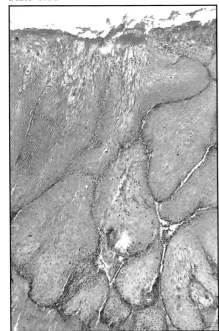

Plate 6.17

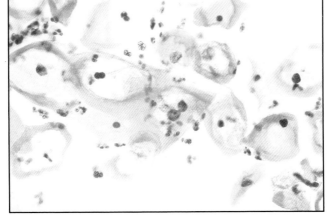

Plate 6.18

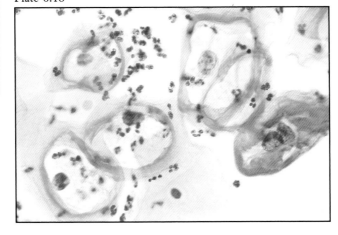

Plate 6.19
The limits of the perinuclear cavity of koilocytes are usually sharply cut and the cytoplasm in the periphery is very dense.

Plate 6.20
Often the cytoplasm of koilocytes shows more than one color (amphophilia). The staining may be patchy. Notice the clean background, which is a common observation in HPV infection in the absence of associated pathogens.

Plate 6.21
Some of these koilocytes show patchy amphophilic staining, while others have a dense, deeply eosinophilic cytoplasm, somewhat hyalinlike in texture.

Plate 6.22
A cluster of koilocytes. Many contain two nuclei.

Plate 6.19

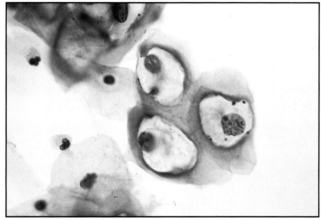

Plate 6.20

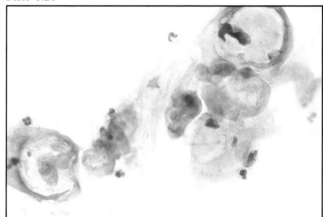

Plate 6.21

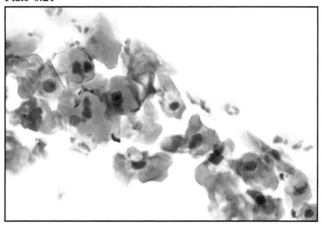

Plate 6.22

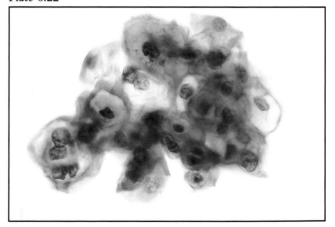

Plate 6.23

Four mature squamous cells on a clean background. One is a normal superficial cell. The others are koilocytes, with typical perinuclear cavities and normal-appearing nuclei.

Plate 6.24

The nuclei in this group of cells from an LGSIL show a smudged chromatin, without any visible detail. This feature is commonly observed in HPV-infected cells.

Plate 6.25

The nuclei of these HPV-infected cells have degenerated and are in the process of karyorrhexis.

Plate 6.26

A field of dyskeratotic cells intermixed with a few koilocytes. Note the brilliant cytoplasmic staining.

Plate 6.23

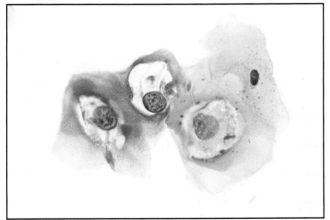

Plate 6.24

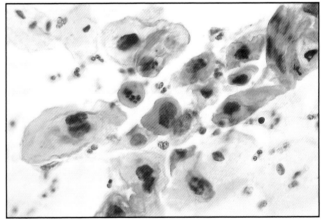

Plate 6.25

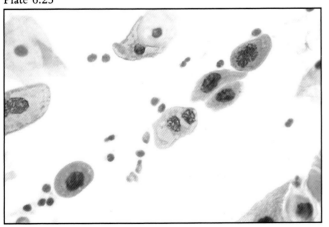

Plate 6.26

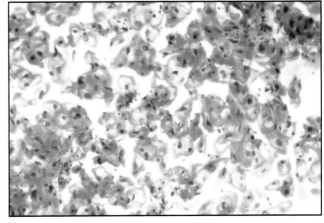

Plate 6.27
Dyskeratocytes often form tiny clusters of overlapping cells. In this case, a few koilocytes are found next to the dyskeratotic cells.

Plate 6.28
At higher magnification the brilliant orangeophilic cytoplasm can be better appreciated. The nuclei have no distinct chromatin pattern.

Plate 6.29
Dyskeratocytes contain one or several—often two—nuclei, whose morphology is identical to that of the nuclei of koilocytes.

Plate 6.30
Cluster of dyskeratotic cells, pathognomonic for HPV infection. Note the dark, somewhat irregular, featureless nuclei, the haphazard arrangement, and the overlapping of the cells.

Plate 6.27

Plate 6.28

Plate 6.29

Plate 6.30

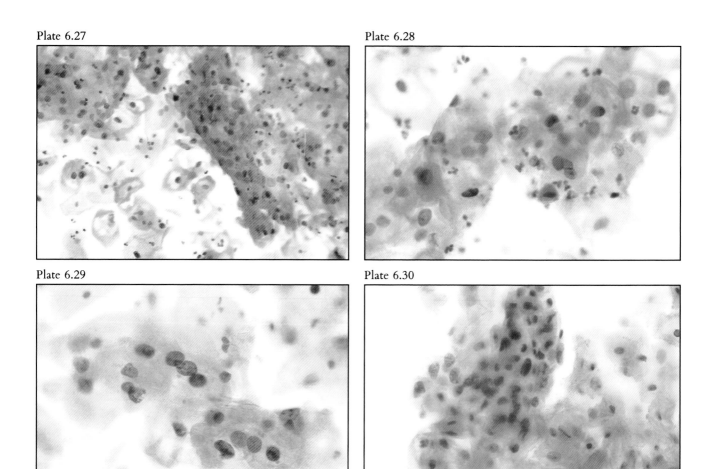

Plate 6.31
A cluster of dyskeratotic cells with a pearl-like formation containing keratin. Most nuclei are darkly stained and lack chromatin detail.

Plate 6.32
A field of miniature squamous cells—small dyskeratocytes. Compare their size with the two superficial cells on the other side of this photomicrograph.

Plate 6.33
This small keratinized pearl formation is not diagnostic for HPV infection.

Plate 6.34
A keratinized pearl formation staining a brilliant orange. This is not diagnostic for HPV infection.

Plate 6.31

Plate 6.32

Plate 6.33

Plate 6.34

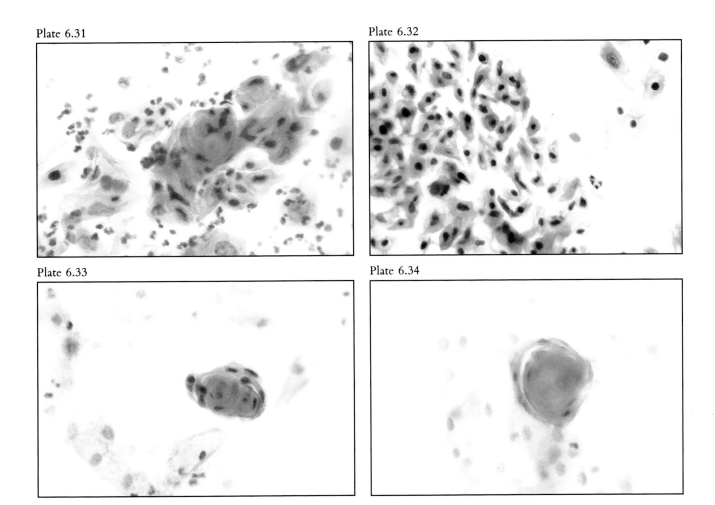

Plate 6.35
These dyskeratotic cells in parallel arrangement are not diagnostic for HPV infection.

Plate 6.36
Elongated, very thin dyskeratotic cells. These cells have no diagnostic significance.

Plate 6.37
The parallel arrangement of these dyskeratotic cells and the lack of overlapping differentiates these cells from the dyskeratotic clusters seen in HPV infection.

Plate 6.38
The staining of the cytoplasm and the structureless nuclei are reminiscent of cells seen in HPV infections. This pattern by itself is not sufficient to establish the diagnosis.

Plate 6.35

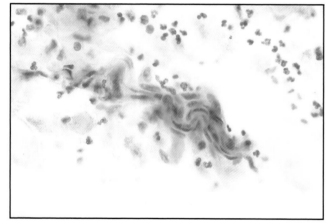

Plate 6.36

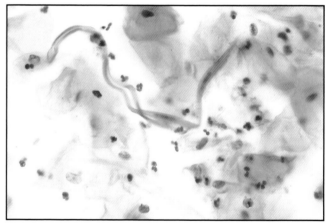

Plate 6.37

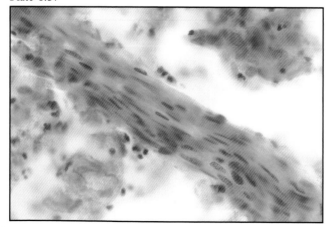

Plate 6.38

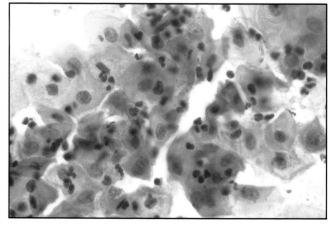

Plate 6.39
Miniature keratinized cells, similar to those depicted in Plate 6.32. Although these cells suggest HPV infection, diagnosis is uncertain without other morphologic signs.

Plate 6.40
Mixed type of association of a high-grade squamous intraepithelial lesion (HGSIL) with signs of HPV infection: the clump of dyskeratotic mature cells contains enlarged, irregular, darkly stained nuclei. Except for the clumping and clean background, the cells resemble those seen in invasive keratinizing squamous carcinoma.

Plate 6.41
HGSIL with signs of HPV infection: mixed association. The dense group of dyskeratotic cells contains large, irregular, darkly stained nuclei.

Plate 6.42
HGSIL with signs of HPV infection: mixed association. Compare the arrangement of the dyskeratotic cells in this grouping with that in Plate 6.40. Although similar, in this case the nuclei are larger, irregular, and show variation in size and shape.

Plate 6.39

Plate 6.40

Plate 6.41

Plate 6.42

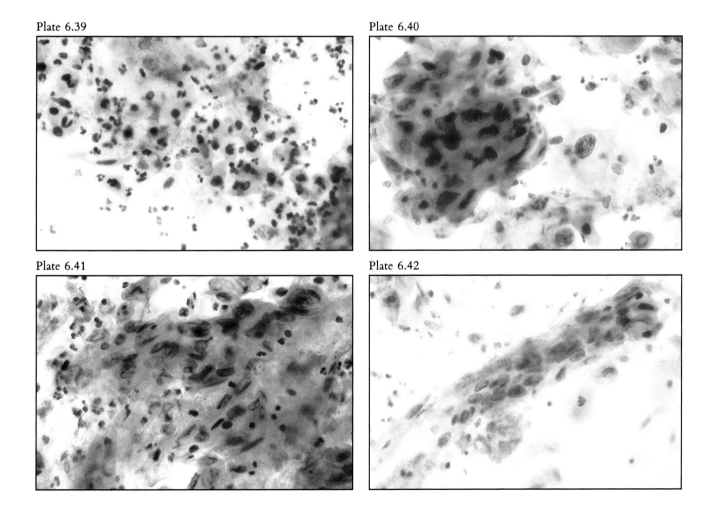

Plate 6.43

HGSIL with discrete signs of HPV infection, mostly evident by the amphophilic cytoplasmic staining. These cells are smaller, the nuclear/cytoplasmic ratio is increased, and the nuclei are darkly stained.

Plate 6.44

Low-power field of a mixed association. The background is clean. The atypical nuclei stand out like ink dots.

Plate 6.45

High-power view of the smear illustrated in Plate 6.44. The darkly stained nuclei are completely featureless and very large (compare with the normal nuclei in the background).

Plate 6.46

HGSIL with HPV infection. These dyskeratotic cells contain large, darkly stained, irregular nuclei.

Plate 6.43

Plate 6.44

Plate 6.45

Plate 6.46

Plate 6.47

HGSIL with HPV infection. The nuclei are considerably enlarged and irregular. The group of dyskeratotic cells is compact and three-dimensional, with much overlapping of the cells.

Plate 6.48

Tissue section from a case of mixed association of HGSIL with HPV infection. Koilocytes can be seen, but atypical nuclei occupy most of the thickness of the epithelium.

Plate 6.49

HGSIL with HPV infection: the mixed association. The squamous epithelium has the general appearance of a HGSIL, but koilocytes can be seen in the middle and upper layers. Nuclei are hyperchromatic, enlarged, and irregular.

Plate 6.50

HGSIL with HPV infection. In contrast to LGSIL (see Plate 6.1), the deeper layers of the epithelium are involved here, and the nuclei are sometimes enlarged and irregular.

Plate 6.47

Plate 6.48

Plate 6.49

Plate 6.50

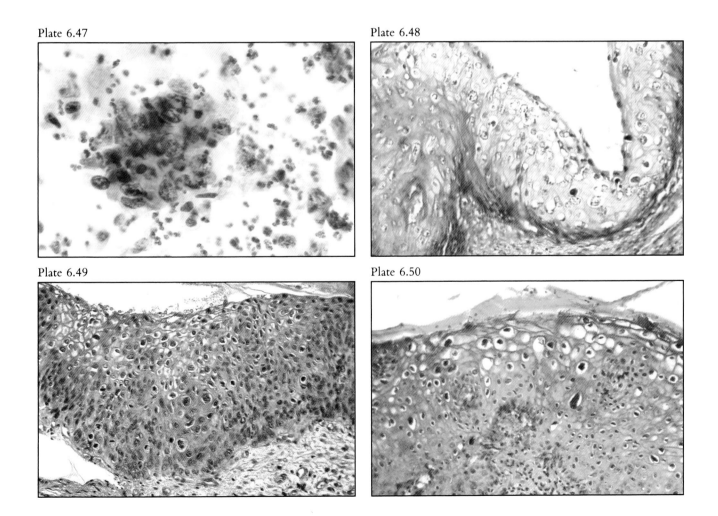

Plate 6.51

HGSIL with HPV infection. Note the enlarged, hyperchromatic, featureless nuclei.

Plate 6.52

HGSIL with HPV infection. This section demonstrates the marked anisokaryosis that is one of the more important signs of the mixed association. Koilocytes can be seen on the surface.

Plate 6.53

HGSIL with HPV infection, showing the horizontal association. This section shows the two lesions situated adjacent to each other.

Plate 6.54

HGSIL with HPV infection, showing two lesions adjacent to each other. Notice the blood vessel coursing through the lesion towards the surface.

Plate 6.51

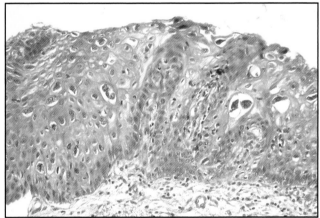

Plate 6.52

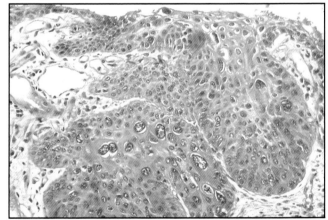

Plate 6.53

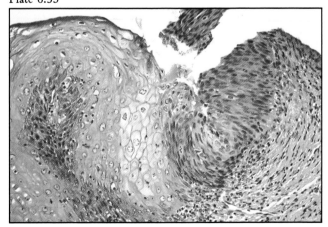

Plate 6.54

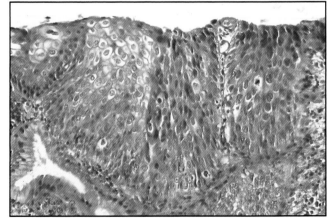

Plate 6.55

HGSIL with HPV infection. Most of the field is pure HGSIL. Adjacent to this lesion is a small area of LGSIL.

Plate 6.56

In this section, the HGSIL can be seen penetrating into a glandular opening, while the LGSIL is observed on the external surface.

Plate 6.57

In this case, the HGSIL is peripheral, and the LGSIL penetrates into the gland openings.

Plate 6.55

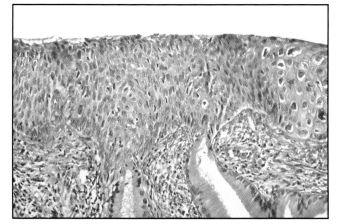

Plate 6.56

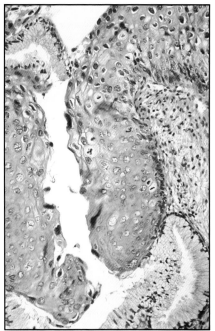

Plate 6.57

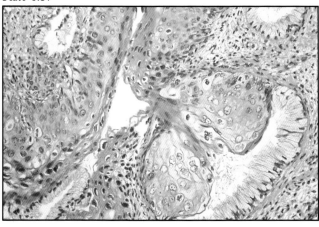

Plate 6.58
Cellular pattern from a case of horizontal association of HGSIL with HPV infection. The dyskeratotic clump of cells on one side of this microphotograph shows the pattern of a mixed association. The smaller, parabasal-like cells are characteristic of HGSIL.

Plate 6.59
HGSIL with HPV, showing the vertical association. The lower layers are typical of HGSIL, and koilocytes appear in the upper layers.

Plate 6.60
The vertical association of HGSIL and HPV infection. Such a lesion may not be readily diagnosed on the smear.

Plate 6.58

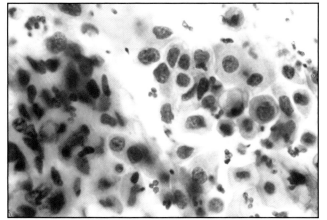

Plate 6.59

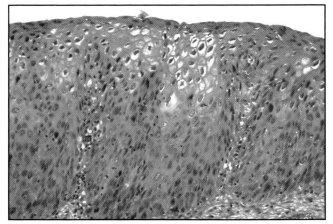

Plate 6.60

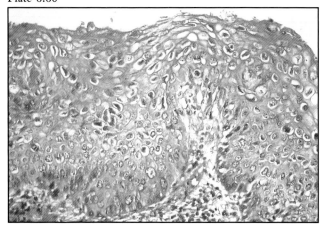

Plate 6.61

HGSIL and HPV infection in vertical association. The surface is keratinized. A smear from such a case may not reveal the underlying HGSIL.

Plate 6.62

A case of vertical association of HGSIL with HPV infection, demonstrating extreme keratinization of the surface layers.

Plate 6.63

HGSIL and HPV infection in vertical association. There is epidermization with a thick keratin layer on the surface. This lesion would not shed significant cells on the smear (see Plate 6.67).

Plate 6.61

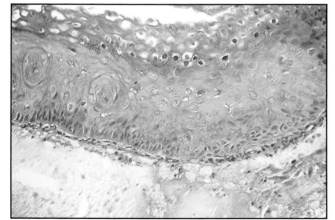

Plate 6.62

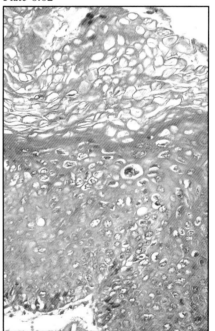

Plate 6.63

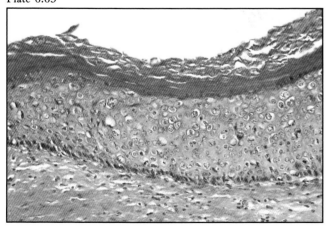

Plate 6.64

Cell spread from the case illustrated in Plate 6.63. Only anucleated squames have been obtained by scraping the surface of this lesion.

Plate 6.65

Detection of papillomavirus antigen in a low-grade intraepithelial lesion of the uterine cervix. Gold-brown nuclei are positive. Peroxidase antiperoxidase technique.

Plate 6.66

A higher magnification of above. Positive nuclei (gold-brown) do contain the capsid antigen of papillomaviruses. Unstained nuclei are negative. Peroxidase antiperoxidase technique.

Plate 6.64

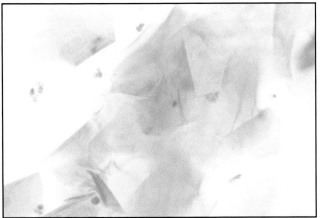

Plate 6.65

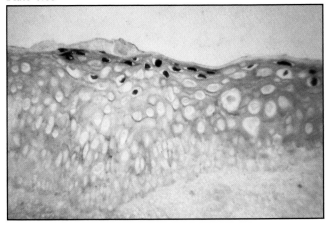

Plate 6.66

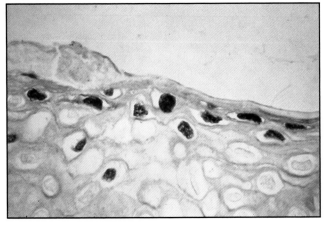

Plate 6.67
Histologic section of an HGSIL hybridized with biotinylated HPV-16 DNA. Intense hybridization is revealed by the brown staining of nuclei, indicating the presence of HPV-16.

Plate 6.68
Histologic section of an LGSIL following in situ hybridization with biotinylated HPV-16 DNA under stringent conditions. Dark brown nuclei are positive for HPV-16.

Plate 6.67

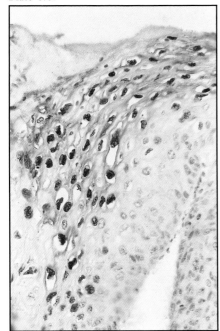

Plate 6.68

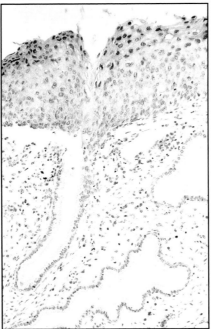

References

1. Ayre, JE: The vaginal smear. "Precancer" cell studies using a modified technique. *Am. J. Obstet Gynecol* 58:1205–1219, 1949.

2. Ayre, JE: Cancer Cytology of the Uterus. New York, Grune & Stratton, 1951.

3. Beaudenon S, Kremsdorf D, Croissant O, Jablonska S, Wain-Hobson S, Orth G: A novel type of human papillomavirus associated with genital neoplasias. *Nature* 321:246–249, 1986.

4. Beaudenon S, Kremsdorf D, Obalek S, Jablonska S, Pehau-Arnaudet G, Croissant O, Orth G: Plurality of genital human papillomaviruses: Characterization of two new types with distinct biological properties. *Virology* 161:374–384, 1987.

5. Beckmann AM, Myerson D, Daling JR, Kiviat NB, Fenoglio CM, McDougall JK: Detection and localization of human papillomavirus DNA in human genital condylomas by in situ hybridization with biotinylated probes. *J Med Virol* 16:265–273, 1985.

6. Boon ME, Deng Z, Baowen G, Ryd W: Koilocyte frequency in positive cervical smears as indicator of sexual promiscuity. *Lancet* iii:205, 1986.

7. Boon ME, Kok LP: Koilocytotic lesions of the cervix: the interrelation of morphometric features, the presence of papillomavirus antigens, and the degree of koilocytosis. *Histopathology* 9:751–763, 1985.

8. Boshart M, Gissmann L, Ikenberg H, Kleinheinz A, Scheurlen W, zur Hausen H: A new type of papillomavirus DNA, its presence in genital cancer biopsies and in cell lines derived from cervical cancer. *Embo J* 3:1151–1157, 1984.

9. Brescia RJ, Jenson B, Lancaster WD, Kurman RJ: The role of human papillomavirus in the pathogenesis and histologic classification of precancerous lesions of the cervix. *Human Pathol* 17:552–559, 1986.

10. Burk RD, Kadish AS, Calderin S, Romney SL: Human papillomavirus infection of the cervix detected by cervicovaginal lavage and molecular hybridization: Correlation with biopsy results and Papanicolaou smears. *Am J. Obstet Gynecol* 154:982–989, 1986.

11. Byrne P, Woodman C, Meanwell C, Kelley K, Jordan K: Koilocytes and cervical human papillomavirus infection (Letter). *Lancet* i(8474):205–206, 1986.

12. Casas-Cordero M, Morin C, Roy M, Fortier M, Meisels A: Origin of the koilocyte in condylomata of the human cervix. Ultrastructural study. *Acta Cytol* 25:383–392, 1981.

13. Chakrabasti RN, Bhattacharya D, Sarkhel T: Detection of human papilloma virus infection in routine Papanicolaou-stained cervical smears. *Eur J Gynaecol Oncol* 8:22–25, 1987.

14. Choo KB, Pan CC, Liu MS, Ng HT, Chen CP, Lee YN, Chao CF, Meng CL, Yeh MY, Han SH: Presence of episomal and integrated human papillomavirus DNA sequences in cervical carcinoma. *J Med Virol* 21:101–107, 1987.

15. Cole ST, Streeck RE: Genome organization and nucleotide sequence of human papillomavirus type 33, which is associated with cervical cancer. *J Virol* 58:991–995, 1986.

16. Dartmann K, Schwartz E, Gissmann L, et: The nucleotide sequence and genome organization of a new human papilloma virus type. *Virology* 151:123–130, 1986.

17. de Brux J, Orth G, Croissant O, Cochard B, Ionesco M: Lésions condylomateuses du col utérin: Evolution chez 2,466 patientes. *Bull Cancer* 70:410–422, 1983.

18. Dekmezian R, Chen X, Kuo T, Ordonez N, Katz RL: DNA hybridization for human papillomavirus (HPV) in cervical lesions. *Arch Pathol Lab Med* 111:22–27, 1987.

19. Deligeorgi-Politi H, Mui KK, Trotta K, Safaii H, An-Foraker SH, Wolfe H, Hutchinson M: Immunocytochemical localization of human papilloma virus and cytomorphologic correlation in smears and biopsies of cervical flat condylomata. *Diag Cytopath* 2:320–325, 1986.

20. Della Torre G, Pilotti S, De Palo G, Rilke F: Viral particles in cervical condylomatous lesions. *Tumori* 64:549–553, 1978.

21. de Villiers EM, Gissmann L, zur Hausen H: Molecular cloning of viral DNA from human genital warts. *J Virol* 40:932–935, 1981.

22. de Villiers EM, Schneider A, Gross G, zur Hausen H: Analysis of benign and malignant urogenital tumors for human papillomavirus infection by labelling cellular DNA. *Med Microbiol Immuno* 174:281–286, 1986.

23. de Villiers EM, Wagner D, Schneider A, Wesch H, Miklaw H, Wahrendorf J, Papendick U, zur Hausen H: Human papillomavirus infections in women with and without abnormal cervical cytology. *Lancet* ii:703–705, 1987.

24. Drake M, Medley G, Mitchell H: Cytologic detection of human papillomavirus infection. *Obstet Gynecol Clin* 14:431–450, 1987.

25. Dürst M, Gissmann L, Ikenberg H, zur Hausen H: A papillomavirus DNA from a cervical carcinoma and its prevalence in cancer biopsy samples from different geographic regions. *Proc Natl Acad Sci* 80:3812–3815, 1983.

26. Dunn J, Weinstein L, Droegemueller W, Meincke W: Immunologic detection of condylomata acuminata-specific antigens. *Obstet Gynecol* 57:351–356, 1981.

27. Dyson JL, Walker PG, Singer A: Human papillomavirus infection of the uterine cervix: histological appearance in 28 cases identified by immunocytochemical technique. *J Clin Pathol* 37:126–130, 1984.

28. Ferenczy A, Braun L, Shah KV: Human papillomavirus (HPV) in condylomatous lesions of cervix. A comparative ultrastructural and immunohistochemical study. *Am J Surg Path* 5:661–670, 1981.

29. Ferenczy A, Mitao M, Nagai M, Silverstein SJ, Crum CP: Latent papillomavirus and recurring genital warts. *New Engl J Med* 313:784–788, 1985.

30. Fletcher S: Histopathology of papilloma virus infection of the cervix uteri: the history, taxonomy, nomenclature and reporting of koilocytotic dysplasias. *J Clin Pathol* 36:616–624, 1983.

31. Gissmann L, zur Hausen H: Partial characterization of viral DNA from human genital warts (condylomata acuminata). *Int J Cancer* 25:605–609, 1980.

32. Gissmann L, Diehl V, Schulz-Caulon HJ, zur Hausen H: Molecular cloning and characterization of human papillomavirus DNA derived from a laryngeal papilloma. *J Virol* 44:393–400, 1982.

33. Gissmann L, Boshart M, Dürst M, Ikenberg H, Wagner D, zur Hausen H: Presence of human papillomavirus in genital tumors. *J Invest Dermatol* 83:25–28, 1984.

34. Gupta J, Gendelman HE, Naghashfar Z, Gupta P, Rosenshein N, Sawada E, Woodruff JD, Shah K: Specific identification of human papillomavirus type in cervical smears and paraffin sections by in situ hybridization with radioactive probes: a preliminary communication. *Intern J Gynecol Pat* 4:211–218, 1985.

35. Gupta JW, Gupta PK, Shah KV, Kelly DP: Distribution of human papillomavirus antigen in cervico-vaginal smears and cervical tissues. *Int J Gynecol Pathol* 2:160–170, 1983.

36. Hills E, Laverty CR: Electron microscopic detection of papilloma virus particles in selected koilocytotic cells in a routine cervical smear. *Acta Cytol* 23:53–56, 1979,

37. Kadish AS, Burk RD, Kress Y, Calderin S, Romney SL: Human papillomaviruses of different types in precancerous lesions of the uterine cervix. Histologic, immunocytochemical and ultrastructural studies. *Human Pathol* 17:384–392, 1986.

38. Kanda T, Furuno A, Yoshiike K: Human papillomavirus type 16 open reading frame E7 encodes a transforming gene for rat 3Y1 cells. *J Virol* 62:610–613, 1988.

39. Karageosov I, Dimova R, Makaveeva V: Electron microscopic detection of viruses in cervix papilloma. *Ztrblt für Gynäkolog* 107:187–191, 1985.

40. Koss LG: Cytologic and histologic manifestations of human papillomavirus infection of the female genital tract and their clinical significance. *Cancer* 60:1942–1950, 1987.

41. Koss LG, Durfee GR: Unusual patterns of squamous epithelium of the uterine cervix: cytologic and pathologic study of koilocytotic atypia. *Ann NY Acad Sci* 63:1245–1261, 1956.

42. Lancaster WD, Kurman RJ, Sanz LE, Perry S, Jenson AB: Human papillomavirus: Detection of viral DNA sequences and evidence for molecular heterogeneity in metaplasias and dysplasias of the uterine cervix. *Intervirology* 20:202–212, 1983.

43. Laverty CR, Booth N, Hills E, Cossart Y, Wills EJ: Noncondylomatous wart virus infection of the postmenopausal cervix. *Pathology* 10:373–378, 1978.

44. Laverty CR, Russell P, Hills E, Booth N: The significance of noncondylomatous wart virus infection of the cervical transformation zone. A review with discussion of two illustrative cases. *Acta Cytol* 22:195–201, 1978.

45. Lorincz AT, Lancaster WD, Temple GF: Cloning and characterization of a new human papillomavirus from a woman with dysplasia of the uterine cervix. *J Virol* 58:225–229, 1986.

46. Lorincz AT, Quinn AP, Lancaster WD, Temple GF: A new type of papillomavirus associated with cancer of the uterine cervix. *Virology* 159:187–190, 1987.

47. Macnab JCM, Walkinshaw SA, Cordiner JW, Clements JB: Human papillomavirus in clinically and histologically normal tissue of patients with genital cancer. *N Engl J Med* 315:1052–1058, 1986.

48. Matsukura T, Kanda T, Furuno A, Yoshikawa H, Kawana T, Yoshiike K: Cloning of monomeric human papillomavirus type 16 DNA integrated within cell DNA from a cervical carcinoma. *J Virol* 58:979–982, 1986.

49. Meisels A: The story of a cell. The George N. Papaniaoloau Award Lecture. *Acta Cytol* 27:584–596, 1983.

50. Meisels A, Alonso de Ruiz P: Human papillomavirus-related changes in the genital tract. In: Human Papillomavirus and Cervical Cancer. Muñoz N, Bosch FX, Jenson OM, eds. IARC Scientific Publication No. 94, International Agency for Research on Cancer, Lyon, 1989. pp. 67–85.

51. Meisels A, Casas-Cordero M, Morin C: Cervical condyloma planum. *Clinics in Dermatol* 3:114–123, 1985.

52. Meisels A, Fortin R: Condylomatous lesions of the cervix and vagina. I. Cytologic patterns. *Acta Cytol* 20:505–509, 1976.

53. Meisels A, Fortin R, Roy M: Condylomatous lesions of the cervix. II. Cytologic, colposcopic and histopathologic study. *Acta Cytol* 21:379–390, 1977.

54. Meisels A, Morin C: Flat condyloma of the cervix: Two variants with different prognosis. In: Viral Etiology of Cervical Cancer. Banbury Report 21:115–119. Cold Spring Harbor Laboratories, Cold Spring Harbor, NY, 1986.

55. Meisels A, Morin C, Casas-Cordero M: Human papillomavirus infection of the uterine cervix. *Int J Gynecol Path* 1:75–94, 1982.

56. Meisels A, Roy M, Fortier M, Morin C: Condylomatous lesions of the cervix. Morphologic and colposcopic diagnosis. *Am J Diag Gynecol Ob* 1:109–116, 1979.

57. Meisels A, Roy M, Fortier M, Morin C, Casas-Cordero M, Shah KV, Turgeon H: Human papillomavirus infection of the cervix: The atypical condyloma. *Acta Cytol* 25:7–16, 1981.

58. Morin C, Braun L, Casas-Cordero M, Shah KV, Roy M, Fortier M, Meisels A: Confirmation of the papillomavirus etiology of condylomatous cervix lesions by the peroxidase antiperoxidase technique. *JNCI* 66:831–835, 1981.

59. Morin C, Meisels A: Human papillomavirus infection of the uterine cervix. *Acta Cytol* 24:82–84, 1980.

60. Nakajima T, Tsumuraya M, Morinaga S, Teshima S, Shimosato Y, Kishi K, Ohmi K, Sonoda T, Tsunematsu R, Tanemura K, Yamada T, Kasamatsu T: The frequency of papillomavirus infection in cervical precancerous lesions in Japan: An immunoperoxidase study. *Jpn J Cancer Res* (Ga 77:891–895, 1986.

61. Okagaki T, Twiggs L, Zachow K, Clark B, Ostrow R, Faras A: Identification of human papillomavirus DNA in cervical and vaginal intraepithelial neoplasia with molecularly cloned virus specific DNA probes. *J Gynecol Pathol* 2:153–159, 1983.

62. Ostrow RS, Manias DA, Clark BA, Okagaki T, Twiggs LB, Faras AJ: Detection of papillomavirus DNA in invasive carcinomas of the cervix by in situ hybridization. *Cancer Res* 47:649–653, 1987.

63. Patten SF: Morphologic subclassification of preinvasive cervical neoplasia. In: Compendium on Diagnostic Cytology, Wied GL, Keebler CM, Koss LG, Reagan JW (editors), The Tutorials of Cytology, Chicago, 1988, pp. 105–113.

64. Pilotti S, Rilke F, De Palo G, Della Torre G, Alasio L: Condylomata of the uterine cervix and koilocytosis of cervical intraepithelial neoplasia. *J Clin Pathol* 34:532–541, 1981.

65. Purola E, Savia E: Cytology of gynecologic condyloma acuminatum. *Acta Cytol* 21:26–31, 1977.

66. Reagan JW, Patten SF: Dysplasia: A basic reaction to injury in the uterine cervix. *Ann NY Acad Sci* 97:662–682, 1962.

67. Reid R, Laverty CR, Coppleson M, Isarangul W, Hills E: Noncondylomatous cervical wart virus infection. *Obstet Gynecol* 55:476–483, 1980.

68. Roy M, Morin C, Casas-Cordero M, Meisels A: Human papillomavirus and cervical lesions. *Clin Obstet Gynecol* 26:949–967, 1983.

69. Saigo PE: Cytology of condyloma of the uterine cervix. *Semin Diagn Pathol* 3:204–210, 1986.

70. Saito J, Yutsudo M, Inoue M, Ueda G, Tanizawa O, Hakura A: New human papillomavirus sequences in female genital tumors from Japanese patients. *Gann* 78:1081–1087, 1987.

71. Saurel J, Laisne M, Rabreau M, Marc J, Morard JL: Les lésions condylomateuses du col utérin. A propos de 2638 cas. *Gynécologie* 34:221–233, 1983.

72. Schneider A, Hotz M, Gissmann L: Increased prevalence of human papillomaviruses in the lower genital tract of pregnant women. *Int J Cancer* 40:198–201, 1987.

73. Stanbridge CM, Mather J, Curry A, Butler BE: Demonstration of papilloma virus particles in cervical and vaginal scrape material: A report of 10 cases. *J Clin Pathol* 34:524–531, 1981.

74. Sterrett GF, Alessandri LM, Pixley E, Kulski JK: Assessment of precancerous lesions of the uterine cervix for evidence of human papillomavirus infection: a histological and immunohistochemical study. *Pathology* 19:84–90, 1987.

75. Stoler MH, Broker TR: In situ hybridization detection of human papillomavirus DNAs and messenger RNAs in genital condyloma and a cervical carcinoma. *Human Pathol* 17:1250–1258, 1986.

76. Syrjänen KJ: Condylomatous epithelial changes in the uterine cervix and their relationship to cervical carcinogenesis. *Int J Gynaecol Obste* 17:415–420, 1980.

77. Syrjänen K, Pyrhonen S: Immunoperoxidase demonstration of human papillomavirus (HPV) in dysplastic lesions of the uterine cervix. *Arch Gynecol* 233:52–61, 1982.

78. Syrjänen K, Pyrhonen S: Demonstration of human papillomavirus (HPV) antigen in the condylomatous lesions of the uterine cervix by immunoperoxidase technique. *Gynecol Obstet Inves* 14:90–96, 1982.

79. Syrjänen K, Väyrynen M, Castrén O, Mäntyjärvi R, Pyrhonen S, Yliskoski M: Morphological and immunohistochemical evidence of human papillomavirus (HPV) involvement in the dysplastic lesions of the uterine cervix. *Int J Gynecol Obstet* 21:77–82, 1983.

80. Syrjänen K, Väyrynen M, Mäntyjärvi R, Holopainen H, Saarikoski S, Syrjänen S, Parkkinen S, Castrén O: Electron microscopy in the assessment of the biological behavior of human papillomavirus infections in the uterine cervix. *Neoplasma* 33:493–505, 1986.

81. Syrjänen S, Syrjänen K, Mäntyjärvi R, Parkkinen S, Väyrynen M, Saarikoski S, Castrén O: Human papillomavirus (HPV) DNA sequences demonstrated by in situ DNA hybridization in serial paraffin-embedded cervical biopsies. *Arch Gynecol* 239:39–48, 1986.

82. Takebe N, Tsunokawa Y, Nozawa S, Terada M, Sugimura T: Conservation of E6 and E7 regions of human papillomavirus types 16 and 18 present in cervical cancers. *Biochem Byophys Res* 143:837–844, 1987.

83. Toki T, Oikawa N, Tase T, Wada Y, Yajima A, Suzuki M, Higashiiwai H: Immunoperoxidase demonstration of papillomavirus antigen in dysplasia of the uterine cervix. *Acta Obstet et Gynae* 37:411–415, 1985.

84. Toki T, Oikawa N, Tase T, Sato S, Wada Y, Yajima A, Higashiiwai H: Immunohistochemical and electronmicroscopic demonstration of human papillomavirus in dysplasia of the uterine cervix. *Tohoku J Exp Med* 149:163–167, 1986.

85. Toon PG, Arrand JR, Wilson LP, Sharp DS: Human papillomavirus infection of the uterine cervix of women without cytological signs of neoplasia. *Brit Med J* 293:1261–1264, 1986.

86. Wagner D, de Villiers EM, Gissmann L: Detection of various papillomavirus types in cytologic smears of precancerous conditions and cancers of the uterine cervix. *Geburtsh u Frauenh* 45:226–231, 1985.

87. Wickenden C, Steele A, Malcolm AD, Coleman DV: Screening for wart virus infection in normal and abnormal cervices by DNA hybridization of cervical scrapes. *Lancet* ii:65–67, 1985.

88. Woodruff JD, Braun L, Cavalieri R, Gupta P, Pass F, Shah KV: Immunologic identification of papillomavirus antigen in condyloma tissues from the female genital tract. *Obstet Gynecol* 56:727–732, 1980.

89. Woodruff JD, Peterson WF: Condylomata acuminata of the cervix. *Am J Obstet Gynecol* 75:1354–1362, 1958.

90. zur Hausen H: Human papillomavirus and their possible role in squamous carcinomas. *Curr Top Microbiol Immunol* 78:1–30, 1977.

91. zur Hausen H, Gissmann L, Steiner W, Dippold W, Dreger J: Human papillomaviruses and cancer. Clemmensen J, Voln DS, eds. *Bibl Haematologica* 43:569–571, 1975.

CHAPTER SEVEN

The Human Papillomaviruses and Cancer of the Uterine Cervix

During the past decade the papillomaviruses (PV) have attracted considerable attention, mainly because of their possible involvement in carcinoma of the uterine cervix. In 1975, only a few groups located in England, France, Germany, Scotland, and the United States were involved in the study of animal and human papillomaviruses. These viruses were believed to be inoffensive agents producing benign proliferative tumors of the skin or mucosa, known as warts, and capable of spontaneous regression in most instances. Today clinical and fundamental biologic research studies on papillomaviruses are going on in more than 20 countries around the world and in some of these countries more than one group are interested in these viruses and their corresponding pathology. Since 1976, more than 400 scientific publications have been specifically devoted to papillomaviruses and cervical lesions.

A large amount of knowledge has been accumulated concerning the relationship of papillomaviruses to human and animal diseases, their biologic, chemical, and physical characterization, the molecular cloning of their genomes, their transformation capability in vitro and in vivo, the expression of their genomes in the host cell, the entire nucleotide sequencing of several types, and the difficulty of replicating them in vitro. In this chapter, we intend to review some of the current knowledge on papillomaviruses. Most of the sections will deal with human papillomaviruses, although animal papillomaviruses will be briefly discussed to emphasize the suspected role of PV in carcinogenesis.

Historical Review

Genital warts were described in the literature of antiquity. They were believed to be a sexually transmitted disease limited mainly to the homosexual population.[6] From the Roman—Hellenistic period to the fifteenth century, references to this disease are almost nonexistent, and description inaccurate. During the period from the fifteenth to the eighteenth century, the belief that genital warts were a manifestation of syphilis was first suggested and subsequently abandoned; they were then linked to gonorrhea. But this idea was also abandoned in the nineteenth century, when it was thought that genital warts were caused by skin irritants. A few observers reported that these irritants could be sexually transmitted and secreted by warts.[114]

Unitary Theory

In 1893, it was suggested[114] that genital warts might be related to skin warts because of histologic similarity in both conditions. Experimental inoculations[27,65,77,78,87,109,150,151,163] of unfiltered and filtered extracts of skin and genital warts, made in the first two decades of the twentieth century, tended to support Gemy's postulate, which is discussed in detail in reference 114. These inoculation tests also supported the theory that laryngeal papilloma was caused by the same agent. The viral etiology of skin warts was established by Ciuffo[27] in 1907 following the development of warts on one of his fingers at the site of inoculation with a cell-free filtrate of wart tissue. One must remember here that a tissue extract filtered through a bacterial filter (ie, a filter that can retain bacteria but allow small submicroscopic particles to pass through) without losing its pathogenic potential following inoculation into a susceptible host was supposed to contain a filterable virus. At that time, filtration was the only tool to study viral diseases. The viral etiology of genital warts was subsequently confirmed by Serra (1924),[151] who used filtered extracts of penile condylomata to produce skin warts in volunteers. These experiments were convincing enough to bring medical observers to believe that genital and skin warts were caused by the same virus (for review, see Rowson and Mahy).[136] Almost at the same period, Shope[153] found that papilloma of wild cottontail rabbit is caused by a filterable agent and that it could be transmitted easily by rubbing the filtrate into the scarified skin of rabbits. This virus was the first recognized papillomavirus.

With the advent of electron microscopy, it became possible to visualize the filterable particles. Beginning in 1949, electron microscopy studies[4,21,24,25,85,86,159] of warts brought more evidence (although incorrect) to the devotees of the unitary theory suggesting that skin warts, genital warts, and laryngeal papillomata are caused by the same harmless (related to benign conditions) agent. Viral particles of the same morphology were detected in skin[4,24,25] and genital warts[5,39,113] as well as in laryngeal papillomata.[16,160]

Plurality of Papillomaviruses

But in 1969, the study of Almeida et al[5] using immune electron microscopy showed that the virus of genital warts appears to be antigenically different from the virus present in skin warts. To explain this finding, the authors stated, "The most likely explanation is that genital wart virus is an established mutant, better adapted to the genital epithelium than to the skin in other regions." By this observation, Almeida et al were initiating the concept of the plurality of papillomaviruses. Furthermore, they concluded ". . . electron microscope and complement fixation studies have led us to believe that there is a one-way antigenic cross between the virus of the human common wart and that of the human genital wart . . ." with a proof that both viruses are part of the same group of viruses. This observation was further corroborated and better understood by the studies of Orth et al[116] and Jenson et al,[79] showing an immunologic relatedness of papillomaviruses from different animal species. Both groups showed that papillomaviruses share a common antigenic determinant indicating that these viruses have a common evolutionary origin.

The question is raised, "Is the virus of genital warts, skin warts, and laryngeal papillomata exactly the same virus or different viruses?" In his study on the natural history of genital warts, Oriel[114] concluded, "No epidemiologic evidence was found of a close relationship between genital warts and skin warts." In their epidemiologic surveys, zur Hausen et al[174] showed a different age distribution in the incidence of skin warts, genital warts, and laryngeal warts, respectively. The age distribution of patients with genital warts correlates with the ages in which sexual activity is most frequent. Genital warts appear to be sexually transmitted and are more prevalent in populations of high sexual promiscuity. The malignant conversion of genital warts and laryngeal papillomata is reported many times in the literature.[175] In contrast to genital warts, the age distribution for occurrence of verruca vulgaris and plantar warts extends from childhood to old age. Furthermore, verruca vulgaris and plantar warts have not been associated with malignant proliferation. These observations brought zur Hausen et al[174,175] to say, "The epidemiological pattern suggests the existence of strain differences among human papillomaviruses."

In 1974, the use of a new biochemical instrument, the molecular hybridization, was introduced to study cross hybridization between DNA samples extracted from different wart lesions. This instrument permitted experiments designed to study the nucleic acid homology between two DNA strands. Almost at the same time, detailed analysis of wart virus DNA became available with the use of different enzymes (the restriction endonucleases) capable of cleaving DNA into fragments which could then be analyzed by gel electrophoresis.

Soon it was found that DNA extracted from plantar warts revealed no cross hybridization with DNA extracted from condylomata or laryngeal warts.[173] This finding added more evidence of the existence of different viral types in wart lesions. The heterogeneity of papillomavirus was confirmed following the analysis of wart viral DNA isolates after digestion with restriction endonucleases.[47,59]

The lack of a permissive tissue culture system (for review see Rowson and Mahy[136]) slowed advancement in the knowledge of the genetic information of papillomaviruses because most of the lesions contain too little viral DNA to permit their complete analysis. But this difficulty was circumvented with the development of the technique of molecular cloning of recombinant papillomavirus DNAs in *Escherichia coli*. By combining all of these techniques (molecular cloning, molecular hybridization, and restriction endonuclease analysis of DNA) the number of human papillomavirus types discovered has increased markedly. In 1976, 4 types were identified; in 1980, 6 types; in 1982, 13 types; in 1983, 24 types; in 1986, 40 types; in 1989, more than 60 types of human papillomaviruses. In the anogenital tract alone, 20 types have been identified, confirming the genetic diversity of papillomaviruses.

Papillomavirus Infection of the Uterine Cervix

Until 1976, it was known that genital warts (caused by papillomavirus infection) were found mostly on the external anogenital organs of men and women: penis, scrotum, anus, vulva, and more rarely, on the vaginal wall and the uterine cervix.

At the time the plurality of HPV was being recognized, a very important observation was made in clinical cytology. Meisels and Fortin[107] noted for the first time that papillomavirus infection of the cervix is much more frequent than previously observed. For many years, this infection tended to be misdiagnosed as an intraepithelial lesion of low grade, without any reference to papillomaviruses. This observation was probably the most important information in the field of exfoliative cytology after the introduction of cytology as a diagnostic tool.

In 1978, electron microscopy[38,72] confirmed that the cells diagnostic for papillomavirus infection, the koilocytes, observed in histologically flat and papillary lesions, were harboring viral particles in their nuclei. These particles were identical to those found in condylomata acuminata.

In 1980 and 1981, immunohistochemists,[48,110,167] using a serum broadly cross reactive to a capsid papillomavirus antigen of all animal species added confirmation to the work of Meisels and Fortin.

First attempts[37,60,115] to selectively purify and characterize virus particles from human genital warts were partially successful because of the scarcity of virus-producing cells within such lesions. The cloning of the first HPV DNA from genital warts was done by de Villiers et al[35] in 1981. This HPV DNA was classified as HPV-6. A very high percentage of condylomata acuminata were found to harbor HPV-6 DNA. One year later, in 1982, a second HPV DNA was cloned from a laryngeal papilloma and it was designated HPV-11 by Gissmann and his coworkers.[61] This new HPV type was also recovered from condylomata acuminata, flat cervical lesions, malignant cervical tumors, and Buschke-Lowenstein tumors.[62] These data were supporting a genital origin for laryngeal papillomata.

In 1983, a third variety of papillomavirus DNA from a genital tumor (a cervical carcinoma), was cloned and classified as HPV-16.[41] This HPV type was then used as a probe and was detected in a high number of cervical cancer samples from German patients (61.1%). HPV-16 DNA sequences were also detected in Bowen's disease, bowenoid papulosis, and in vulval and penile cancer biopsy samples. Another new papillomavirus (subsequently named type 18) was cloned and partially characterized from a cervical carcinoma biopsy by Boshart et al.[14] HPV-18 DNA was found in cervical and penile cancer biopsy specimens and also in cell lines established from cervical cancer, that is, the cells of the HeLa, KB and C4-1 lines. Since then, it has become evident that HPV-16 and HPV-18 exhibit a remarkable association with malignant genital tissues. Subsequently, other HPV types classified as HPV-31, HPV-33, HPV-35, and HPV-39 were cloned from intraepithelial lesions and genital neoplasia.[8,9,100,101]

Classification

The papillomaviruses (genus A) and polyomaviruses (genus B) are both members of the Papovaviridae family. Following the suggestion of Melnick,[108] the name PaPoVavirus was obtained by taking the first two letters from the name of the viruses in the order in which they were discovered: the papillomavirus of rabbit,[153] the polyomavirus of mice,[67] and the vacuolating virus of monkeys (SV40).[161] Melnick grouped these viruses together because they were small, oncogenic, lipid-free DNA viruses that appeared similar in structure on electron microscopy. But recent molecular and biologic studies strongly confirm that these two genera are distinct from one another. The International Committee on Taxonomy of Viruses should revise this classification in order to recognize papillomaviruses as a distinct group.

Papillomaviruses are found in mammals generally and in only one avian species: the chaffinch. Shope[153] (1933) was the first to confirm that cottontail rabbits in Kansas and Iowa carry large horny warts of the skin caused by a filterable agent. Papillomaviruses were subsequently detected from a variety of commonplace mammalian species, including cattle, coyote, deer, dog, elk, goat, horse, monkey, mouse, opossum, pig, rabbit, and sheep, without forgetting the human species. The cottontail rabbit papillomavirus and bovine papillomaviruses are probably the most thoroughly studied viral types in animal groups, mainly in relation to their oncogenic potential in natural and experimental conditions.[92]

Classification Scheme for Papillomaviruses

The scheme and criteria for the classification of papillomaviruses were proposed at a conference on papillomaviruses and cancer held in 1978 at the University of South Alabama College of Medicine.[28] The present propositions for the nomenclature of PV are the following:

1. Each virus must be classified first according to its natural host.
2. The virus must be abbreviated by the first two letters of the English name of the animal that is the natural host of the virus: the first letter is upper case, the second lower case. Human and bovine papillomaviruses (for which the abbreviations HPV and BPV have become standard in the literature) are exceptions. (Note: From the literature, it is evident that proposition 2 has not always been respected in the classification of animal papillomaviruses.)
3. Viruses from a given species will be classified as types and subtypes according to their nucleotide sequence homology. Definition: new viral isolates are considered a subtype of a previous isolate if there is more than 50% nucleotide sequence homology after S1 nuclease digestion as determined by reassociation of heterologous DNA in liquid phase. Independent types will show less than 50% sequence homology in the same conditions.
4. Each virus type should be numbered sequentially, and each subtype should be designated in alphabetical sequence in lower case. Example: HPV-6a for human papillomavirus type 6, subtype a.

In the future, it is not improbable that papillomaviruses will be classified according to another scheme, based upon their serologic properties, or the degree of amino acid homology between their proteins. Such a new reclassification scheme should have the advantage of reducing the growing number of HPV types that have a closer DNA sequence homology than predicted by reassociation kinetics.

Diversity of Human Papillomaviruses and Associated Lesions

More than 60 types of human papillomaviruses have been identified to date as determined by the degree of homology following reassociation kinetics (see Table 6.1, page 90). The first explanation for such diversity should be a high rate of mutation. But it appears that HPV are rather stable as demonstrated by the sequence data of viruses identified in different geographic locations and after many years of propagation of viral DNA in animals and in cell lines.[58] The plurality of HPV remains unexplained.

However, one must be aware that the classification of HPV based on the homology determined by reassociation kinetics does not take into account the real homology between various HPV types. Complete DNA sequence analysis and transmission electron microscopy of DNA-DNA heteroduplex of cloned DNA[20] clearly demonstrate that there is much more homology between different HPV types than previously determined by reassociation kinetics.

Different HPV types have been isolated from cutaneous and mucosal (genital, oral, and respiratory mucosae) epithelia: plantar and palmar myrmecia, plantar warts, common warts, flat warts, lesions of epidermodysplasia verruciformis, oral focal epithelial hyperplasia, laryngeal papillomata, anogenital condylomata, keratoacanthoma, Bowen's disease, bowenoid papulosis, intraepithelial neoplasia and carcinoma (cervix, vagina, vulva, penis, anus), and melanoma, (see Chapter Six). Human papillomavirus DNA has also been extracted from primary as well as metastatic sites.[93]

Specific Anatomic Tropism of HPV

Papillomaviruses have a specificity for the anatomic site that they infect. For instance, certain HPV (types 1 and 2) replicate preferably in thick epithelium, such as the sole of the foot or the palm of the hand. Other types (namely HPV-16 and HPV-18) preferably infect the genital epithelium, such as the uterine cervix or the penis. To explain such a specificity, Howley and Schlegel[75] speculated: "Keratinocytes from different anatomic sites may be in different states of differentiation, evident from the distinct types of keratin proteins that they synthesize and from the pattern of synthesis of other epithelial specific proteins, such as involucrin. The ability of HPVs to proliferate at a particular anatomic site may, therefore, reflect a very specific interaction between viral and cellular gene expression."

High- and Low-Risk Papillomaviruses

According to the results obtained by Lorincz et al,[99] it seems that individual HPV types that infect the cervix have varying degrees of oncogenic association: HPV-6 and HPV-11 appear to have very little oncogenic association, HPV-31 has low oncogenic association, and HPV-16 and HPV-18 have high oncogenic association. They also noted that the frequency of detection of HPV-16 increases with increasing grade of the intraepithelial lesion, from 20% in lesions Grade 1, to 43% in lesions Grade 2, and 50% in lesions Grade 3. The same authors found that 47% of squamous carcinoma contained HPV-16, suggesting that cervical cancer may develop in a stepwise fashion through increasing grades of intraepithelial lesions. Infections with HPV-6 or HPV-11 result in a benign lesion that can persist or regress but very rarely progresses to cancer. This is why certain types of HPV are considered low- or high-risk factors for the development of cervical cancer. Further studies are mandatory to elucidate the real degree of oncogenicity of each HPV type. In fact, more recent studies suggest HPV-6 and HPV-11 may be associated with the initiation of malignant epithelial neoplasms.[10,104] Other findings[165] indicate that HPV-18–containing tumors have a more aggressive clinical course than do similar cervical cancers with HPV-16 DNA. This report tends to demonstrate that the HPV genotype can influence the clinical outcome for women with cervical cancer. This suggests that HPV genotype could be a prognostic indicator in carcinoma of the uterine cervix. It was also reported that patients with HPV-16/18 had significantly more recurrences after laser therapy than patients with HPV 6/11.[54]

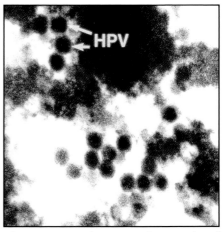

Figure 7.1 Electron micrograph of papillomavirus particles (HPV) observed in a nucleus of a lesion of the uterine cervix. Note that intranuclear particles are uniform in size and shape. Each particle appears as a dense central core surrounded by a less dense material. Uranyl acetate and lead citrate staining, 147,000×.

Morphologic, Physical, and Chemical Properties of PV

Electron microscopy shows that papillomavirus particles isolated from man and animals harbor the same morphology: they are nonenveloped icosahedral capsids composed of 72 capsomers, whose diameters range from 44–55 nm.[85,86,108] A core of a DNA chromosome is encapsulated inside the capsid (Figures 7.1 and 7.2). Papillomaviruses do not contain lipid. The capsid harbors two protein species: a major protein with a molecular weight of about 54,000 daltons and a minor protein with a molecular weight of about 76,000 daltons. The DNA is a covalently closed, circular, double-stranded molecule. The molecular length of the chromosome is about 7,900 base pairs with a molecular weight of about 5.0×10^6 daltons. The DNA molecules represent around 12% of the virion by weight.

Antigenic Cross Reactivity

The denatured major capsid proteins of animal or human papillomaviruses induce in animals the production of antiserum that is cross reactive with different papillomavirus types. It is believed that this group-specific antibody recognizes a nonaccessible antigenic site that is revealed only by disruption of the virus capsid. This property was clearly demonstrated by Orth et al[116] and Jenson et al.[79] The use of this antiserum and immunohistochemistry has shown that about 50% of genital condylomata[48,110,167] contain the cross-reactive PV antigen. But this antiserum detects only productive infection, not latent infection. Furthermore, it was demonstrated more recently that the commercial antiserum raised against sodium-dodecyl-sulphate–denatured BPV virions do not recognize all human papillomavirus types equally well. As a matter of fact, Firzlaff et al[49] have observed cases in which the commercial antiserum could not detect the capsid antigen seen with polyclonal antisera raised against the HPV-16 L1 fusion protein. The genus-specific epitope of the major capsid antigen is more closely conserved between bovine papillomavirus type 1 (BPV-1) and HPV-6 than between BPV-1 and HPV-16. Thus, lesions containing HPV-6 and related types will be stained by the cross-reacting antiserum more frequently than HPV-16 lesions.

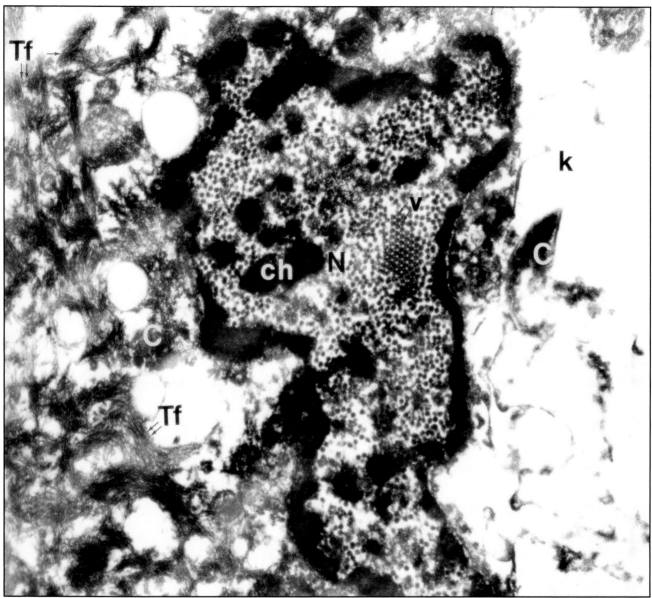

Figure 7.2 Electron micrograph of a part of a koilocyte. The nucleus (N) is filled by papillomavirus particles (v) forming in one area a paracrystalline array. Chromatin (ch) is mainly located in the periphery of the nucleus. On the right of the nucleus, a large cavity (k = koilocytotic area) is seen. On the left, bundles of tonofilaments (Tf) are visible in the cytoplasm (C). Uranyl acetate and lead citrate staining, 22,500×.

Genomic Organization of PV

The complete DNA sequences of many papillomaviruses have been determined.[29,30,32,33,64,147,148] Comparing their sequences reveals that they all possess a similar genetic organization. Different regions, called open reading frames (ORFs), are capable of coding for proteins. But unlike other viruses, synthesized proteins are encoded by only one of the two strands of viral DNA. This means that all messenger RNAs are copied from one strand. The PV genome is organized into three distinct regions:

1. the early region: encoding for proteins involved in viral DNA replication, transcription, and cellular transformation. The genes located in this early region are designated E1, E2, E3, E4, E5, E6, E7, and E8 (note that E3, E5, and E8 ORFs may not be present in all papillomavirus genomes).
2. the late region: encoding for the viral capsid proteins. The genes located in the late region are designated L1 and L2.
3. the noncoding region (NCR) known as the upstream regulatory region (URR) or the long control region (LCR).

The E6 and E7 ORFs appear to be important for the replication and maintenance of a high number of copies of viral DNA in the cells. The E6 region is involved in cellular transformation and alteration of growth properties of cells in culture. The E6 ORF is retained and actively transcribed in cervical carcinoma cell lines and in tumor biopsies.[97,106,145,146,164] The E7 protein was present in cervical cancer cell lines containing HPV-16 or HPV-18.[149,155] For more information concerning the role of each ORF, see reference 119.

HPV and Human Chromosomes

In benign lesions (warts, condylomata), the viral DNA appears to be episomal, ie, an unintegrated or extrachromosomal plasmid floating freely within the cellular nucleoplasm.[14,40] On the other hand, invasive cancers often contain integrated viral sequences (ie, viral DNA is inserted within human chromosomes)[106,164] although extrachromosomal HPV DNA can also be found in some carcinomas. For instances, HPV-33 was found to persist extrachromosomally in cervical cancers, suggesting that integration may not be a prerequisite of malignant transformation.[9,26]

The integration of HPV-16 and HPV-18 DNA in cervical cancer cells does not appear to be specific to particular host chromosome sites[42,126] even though integration has been mapped to chromosome 8 in the close proximity of the myc oncogene in two cell lines. However, integration seems to involve specific regions of the viral genome, namely the E6 and E7 ORFs, which remain intact within the host genome of cancerous cells.

Pathogenesis and Transmission of Warts

Under natural conditions, cross-species infections do not occur. However, under experimental conditions, PVs that induce a fibroblastic proliferation such as BPV-1 and BPV-2 are able to induce infections in horses and mice.[92] Up to now, no human beings have been found to be infected by animal papillomaviruses.

It is presumed that PV infections are transmitted from one human to another. Thick epithelia (surface of hands and plantar surface of feet) as well as thin epithelia (abdomen, vagina, cervix) are susceptible to harboring PV infections. In normal conditions, epithelia are barriers to outside invaders. A wound or abrasion of the epithelium is, therefore, necessary to provide the virus access to the basal cells. These cells are capable of division. Under the papillomavirus stimuli controlled by specific viral genes, hyperproliferation of cells occurs in the intermediate cell layers. The cells differentiate progressively as the cells move outward in the epithelium. Abnormal keratinization, cytoplasmic vacuolization, and nuclear degeneration become visible. In the more superficial cells, there is synthesis of new viral DNA and capsid protein production as revealed by in situ hybridization, immunohistochemistry, and electron microscopy.[11,23,44,48,69,82,110,118] This synthesis is the vegetative replication of HPV. The complete virions can be transmitted to another wounded epithelium.

The study of Oriel[114] has shown that 60% of partners of persons with genital warts developed genital warts after an average of 3 months. Rosemberg et al[131] have found that 73% of the partners of women with human papillomavirus–associated disease of the lower genital tract have evidence of HPV infection. Barrasso et al[7] have shown that 64.4% of male partners of women with cervical condylomata or cervical intraepithelial neoplasia have evidence of penile HPV infections. Several lesions in men are subclinical, ie, entirely invisible without the aid of acetic acid soaking and androscopy.[7,12,13,131] All these findings support the sexual transmission of genital HPV.

Nonsexual transmission of HPV and vertical transmission from the mother to the child has been reported (for review see Koutsky et al).[88] Iatrogenic transmission of HPV has not been documented in the literature. The detection of naked HPV DNA in vapors generated during laser therapy has not yet been proven dangerous for the patients or for the clinician.[55]

PV and Tissue Culture

Complete maturation of papillomaviruses in host tissues appears in the uppermost layers of the squamous epithelium (including the upper stratum spinosum and the stratum granulosum), suggesting that the keratinocyte is the target cell for the replication of papillomaviruses. As the cells of the epidermis migrate from the basal layer to the surface, they undergo a program of differentiation. The control of papillomavirus late gene expression, encoding for capsid proteins and virion assembly, appears tightly linked to the program of differentiation of the squamous epithelial cells.

Many attempts to propagate papillomaviruses in tissue culture have failed (for review see Rowson and Mahy;[136] Reilly and Taichman).[128] No evidence of vegetative viral synthesis (ie, no production of detectable virus particles) has been obtained in the most sophisticated culture models using human keratinocytes capable of differentiating in vitro to form a stratified squamous epithelium.

In these systems, cells of the outer layer become cornified as they do in vivo, but keratins indicative of terminally differentiated epidermal cells are not synthesized, providing no support for the productive infection.[15] However, there is, apparently, an exception. Bossens[15] et al in 1989 reported in an abstract that they were able to replicate HPV-1 in more physiological conditions. Their culture system was composed of de-epidermized human vaginal submucosa on which keratinocytes were cultured at an air-liquid interface. These observations remain to be repeated for confirmation. If HPV particles do not mature easily in cultured keratinocytes, HPV-DNA replicates in these cells and some viral transcription takes place. But eventually, during successive passage of the infected cells, HPV DNA is progressively lost.[22,94] Further studies are needed to understand the molecular basis controlling the program of differentiation of the squamous epithelial cells and consequently to understand the vegetative synthesis of papillomaviruses.

Papillomaviruses and Transformation in Vitro

HPV-16 is the most frequent type of papillomavirus found in cervical cancers. HPV-16 has been shown to transform mouse 3T3 cells[164,169] and to immortalize human fibroblasts and keratinocytes.[43,125] The whole viral genome is not necessary for inducing transformation. The data obtained by Kanda et al[83] indicate that expression of the HPV-16 E7 ORF is sufficient to induce focal transformation of rat cells. It is interesting to note here that cervical cancer lines CaSki and SiHa contain a large quantity of E7 protein. This may suggest that the E7 ORF is involved in generation or maintenance of human cervical cancers. The interrelation between viral gene and oncogene is reported by Matlashewski et al,[105] who have found that HPV-16 can cooperate with activated rat gene in transforming primary rat kidney cells. Not all HPVs possess the capability of transforming cells: HPV-6, and HPV-11, which are considered low-risk factors for cancer, are not capable of converting foreskin or cervical keratinocytes[121,141,168] to the tumorigenic state.

HPV and Tumor Suppressor Genes

It was first believed that activated oncogenes could suffice to create a cancerous cell. However, different studies have shown that hybrid cells formed by fusion of a malignant cell with a normal cell are nontumorigenic.[156,157] These observations have indicated that a gene from the normal cell might restore a defective function in the cancer cell. In other words, the malignant cell becomes responsive to the cell growth regulator genes of the normal cell when hybrids are formed.

These genes were termed "tumor suppressor genes."[84] The importance of such "genes" was first demonstrated in retinoblastoma cells, which lack a functional protein—p105-Rb.[50,51,96] The introduction of the "Rb1 gene" into these cancerous cells proved to inhibit the tumor formation.[76] The Rb1 gene seems to play a major role in the control of the cell cycle of many tumors.[50] Tumor suppressor genes are probably a determinant mechanism for cancer protection.

When suppressor gene(s) are inactivated (by methylation, deletion, or point mutation) or when their product (specific protein, for instance, the Rb protein) is inactivated or lowered, cells are then submitted to abnormal proliferation. Thus it was found that the transforming proteins of adenoviruses[166] or SV40 virus[34] form protein complexes with the p105-Rb protein. It was therefore speculated that the formation of these complexes inactivates the RB protein, mimicking the loss of the Rb1 gene and possibly leading to cell proliferation.

Very interestingly, Dyson et al[45] have shown that the E7 oncoprotein of HPV-16 can also form complexes in vitro with the p105-retinoblastoma protein. It is believed that the alteration or the inactivation of the retinoblastoma gene product by the HPV-16 E7 protein may favor the initiation of cervical cancer. On the other hand, the E7 proteins of the nononcogenic HPV-6b and 11 bind with lower affinity with the product of the retinoblastoma tumor-suppressor gene.[53] This may explain why HPV-6b and HPV-11 are very rarely seen in cancerous tissues.

These observations point out that Rb protein binding may be a possible step in HPV carcinogenesis. The possible interactions between positive factors (oncogens) and negative factors (anti-oncogens: tumor suppressor genes) appear to be an important key for understanding the carcinogenesis of the uterine cervix.

The fusion of HeLa cells with normal fibroblasts or keratinocytes also results in the suppression of the malignant phenotype.[156] Such hybrids have been termed the "nonmalignant HeLa hybrids." These nonmalignant HeLa-fibroblast or HeLa-keratinocyte hybrids are relatively stable. But occasionally, when chromosome 11, originating from the normal cells (fibroblasts or keratinocytes) is lost, reconversion to the malignant phenotype happens.[138] These malignant hybrids have been termed "malignant revertants (or segregants)."

It is interesting to recall here that HeLa cells are a cell line derived from an adenocarcinoma of the uterine cervix and were established by Gey in 1951.[57,81] This cell line was proved by Boshart et al in 1984[14] to contain HPV-18 DNA integrated within the cell genome. HeLa cells express transcription of HPV-18–DNA into HPV-18–RNA.

The group of zur Hausen, in Germany, has analyzed HPV-18–DNA transcription in nonmalignant HeLa hybrids as well as in their malignant revertants.[132,170] The in vitro rate of HPV transcription did not differ significantly in nonmalignant hybrids and their malignant segregants from that of the parental HeLa line. However, heterografting of these cells into nude mice significantly reduces HPV transcription within the nonmalignant hybrids. These data have indicated to zur Hausen's group that HPV transcription is regulated differently in nonmalignant hybrids kept under in vivo or in vitro conditions. Also, the German group has suspected that the selective downregulation of HPV transcription in vivo is possibly triggered by a humoral factor. Following all these observations, zur Hausen has submitted a hypothetical mechanism to explain the intracellular surveillance of persisting viral infections.[176]

A rapid and selective switchoff of HPV-18 transcription in nonmalignant hybrids can be obtained in vitro using a demethylating compound—5-azacytidine.[132] The down regulation of transcription is accompanied by a rapid growth inhibition. Cells from "malignant segregants" remain unaffected, ie, the HPV-18 transcription remains switched on. The switch off effect is reversible by cycloheximide treatment, pointing to a protein factor involved in its induction. As stated by zur Hausen,[170] this protein factor should be supplied by activated cellular genes originating from the normal fusion partner (normal fibroblast or normal keratinocyte). It is tempting to speculate that these activated cellular genes could be tumor suppressor genes.

PV Detection Tests

Clinical and laboratory diagnostic tests, including colposcopy, exfoliative cytology, and histopathology, are unable to provide information about the type of HPV in associated lesions. Electron microscopy and immunohistochemistry allow, respectively, the detection of viral particles and the genus-specific antigen present within productive infections, but both methods miss around 50% of frankly HPV-associated lesions. Furthermore, electron microscopic and immunohistochemical analysis do not shed light on the specific HPV type found in a given lesion. Although most human viruses (herpesviruses, adenoviruses) are directly diagnosed by serologic or cell culture methods, papillomaviruses cannot be in routine practice. But a gleam of hope has recently emerged with the work of Jochmus-Kudielka et al[80] concerning the first attempt in seroepidemiology of antibody responses against specific HPV-16–coded protein. Moreover, HPV-16 E7 and HPV-18 E7 monoclonal antibodies developed by Triton Biosciences are now available for research use in Western blot and immunoprecipitation analyses.

Consequently, HPVs must be typed by the following DNA hybridization tests: in situ, filter in situ, dot blot, Southern blot, or by PCR (polymerase chain reaction). All these techniques and related principles are fully described in Chapter Fifteen.

HPV and Cancer

According to Pfister,[123] only one in 100 HPV-16–infected women will develop cervical cancer. His calculations are roughly based on the ratio of the prevalence of a given type in the normal population versus the prevalence of HPV-positive cancers. The risk of malignant progression of HPV-16 lesions appears to be fivefold to tenfold higher than for HPV-6, HPV-11, or HPV-31, suggesting that specific HPV types are more aggressive than others.

Table 7.1
Cofactors Possibly Involved in the Genesis of Uterine Cancer

1. **Carcinogenic and mutagenic substances from tobacco:** Women who smoke reveal an increased risk for developing cancer, as revealed by epidemiological studies.[19,66,91] Mutagenic substances have been isolated from cervical secretions of female smokers,[71,73,137,140] and DNA damage reported in cervical cells.[124]

2. **Other carcinogens or mutagens** of known or unsuspected origin. Certain vagino-cervical microorganisms can produce mutagenic substances, such as dimethylnitrosamine.[70] Treatment of cells with the carcinogen 4-nitroquinoline-1-oxide has induced a fivefold to tenfold amplification of HPV-18 sequences.[17] The notion that chemical carcinogens (tar or methylcholanthrene) produce a synergistic effect on the malignant conversion of rabbit warts was intensively studied.[134,135] Simultaneous application of CRPV (cottontail rabbit papillomavirus) and DMBA (dimethylbenzenthracene) on the rabbit skin increases the malignant conversion of warts.[130]

3. **Coexisting viral and microbial infections:** Different studies have shown that amplification of HPV sequences ranged from twofold to eightfold in herpesvirus-infected cells.[17] Furthermore, herpesviruses were proven mutagenic within the host cell genome.[142,172] Different microorganisms (*Trichomonas vaginalis, Chlamydia trachomatis, Treponema pallidum, Neisseria gonorrhoeae*) have been suspected of playing a role in the genesis of cervical cancer.[2,52,139,162] All these agents were also found in association with HPV infection.

4. **Natural and contraceptive hormones:** Oral contraceptives are suspected to be a risk factor for cervical cancer.[18,46,90,133] Comparison of the prevalence of HPV infection in sexually active women (10%–12%)[36] and in pregnant women (30%)[143] strongly suggests that hormone use may contribute to an increase of HPV production. Gloss et al[63] and Pater et al[120] have shown that glucocorticoid hormones are able to activate a specific region of HPV-16 that contains an E2 protein independent enhancer that is specific for cervical carcinoma cells.

5. **Host immune status:** Immunodeficiency plays an important role in the pathogenesis of HPV infection and neoplasia. Most of the immunosuppressed women with HPV infection do develop a clinical manifestation, such as warts and condylomata. Warts are seen in 43% of renal transplant patients with frequent involvement of the anogenital region.[3,122,144,154] On the contrary, the majority of women with intact immunity do not present clinical signs of HPV despite the fact they are infected with the virus. Progression to invasion from intraepithelial lesions occurs more frequently and at a more rapid rate in immunosuppressed patients than in the general population.[154]

6. **Oncogene activation:** Both viruses and cellular oncogenes are involved in animal carcinogenesis. For instance, HPV-18 was found to be integrated in the vicinity of the c-myc gene in HeLa cell lines. Furthermore this oncogene was overexpressed in a large number of cervical cancers.[56,95,112,129]

7. **Dietary deficiencies:** Several epidemiological studies have suggested that vitamin A (or its precursor, Beta-carotene) may have a protective effect against cancer.[89,102,152] Considerable evidence points to the efficacy of retinoids in inducing the regression of PV lesions (warts, oral leukoplakia).[68,74,158] Li et al[98] have shown that retinoic acid treatment of a transformed cell line (C127) reduced the number of viral BPV-DNA copies from 60 to an average of less than one per cell within 5 weeks. Furthermore, the RA-treated cell populations that contained less than one BPV-DNA copy lost the transformed phenotype.

8. **Radiation exposure:** Ultraviolet light and x-rays were also proved to favor malignant progression of HPV-infected lesions. In patients suffering from epidermodysplasia verruciformis, lesions infected specifically with HPV-5 or HPV-8 develop into cancers most often upon parts of the skin most exposed to the sun.[103,117] There was also an interaction between laryngeal papillomata that resulted in the development of squamous cell carcinoma when therapeutic x-ray irradiation was used a few decades ago.[171,175]

9. **Other factors:** Chronic irritation and inflammation that results in frequent recurrence of wounded epithelium can exert a less specific effect.

The presence of a suspected carcinogenic (or aggressive) HPV (ie, HPV-16 or HPV-18), does not seem to suffice to induce a low-grade intraepithelial lesion to progress to a high-grade lesion or to a frank cancer.[1,127] This hypothesis is reinforced by the fact that only a subset of the patients with a low-grade lesion who are infected with suspected aggressive viruses will eventually develop a carcinoma. Furthermore, it was recently proven that men are more frequently infected than previously suspected with the same aggressive HPV[7,131] as found in their sexual partner(s), without experiencing a high level of progression to cancer. Another observation that may suggest that cervical cancer results from multifactorial events is the long period of time that occurs between the first sign of intraepithelial lesion and the development of invasive cancer. Different cofactors are suspected to participate in the genesis of the uterine cervix cancer. Table 7.1 lists those cofactors.

Many experimental and clinical studies have reported arguments favoring the role of HPV in cervical carcinogenesis (Table 7.2). But does human papillomavirus cause or contribute to the development of cervical cancer? Muñoz et al[111] answers, "Whereas there is an impressive body of experimental evidence suggesting an oncogenic potential for certain HPV types, no epidemiological study has convincingly demonstrated that HPV causes cervical cancer."

"The association of a virus with a tumour may occur for a variety of reasons other than the virus being the cause of the tumour," said Crawford,[31] But it is clear that a causal relationship requires that the virus should always be found at some stage in every case where the tumor occurs. This premise is well demonstrated by a close association between papillomavirus DNA and intraepithelial lesions that lead to cervical cancer. However, the question concerning the oncogenicity of human papillomaviruses remains, even though the production of tumors in animals and the transformation in vitro tests are good circumstantial evidence suggesting the virus is tumorigenic.

Table 7.2

Arguments in Favor of the Role of HPV in Cervical Cancer

1. Many intraepithelial lesions and carcinomas of the uterine cervix are infected by HPVs. More than 90% of malignant tumors contain PV genomes.
2. Metastatic tumors harbor the same virus type as the primary cervical tumor.[93]
3. Cell lines derived from cervical cancers such as HeLa, CaSki, and SiHa contain carcinogenic HPV (HPV-16, HPV-18, or related types).
4. Specific portions of the viral genomes become integrated within the host genome; and the viral genes are actively transcribed.
5. Members of the papillomavirus group are tumorigenic in animals.
6. Specific HPV types prevail in benign and malignant tumors.
7. Transformation in vitro is often reported.

References

1. Acs J, Hildesheim A, Reeves WC, Brenes M, Brinton L, Lavery C, de la Guardia ME, Godoy J, Rawls WE: Regional distribution of human papillomavirus DNA and other risk factors for invasive cervical cancer in Panama. *Cancer Res* 49:5725–5729, 1989.

2. Allerding TJ, Jordan SW, Boardman RE: Association of human papillomavirus and Chlamydia infections with incidence cervical neoplasia. *Acta Cytol* 29:653–660, 1985.

3. Alloub MI, Barr BBB, McLaren KM, Smith IW, Bunney MH, Smart GE: Human papillomavirus infection and cervical intraepithelial neoplasia in women with renal allografts. *Brit Med J* 298:153–156, 1989.

4. Almeida JD, Howatson AF, Williams MG: Electron microscope study of human warts; sites of virus production and nature of the inclusion bodies. *J Invest Dermatol* 38:337–345, 1962.

5. Almeida JD, Oriel JD, Stannard LM: Characterization of the virus found in human genital warts. *Microbios* 3:225–232, 1969.

6. Bafverstedt B: Condylomata acuminata—Past and present. *Acta Dermatol Venereol* 47:376–381, 1967.

7. Barrasso R, de Brux J, Croissant O, Orth G: High prevalence of papillomavirus-associated penile intraepithelial neoplasia in sexual partners of women with cervical intraepithelial neoplasia. *N Engl J Med* 317:916–923, 1987.

8. Beaudenon S, Kremsdorf D, Obalek S, et al: Plurality of genital human papillomaviruses: Characterization of two new types with distinct biological properties. *Virology* 161:374–384, 1987.

9. Beaudenon S, Kremsdorf D, Croissant O, Jablonska S, Wain-Hobson S, Orth G: A novel type of human papillomavirus associated with genital neoplasias. *Nature* 321:246–249, 1986.

10. Beckmann AM, Daling JR, Sherman KJ, Maden C, Miller BA, Coates RJ, Kiviat NB, Myerson D, Weiss NS, Hislop TG, Beagrie M, McDougall JK: Human papillomavirus infection and anal cancer. *Int J Cancer* 43:1042–1049, 1989.

11. Beckmann AM, Myerson D, Daling JR, Kiviat NB, Fenoglio CM, McDougall JK: Detection and localization of human papillomavirus DNA in human genital condylomas by in situ hybridization with biotinylated probes. *J Med Virol* 16:265–273, 1985.

12. Boon ME, Susanti I, Tasche MJA, Kok LP: Human papillomavirus (HPV)-associated male and female genital carcinomas in a Hindu population. The male as vector and victim. *Cancer* 64:559–565, 1989.

13. Boon ME, Schneider A, Hogewoning CJA, van der Kwast TH, Bolhuis P, Kok LP: Penile studies and heterosexual partners. Peniscopy, cytology, histology, and immunocytochemistry. *Cancer* 61:1652–1659, 1988.

14. Boshart M, Gissmann L, Ikenberg H, Kleinheinz A, Scheurlen W, zur Hausen H: A new type of papillomavirus DNA and its presence in genital cancer biopsies and in cell lines derived from cervical cancer. *Embo J* 3:1151–1157, 1984.

15. Bossens M, Heenen M, Tuyndet M, Faures A, Rommelaere J: In vitro production of human papillomavirus type 1 virions in a highly differentiated keratinocytes culture system. (Abstract) *J Invest Dermatol* 92:406, 1989.

16. Boyle WF, Riggs JL, Oshiro LS, Lennette EH: Electron microscopic identification of Papova virus in laryngeal papilloma. *Laryngoscope* 83:1102–1108, 1973.

17. Brant CR, McDougall JK, Galloway DA: Synergistic interactions between human papillomavirus type-18 sequences, herpes simplex virus infection, and chemical carcinogen treatment. In Steinberg, Brandsma JL, Taichman LB, eds; Cancer Cells: Papillomaviruses Vol 5: 179–186. Cold Spring Harbor Laboratory, Cold Spring Harbor, NY, 1987.

18. Brinton LA, Huggins GR, Lehman HF, Mallin K, Savitz DA, Trapido E, Rosenthal J, Hoover R: Long term use of oral contraceptives and risk of invasive cervical cancer. *Int J Cancer* 38:339–344, 1986.

19. Brinton LA, Schairer C, Haenszel W, Stolley P, Lehman HF, Levine

R, Savitz DA: Cigarette smoking and invasive cervical cancer. *JAMA* 255:3265–3269, 1986.

20. Broker TR, Chow LT: Human papillomaviruses of the genital mucosa: electron microscopic analysis of DNA heteroduplexes formed with HPV types 6, 11 and 18. *In* Botchan M, Grodzicker T, Sharp PA. eds. DNA Tumor Viruses: Control of gene expression and replication. *In* Cancer Cells Vol. 4:589–594. Cold Spring Harbor Laboratory, Cold Spring Harbor, NY, 1986.

21. Bunting H: Close-packed array of virus-like particles within cells of a human skin papilloma. *Proc Soc Exp Biol Med* 84:327–332, 1953.

22. Burnett TS, Gallimore PH: Establishment of a human keratinocyte cell line carrying complete human papillomavirus type 1 genomes: Lack of vegetative viral DNA synthesis upon keratinization. *J Gen Virol* 64:1509–1520, 1983.

23. Casas-Cordero M, Morin C, Roy M, Fortier M, Meisels A: Origin of the koilocyte in condylomata of the human cervix. Ultrastructural study. *Acta Cytol* 25:383–392, 1981.

24. Chapman GB, Drusin LM, Toff JE: Fine structure of the human wart. *Am J Pathol* 42:619–642, 1963.

25. Charles A: Electron microscope observations on the human wart. *Dermatologica* 121:193–203, 1960.

26. Choo KB, Pan CC, Liu MS, NG HT, Chen CP, Lee YN, Chao CF, Meng CL, Yeh MY, Han SH: Presence of episomal and integrated human papillomavirus DNA sequences in cervical carcinoma. *J Med Virol* 21:101–107, 1987.

27. Ciuffo G: Innesto positivo con filtrate di verruca vulgare. *Giornale Italiano delle Malattie Veneree* 42:12–17, 1907.

28. Coggin JR, zur Hausen H: Workshop on papillomaviruses and cancer. *Cancer Res* 39:545–546, 1979.

29. Cole ST, Streeck RE: Genome organization and nucleotide sequence of human papillomavirus type 33, which is associated with cervical cancer. *J Virol* 58:991–995, 1986.

30. Cole ST, Danos O: Nucleotide sequence and comparative analysis of the human papillomavirus type 18 genome. Phylogeny of papillomaviruses and repeated structure of the E6 and E7 gene products. *J Mol Biol* 193:599–608, 1987.

31. Crawford L: Criteria for establishing that a virus is oncogenic. *In* Papillomaviruses. Ciba Foundation Symposium 120:104–116; John Wiley, Chichester, 1986.

32. Danos O, Katinka M, Yaniv M: Human papillomavirus 1a complete DNA sequence: A novel type of genome organization among papovaviridae. *Embo J* 1:231–236, 1982.

33. Dartmann K, Schwarz E, Gissmann L, zur Hausen H: The nucleotide sequence and genome organization of human papilloma virus, type 11. *Virology* 151:124–130, 1986.

34. DeCaprio JA, Ludwow JW, Figge J, Shew J-Y, Huang C-M, Lee W-H, Marsilio E, Paucha E, Livingstone DM: SV40 large tumor antigen forms a specific complex with the product of the retinoblastoma susceptibility gene. *Cell* 54:275–283, 1988.

35. de Villiers E-M, Gissman L, zur Hausen H: Molecular cloning of viral DNA from human genital warts. *J Virol* 40:932–935, 1981.

36. de Villiers E-M, Wagner D, Schneider A, Wesch H, Miklaw H,

Wahrendorf J, Papendick U, zur Hausen H: Human papillomavirus infections in women without and with abnormal cervical cytology. *Lancet* ii:703–706, 1987.

37. Delap R, Frieman-Kien A, Rush MG: The absence of human papilloma viral DNA sequences in condylomata acuminata. *Virology* 74:268–272, 1976.

38. Della Torre G, Pilotti S, de Palo G, Rilke F: Viral particles in cervical condylomatous lesions. *Tumori* 64:549–553, 1978.

39. Dunn AEG, Ogilvie MM: Intranuclear virus particles in human genital wart tissue: observations on the ultrastructure of the epidermal layer. *J Ultrastruct Res* 22:282–295, 1968.

40. Durst M, Kleinheinz A, Hotz M, Gissmann L: The physical state of human papillomavirus type 16 DNA in benign and malignant genital tumors. *J Gen Virol* 66:1515–1522, 1985.

41. Durst M, Gissmann L, Ikenberg H, zur Hausen H: A papillomavirus DNA from a cervical carcinoma and its prevalence in cancer biopsy samples from different geographic regions. *Proc Natl Acad Sci* 80:3812–3815, 1983.

42. Durst M, Croce CM, Gissmann L, Schwarz E, Huebner K: Papillomavirus sequences integrate near cellular oncogenes in some cervical carcinomas. *Proc Natl Acad Sci* 84:1070–1074, 1987.

43. Durst M, Dzanlieva-Petrusevska RT, Boukamp P, Fusenig NE, Gissmann L: Molecular and cytogenetic analysis of immortalized human primary keratinocytes obtained after transfection with human papillomavirus type 16-DNA. *Oncogene* 1:251–256, 1987.

44. Dyson JL, Walker PG, Singer A: Human papillomavirus infection of the uterine cervix: histological appearance in 28 cases identified by immunocytochemical technique. *J Clin Pathol* 37:126–130, 1984.

45. Dyson N, Howley PM, Munger K, Harlow E: The human papilloma virus-16 E7 onco-protein is able to bind to the retinoblastoma gene product. *Science* 243:934–937, 1989.

46. Ebeling K, Nischan P, Schindler C: Use of oral contraceptives and risk of invasive cervical cancer previously screened women. *Int J Cancer* 39:427–430, 1987.

47. Favre M, Orth G, Croissant O, Yaniv M: Human papilloma virus DNA: physical map. *Proc Nat Acad Sci* 72:4810–4814, 1975.

48. Ferenczy A, Braun L, Shah KV: Human papillomavirus (HPV) in condylomatous lesions of cervix. A comparative ultrastructural and immunohistochemical study. *Am J Surg Path* 5:661–670, 1981.

49. Firzlaff JM, Kiviat NB, Beckmann AM: Detection of human papillomavirus capsid antigens in various squamous epithelial lesions using antibodies directed against the L1 and L2 open reading frames. *Virology* 164:467–477, 1988.

50. Friend SH, Bernards R, Rogelj S, Weinberg R, Rapoport JM, Albert DM, Dryja TP: A human DNA segment with properties of the gene that predisposes to retinoblastoma and osteosarcoma. *Nature* 323:643–646, 1986.

51. Fung YK, Murphree AL, T'Ang A qian J, Hinrichs SH, Benedict WF: Structural evidence for the authenticity of the human retinoblastoma gene. *Science* 236:1657–1661, 1987.

52. Furgyik S, Astedt B: Gonorrheal infection followed by an increased frequency of cervical carcinoma. *Acta Obstet Gynecol Scand* 59:521–524, 1980.

53. Gage JR, Meyer C, Wettstein FO: The E7 proteins of the nononcogenic human papillomavirus type 6b (HPV6b) and the oncogenic HPV 16 differ in retinoblastoma protein binding and other properties. *J Virol* 64:723–730, 1990.

54. Gal D, Friedman M, Mitrani-Rosenbaum S: Transmissibility and treatment failures of different types of human papillomavirus. *Obstet Gynecol* 73:308–311, 1989.

55. Garden JM, O'Banion MK, Shelnitz LS, Pinski KS, Bakus AD, Reichmann ME, Sunberg JP: Papillomavirus in the vapor of carbon dioxide laser-treated verrucae. *JAMA* 259:1199–1202, 1988.

56. Gariglio P, Ocadiz R, Sauceda R: Human papillomavirus DNA sequences and c-myc oncogene alterations in uterine cervix carcinoma. *In* Steinberg M, Brandsma JL, Taichman LB, eds; Cancer Cells: Papillomaviruses, Vol 5:343–348, Cold Spring Harbor Laboratory, Cold Spring Harbor, NY, 1987.

57. Gey GO, Coffman WD, Kubicek MT: Tissue culture studies of the proliferative capacity of cervical carcinoma and normal epithelium. *Cancer Res* 12:264–265, 1952.

58. Giri I, Danos O: Papillomavirus genomes: from sequence data to biological properties. *Trends Genet* 2:227–232, 1986.

59. Gissmann L, zur Hausen H: Human papilloma viruses: physical mapping and genetic heterogeneity. *Proc Natl Acad Sci* 73:1310–1313, 1976.

60. Gissmann L, zur Hausen H: Partial characterization of viral DNA from human genital warts (Condylomata acuminata). *Int J Cancer* 25:605–609, 1980.

61. Gissmann L, Diehl V, Schulz-Coulon HJ, zur Hausen H: Molecular cloning and characterization of human papilloma virus DNA derived from a laryngeal papilloma. *J Virol* 44:393–400, 1982.

62. Gissmann L, Wolnik L, Ikengerg H, Koldovsky U, Schnurch HG, zur Hausen H: Human papillomavirus types 6 and 11 DNA sequences in genital and laryngeal papillomas and in some cervical cancers. *Proc Natl Acad Sci* 80:560–563, 1983.

63. Gloss B, Bernhard HU, Seedorf K, Klock G: The upstream regulatory region of human papillomavirus 16 contains an E2 protein independent enhancer which is specific for cervical carcinoma cells and regulated by glucocorticoid hormones. *Embo J* 6:3735–3743, 1987.

64. Goldsborough MD, Disilvestre D, Temple GF, Lorincz AT: Nucleotide sequence of human papillomavirus type 31: A cervical neoplasia-associated virus. *Virology* 171:306–311, 1989.

65. Goldschmidt H, Kligman AM: Experimental inoculation of humans with ectodermotropic viruses. *J Invest Dermat* 31:175–182, 1958.

66. Greenberg ER, Vessey M, McPherson K, Yeaates D: Cigarette smoking and cancer of the uterine cervix. *Brit J Cancer* 51:139–141, 1985.

67. Gross L: A filterable agent, recovered from Ak leukemic extracts, causing salivary gland carcinomas in C3H mice. *Proc Soc Exp Biol Med* 83:414–421, 1953.

68. Gross G, Pfister H, Hagdorn M, et al: Effect of oral aromatic retinoid (Ro 10–9359) on human papillomavirus 2-induced common warts. *Dermatologica* 166:48–53, 1983.

69. Gupta JW, Gupta PK, Shah KV, Kelly DP: Distribution of human

papillomavirus in cervico-vaginal smears and cervical tissues. *Int J Gynecol Pathol* 2:160–170, 1983.

70. Harrington JS, Nunn JR, Irwig L: Dimethyl-nitrosamine in the human vaginal vault. *Nature* 241:49–50, 1973.

71. Hellberg D, Nilsson S, Haley NJ, Hoffman D, Wynder E: Smoking and cervical intraepithelial neoplasia: Nicotine and cotinine in serum and cervical mucus in smokers and nonsmokers. *Am J Obstet Gynecol* 158:910–913, 1988.

72. Hills E, Laverty CR: Electron microscopic detection of papilloma virus particles in selected koilocytotic cells in a routine cervical smear. *Acta Cytol* 23:53–56, 1979.

73. Holley EA, Petrakis NL, Friend NF, Sarles DL, Lee RE, Flander LB: Mutagenic mucus in the cervix of smokers. *J Natl Cancer Inst* 76:983–986, 1986.

74. Hoon WK, Endicott J, Itri LM, et al: 13-cis-retinoic acid in the treatment of oral leukoplakia. *N Engl J Med* 315:1501–1505, 1986.

75. Howley PM, Schlegel R: The human papillomaviruses. *Am J Med* 85 (Suppl 2A):155–158, 1988.

76. Huang H-JS, Yee J-K, Shew J-Y, Chen P-L, Bookstein R, Friedmann T, Lee EY-HP, Lee W-H: Suppression of the neoplastic phenotype by replacement of the RB gene in human cancer cells. *Science* 242:1563–1566, 1988.

77. Ishikawa K: Klinische und experimentelle Untersuchungen uber die Entstehungsussachen der Papillome. *Fukuoka Acta Med* 29:87–88, 1936.

78. Jadassohn J: Sind die Verrucae vulgares ubertragbar? *Verhandl Deut Dermatol Ges* 5:497–512, 1896.

79. Jenson AB, Rosenthal JD, Olson C, Pass F, Lancaster WD, Shah K: Immunologic relatedness of papillomaviruses from different species. *J Natl Cancer Inst* 64:495–500, 1980.

80. Jochmus-Kudielka I, Schneider A, Braun R, Kimmig R, Koldovsky U, Schneweis KE, Seedorf K, Gissmann L: Antibodies against the human papillomavirus type 16 early proteins in human sera: correlation of anti-E7 reactivity with cervical cancer. *JNCI* 81:1698–1704, 1989.

81. Jones HW, McKusick VA, Harper PS, Wuu KD: The HeLa cell and a reappraisal of its origin. *Obstet Gynecol* 38:945–949, 1971.

82. Kadish AS, Burk RD, Kress Y, Calderin S, Romney SL: Human papillomaviruses of different types in precancerous lesions of the uterine cervix. Histologic, immunocytochemical and ultrastructural studies. *Human Pathol* 17:384–392, 1986.

83. Kanda T, Furuno A, Yoshiike K: Human papillomavirus type 16 open reading frame E7 encodes a transforming gene for rat 3Y1 cells. *J Virol* 62:610–613, 1988.

84. Klein G: The approaching era of the tumor suppressor genes. *Science* 238:1539–1545, 1987.

85. Klug A, Finch JT: Structure of viruses of the papilloma-polyoma type. I. human wart virus. *J Mol Biol* 11:403–423, 1965.

86. Klug A: Structure of viruses of the papilloma-polyoma type. II. Comments on other works. *J Mol Biol* 11:424–431, 1965.

87. Koller LD, Olson C: Attempted transmission of warts from man,

cattle, and horses and of deer fibroma, to selected host. *J Invest Dermatol* 58:366–368, 1972.

88. Koutsky LA, Galloway DA, Holmes KK: Epidemiology of genital human papillomavirus infection. *Epidem Rev* 10:122–163, 1988.

89. La Vecchia C, Franceschi S, Decarli A, Gentile A, Fasoli M, Pampallona S, Tognoni G: Dietary vitamin A and the risk of invasive cervical cancer. *Int J Cancer* 34:319–322, 1984.

90. La Vecchia C, Decarli A, Fasoli M, Franceschi S, Gentile A, Negri E, Parazzini F, Tognoni G: Oral contraceptives and cancers of the breast and of the female genital tract. Interim results from a case-control study. *Bri J Cancer* 54:311–317, 1986.

91. La Vecchia C, Franceschi S, Decarli A, Fasoli M, Gentile A, Tognoni G: Cigarette smoking and the risk of cervical neoplasia. *Am J Epidemiol* 123:22–29, 1986.

92. Lancaster WD, Olson C: Animal papillomaviruses. *Microbiological Rev* 46:191–207, 1982.

93. Lancaster WD, Castellano C, Santos C, Delgado G, Kurman RJ, Jenson AB: Human papillomavirus deoxyribonucleic acid in cervical carcinoma from primary and metastatic sites. *Am J Obstet Gynecol* 154:115–119, 1986.

94. LaPorta RF, Taichman LB: Human papilloma viral DNA replicates as a stable episome in cultured epidermal keratinocytes. *Proc Natl Acad Sci* 79:3393–3397, 1982.

95. Lazo PA, DiPaolo JA, Popescu NC: Amplification of the integrated viral transforming genes of human papillomavirus 18 and its 5'-flanking cellular sequence located near the myc protooncogene in HeLa cells. *Cancer Res* l49:4305–4310, 1989.

96. Lee WH, Bookstein R, Hong F, Young LJ, Shew JY, Lee EY-HP: Human retinoblastoma susceptibility gene: cloning, identification, and sequence. *Science* 235:1394–1399, 1987.

97. Lehn H, Drieg P, Sauer G: Papillomavirus genomes in human cervical tumors: analysis of their transcriptional activity. *Proc Natl Acad Sci* 82:5540–5544, 1985.

98. Li G, Tsang SS, Stich HF: Changes in DNA copy numbers of bovine papillomavirus type 1 after termination of retinoic acid treatment. *J Natl Cancer Inst* 80:1567–1570, 1988.

99. Lorincz AT, Temple GF, Kurman RJ, Jenson AB, Lancaster WD: Oncogenic association of specific human papillomavirus types with cervical neoplasia. *J Natl Cancer Inst* 79:671–677, 1987.

100. Lorincz AT, Quinn AP, Lancaster WD, Temple GF: A new type of papillomavirus associated with cancer of the uterine cervix. *Virology* 159:187–190, 1987.

101. Lorincz AT, Lancaster WD, Temple GF: Cloning and characterization of the DNA of a new human papilloma virus from a woman with dysplasia of the uterine cervix. *J Virol* 58:225–229, 1986.

102. Lotan R: Effects of vitamin A and its analogs (retinoids) on normal and neoplastic cells. *Biochem Biophys Acta* 605:33–91, 1980.

103. Lutzner MA: Epidermodysplasia verruciformis: an autosomal recessive disease characterized by viral warts and skin cancer. A model for viral oncogenesis. *Bull Cancer* 65:169–182, 1978.

104. Manias DA, Ostrow RS, McGlennen RC, Estensen RD, Faras AJ: Characterization of integrated human papillomavirus type 11 DNA

in primary and metastatic tumors from a renal transplant recipient. *Cancer Res* 49:5514–5519, 1989.

105. Matlashewski G, Schneider J, Banks L, et al: Human papillomavirus type 16 DNA cooperates with activated ras in transforming primary cells. *Embo J* 6:1741–1746, 1987.

106. Matsukura T, Kanda T, Furuno A, Yoshikawa H, Kawana T, Yoshiike K: Cloning of monomeric human papillomavirus type 16 DNA integrated within cell DNA from a cervical carcinoma. *J Virol* 58:979–982, 1986.

107. Meisels A, Fortin R: Condylomatous lesions of the cervix and vagina. I. Cytologic patterns. *Acta Cytol* 20:505–509, 1976.

108. Melnick JL: Papova virus group. *Science* 135:1128–1130, 1962.

109. Merian L: Spontaner Schwund der Warzen des Gesichtes nach Chirurgfischer Entfernung solcher der Handrucken. *Dermatol Wochschr* 57:1001–1003, 1913.

110. Morin C, Braun L, Casas-Cordero M, Shah KV, Roy M, Fortier M, Meisels A: Confirmation of the papillomavirus etiology of the condylomatous cervix lesions by the peroxidase antiperoxidase technique. *J Natl Cancer Inst* 66:831–835, 1981.

111. Munoz N, Bosch FX, Kaldor JM: Does human papillomavirus cause cervical cancer? The state of the epidemiological evidence. *Br J Cancer* 57:1–5, 1988.

112. Ocadiz R, Sauceda R, Cruz M, Graef AM, Gariglio P: High correlation between molecular alterations of the c-myc oncogene and carcinoma of the uterine cervix. *Cancer Res* 47:4173–4177, 1987.

113. Oriel JD, Almeida JD: Demonstration of virus particles in human genital warts. *Brit J Vener Dis* 46:37–42, 1970.

114. Oriel JD: Natural history of genital warts. *Brit J Vener Dis* 47:1–13, 1971.

115. Orth G, Favre M, Jablonska S, Brylak K, Croissant O: Viral sequences related to a human skin papillomavirus in genital warts. *Nature* 275:334–336, 1978.

116. Orth G, Breitburd F, Favre M: Evidence for antigenic determinants shared by the structural polypeptides of (Shope) rabbit papillomavirus and human papillomavirus type 1. *Virology* 91:243–255, 1978.

117. Orth G, Jablonska S, Jarzalbek-Chorzelska M, Obalek S, Rzesa G, Favre M, Croissant O: Characterizatics of the lesions and risk of malignant conversion associated with the type of human papillomavirus involved in epidermodysplasia verruciformis. *Cancer Res* 39:1074–1082, 1979.

118. Ostrow RS, Manias DA, Clark BA, Okagaki T, Twiggs LB, Faras AJ: Detection of papillomavirus DNA in invasive carcinomas of the cervix by in situ hybridization. *Cancer Res* 47:649–653, 1987.

119. Palefski J: The papillomaviruses: structure and function. In Clinical Practice of Gynecology: Human Papillomavirus infections. B Winkler and RM Richart (Eds). (MS Baggish, Series Editor). Elsevier, NY, Vol. 1 (2), 1989, pages 4–28.

120. Pater MM, Hughes GA, Hyslop DE, Nakshatri H, Pater A: Glucocorticoid-dependent oncogenic transformation by type 16 but not type 11 human papillomavirus DNA. *Nature* 335:832–835, 1988.

121. Pecoraro G, Morgan D, Defendi V: Differential effects of human papillomavirus type 6, 16, and 18 DNAs on immortalisation and

transformation of human cervical epithelial cells. *Proc Natl Acad Sci* 86:563–567, 1989.

122. Penn I: Cancer is a complication of severe immunosuppression. *Surg Gynecol Obstet* 162:603–610, 1986.

123. Pfister H: Relationship of papillomaviruses to anogenital cancer. *Obstet Gynecol Clin N Amer* 14:349–361, 1987.

124. Phillips DH, Hewer A, Malcolm ADB, Ward P, Coleman DV: Smoking and DNA damage in cervical cells. *Lancet* 335:417, 1990.

125. Pirisi L, Yasumoto S, Feller M, Doniger J, DiPaolo JA: Transformation of human fibroblasts and keratinocytes with human papillomavirus type 16 DNA. *J Virol* 61:1061–1066, 1987.

126. Popescu NC, Amsbaugh SC, DiPaolo JA: Human papillomavirus type 18 DNA is integrated at a single chromosome site in cervical carcinoma cell line SW756. *Virol* 51:1682–1685, 1987.

127. Reeves WC, Brinton LA, Garcia M, Brenes MM, Herrero R, Gaitan E, Tenorio F, de Britton RC, Rawls WE: Human papillomavirus infection and cervical cancer in Latin America. *N Engl J Med* 320:1437–1441, 1989.

128. Reilly SS, Taichman LB: Underreplication of human papillomavirus type-1 DNA in cultures of foreskin keratinocytes. In Steinberg BM, Bransma JL, Taichman LB, eds, Cancer Cells: Papillomaviruses Vol 5:159–163. Cold Spring Harbor Laboratory, Cold Spring Harbor, NY, 1987.

129. Riou G, Barrois M, Tordjman I, Dutronquay V, Orth G: Présence de génomes de papillomavirus et amplification des oncogènes c-myc et c-Ha-ras dans des cancers envahissants du col de l'utérus. *CR acad Sci (Paris)* 299:575–580, 1984.

130. Rogers S, Rous P: Joint action of a chemical carcinogen and a neoplastic virus to induce cancer in rabbits. Results of exposing epidermal cells to a carcinogenic hydrocarbon at time of infection with the Shope papilloma virus. *J Exp Med* 93:459–488, 1951.

131. Rosemberg SK, Greenberg MD, Reid R: Sexually transmitted papillomaviral infection in men. *Obstet Gynecol Clin N Amer* 14:495–512, 1987.

132. Rosl F, Durst M, zur Hausen H: Selective suppression of human papillomavirus transcription in non-tumorigenic cells by 5-azacytidine. *Embo J* 7:1321–1328.

133. Rotkin ID: A comparison review of key epidemiological studies in cervical cancer related to current searches for transmissible agents. *Cancer Res* 33:1353–1367, 1973.

134. Rous P, Friedewald WF: The effect of chemical carcinogens on virus induced rabbit papillomas. *J Exp Med* 79:511–537, 1944.

135. Rous P, Kidd JG: The carcinogenic effect of a papilloma virus on the tarred skin of rabbits. I. Description of the phenomenon. *J Exp Med* 67:399–422, 1938.

136. Rowson KEK, Mahy BWY: Human Papova/wart virus. *Bacteriol Rev* 31:110–131, 1967.

137. Sasson IM, Haley NJ, Hoffmann D, Wynder EL, Hellberg D, Nilsson S: Cigarette smoking and neoplasia of the uterine cervix: smoke constituents in cervical mucus (letter). *New Engl J Med* 312:315–316, 1985.

138. Saxon PJ, Srivatsan ES, Stanbridge J: Introduction of human chro-

mosome 11 via microcell transfer controls tumorigenic expression of HeLa cells. *Embo J* 5:3461–3466, 1986.

139. Schachter J, Hill EC, King EB, et al: Chlamydia trachomatis and cervical neoplasia. *JAMA* 248:2134–2138, 1982.

140. Schiffman MH, Haley NJ, Felton JS, Andrews AW, Kaslow RA, Lancaster WD, Kurman RJ, Brinton LA, Lannom LB, Hoffmann D: Biochemical epidemiology of cervical neoplasia: measuring cigarette smoke constituents in the cervix. *Cancer Res* 47:3886–3888, 1987.

141. Schlegel R, Phelps WC, Zhang Y-L, Barbosa M: Quantitative keratinocyte assay detects two biological activities of human papillomavirus DNA and identifies viral types associated with cervical carcinoma. *Embo J* 7:3181–3187, 1988.

142. Schlehofer JR, zur Hausen H: Induction of mutations within the host genome by partially inactivated herpes simplex virus type 1. *Virology* 122:471–475, 1982.

143. Schneider A, Hotz M, Gissmann L: Increased prevalence of human papillomaviruses in the lower genital tract of pregnant women. *Int J Cancer* 40:198–201, 1987.

144. Schneider V, Kay S, Lee HM: Immunosuppression as a high risk factor in the development of condyloma acuminatum and squamous neoplasia of the cervix. *Acta Cytol* 27:220–224, 1983.

145. Schneider-Gadicke A, Schwarz E: Different human cervical carcinoma cell lines show similar transcription patterns of human papillomavirus type 18 early genes. *Embo J* 5:2285–2292, 1986.

146. Schwarz E, Freese UK, Gissmann L, Mayer W, Roggenbuck B: Structure and transcription of human papillomavirus sequences in cervical carcinoma cells. *Nature* 314:111–114, 1985.

147. Schwarz E, Durst M, Demankowski C, Lattermann O, ech R, Wolfsperger E, Suhai S, zur Hausen H: DNA sequence and genome organization of genital human papillomavirus type 6b. *Embo J* 2:2341–2348, 1983.

148. Seedorf K, Krammer G, Durst M, Suhai S, Rowekamp W: Human papillomavirus type 16 DNA sequence. *Virology* 145:181–185, 1985.

149. Seedorf K, Oltersdorf T, Kramer G, Rowekamp W: Identification of early proteins of the human papilloma viruses type 16 (HPV16) and type 18 (HPV18) in cervical carcinoma cells. *Embo J* 6:139–144, 1987.

150. Serra A: Ricerche istologiche e sperimentali sul condiloma acuminato: i papillomi del capo e la verrucca volgare. Contributo all'etiologia, patogenesi, filtrabilita. *Giorn Ital Mal Venereol* 49:11–42, 1908.

151. Serra A: Studi sul virus della verruca, del papilloma, del condiloma acuminato. Etiologia, patogenesi, filtrabilita. *Giornale Italiano delle Mallatie Veneree e della Pelle* 65:1808–1814, 1924.

152. Shamberger RJ: Inhibitory effect of vitamin A on carcinogens. *J Natl Cancer Inst* 47:667–673, 1971.

153. Shope RE: Infectious papillomatosis of rabbits. *J Exp Med* 58:607–624, 1933.

154. Sillman FH, Sedlis A: Anogenital papillomavirus infection and neoplasia in immunodeficient women. *Obstet Gynecol Clinics N Amer* 14:537–558, 1987.

155. Smotkin D, Wettstein FO: Transcription of human papillomavirus type 16 early genes in a cervical cancer and a cancer-derived from cell line and identification of the E7 protein. *Proc Natl Acad Sci* 83:4680–4684, 1986.

156. Stanbridge EJ: Suppression of malignancy in human cells. *Nature* 260:17–20, 1976.

157. Stanbridge JE, Der CJ, Dorsen C-J, Nishimi RY, Peehl DM, Weissman BE, Wilkinson JE: Human cell hybrids: analysis of transformation and tumorigenicity. *Science* 215:252–259, 1982.

158. Stich HF, Hornby AP, Mathew B, et al: Response of oral leukoplakias to the administration of vitamin A: *Cancer Letter* 40:93–101, 1988.

159. Strauss MJ, Shaw EW, Bunting H, Melnick JL: "Crystalline" viruslike particles from skin papillomas characterized by intranuclear inclusion bodies. *Proc Soc Exp Biol Med* 72:46–50, 1949.

160. Svoboda DJ, Kirchner FK, Proud GO: Electron microscopic study of human laryngeal papillomas. *Cancer Res* 23:1084–1089, 1963.

161. Sweet BH, Hilleman MR: The vacuolating virus, SV40. *Proc Soc Exp Biol Med* 105:420–427, 1960.

162. Syrjanen K, Mantyjarvi R, Vayrynen M, Castren O, Yliskoski M, Saarikoski S: Chlamydial cervicitis in women followed-up for human papillomavirus (HPV) lesions of the uterine cervix. 64:467–471, 1985.

163. Templeton HJ: Long incubation period of warts. *Arch Dermatol Syphilol* 32:102–103, 1935.

164. Tsunokawa Y, Takebe N, Kasamatsu T, Terada M, Sugimura T: Transforming activity of human papillomavirus type 16 DNA sequence in a cervical cancer. *Proc Natl Acad Sci* 83:2200–2203, 1986.

165. Walker J, Bloss JD, Liao SY, Berman M, Bergen S, Wilczynski SP: Human papillomavirus genotype as a prognostic indicator in carcinoma of the uterine cervix. *Obstet Gynecol* 74:781–785, 1989.

166. Whyte P, Buchkovich KJ, Howowitz JM, Friend SH, Raybuck M, Weinberg RA, Harlow E: Association between an oncogene and an anti-oncogene: the adenovirus E1A proteins bind to the retinoblastoma gene product. *Nature* 334:124–129, 1988.

167. Woodruff JD, Braun L, Cavalieri R, Gupta P, Pass F, Shah KV: Immunologic identification of papillomavirus antigen in condyloma tissues from the female genital tract. *Obstet Gynecol* 56:727–732, 1980.

168. Woodworth CD, Doniger J, DiPaolo JA: Immortalisation of human foreskin keratinocytes by various human papillomavirus DNAs corresponds to their association with cervical epithelial cells. *J Virol* 63:159–164, 1989.

169. Yasumoto S, Burkhardt AL, Doniger J, DiPaolo JA: Human papillomavirus type 16 DNA-induced malignant transformation of NIH3T3 cells. *J Virol* 57:572–577, 1986.

170. zur Hausen H: Papillomaviruses in anogenital cancer as a model to understand the role of viruses in human cancers. *Cancer Res* 49:4677–4681, 1989.

171. zur Hausen H, Gissmann L: Papillomaviruses. *In* Klein G ed; Viral Oncology, Raven Press, NY, 1980:433–445.

172. zur Hausen H: Human genital cancer: Synergism between two virus

infection or synergism between a virus infection and initiating events. *Lancet* ii:1370–1372, 1982.

173. zur Hausen, H, Meinhof W, Scheiber W, Bornkamm GW: Attempts to detect virus specific DNA sequences in human tumors: I. Nucleic acid hybridizations with complementary RNA of human wart virus. *Int J Cancer* 13:650–656, 1974.

174. zur Hausen H, Gissmann L, Steiner W, Dippold W, Dreger J: Human papilloma viruses and cancer. Clemmensen J and Yohn DS, eds. *Bibl Haematologica* 43:569–571, 1975.

175. zur Hausen H: Human papillomaviruses and their possible role in squamous carcinomas. *Curr Top Microbiol Immunol* 78:1–30, 1977.

176. zur Hausen H: Intracellular surveillance of persisting viral infections. Human genital cancer results from deficient control of papillomavirus gene expression. *Lancet* ii:489–491, 1986.

CHAPTER EIGHT

Squamous Intraepithelial Lesions

Case control studies have confirmed that the risk of contracting squamous intraepithelial lesions (SIL) is related strongly to the number of sexual partners: women who had seven or more sexual partners in a lifetime were found in a study from Sydney, Australia, to have a sixfold increased risk compared to those with one or no partner.[11] That study also showed that early age at first sexual intercourse is a risk factor. This factor, however, is reduced considerably after adjusting for the number of partners, with only a twofold increase persisting for those whose first intercourse takes place before age 16, compared with those whose first sexual intercourse takes place at age 25 or later. The long-term use of contraceptive agents is associated with an elevated risk (2.3 times for more than 6 years of use). There is a decreased risk for women who have had a tubal ligation, for those who practice the rhythm method of birth control, and for women who breastfeed. Another case control study from the People's Republic of China showed similar results.[24] These, and many other similar epidemiologic investigations, suggest that a sexually transmitted agent plays an important role in the development of SIL. At the time of this writing, human papillomaviruses are thought to be the culprit, not only for SIL, but also for invasive squamous and glandular cervical carcinomas.[3,15–18,21–23]

Cellular Patterns of SIL

Historically, cytologic screening was designed to discover intraepithelial lesions of the cervix in an asymptomatic population. Since these lesions are not invasive, they do not represent real cancer and do not immediately endanger the life of the patient. However, as has often been demonstrated, a significant proportion of the lesions eventually progress to invasive cancer. The rate of progression varies in different studies, but it has been stated that no cancer of the cervix appears without first going through an intraepithelial stage. This stage is, therefore, the last chance to actually prevent invasion, by local destruction of the SIL. Cytology has proven particularly successful in diagnosing these early changes in the course of routine screening. A single smear may miss the lesion in up to 20% of cases, but if smears are obtained at regular intervals, the probability of a false negative diagnosis soon becomes vanishingly small. For this reason, routine screening is recommended at yearly intervals, at least during the reproductive years. Several mathematical models have been proposed, suggesting that no great benefit is derived from yearly screening. According to these models, an interval of 2 to 3 years would be adequate. However, in recent years, invasive carcinoma is occurring in younger women, and seems to progress more rapidly than was the case 20 years ago.[1,4–7,9,10,19,20] The relaxation of sexual mores and exposure to the papillomavirus have increased the risk of cancer of the cervix in the younger generation.[2]

Low-Grade Squamous Intraepithelial Lesion

The low-grade squamous intraepithelial lesion (LGSIL) category of the Bethesda System encompasses cellular changes due to HPV infection (see Chapter Six) and mild or slight dysplasia (cervical intraepithelial neoplasia Grade 1, or CIN 1). Classical descriptions of mild dysplasia (CIN 1) refer to mature superficial or intermediate cells containing enlarged, somewhat irregular nuclei, with a regular, granular, or reticular chromatin. Nucleoli are not visible. The nuclear membrane may be slightly convoluted, but generally appears smooth. Binucleation can be seen. The nuclear/cytoplasmic (N/C) ratio is moderately increased. The cytoplasm often appears normal; sometimes the staining is amphophilic and a perinuclear halo can be observed occasionally (Plates 8.1–8.3).

When we (Meisels, Fortin, and Roy) first described the cellular manifestations of HPV infection,[12,13] we reviewed about 3,000 cases that had previously been diagnosed as mild dysplasia. We found at that time that over 70% of these cases represented HPV infection, and most of the remaining cases could have been classified either as inflammation or repair, or as atypical cells of undetermined significance that would have required only a cytologic followup within 6 months.

It is probable that the terms "mild dysplasia" and "CIN 1" have been used in the past to describe cellular changes that fall within the range of HPV-related patterns. Because of the importance of HPV infections, it would therefore seem advisable to reserve the term "low-grade squamous intraepithelial lesion" to the cellular manifestations of HPV infection described in Chapter Six.

High-Grade Squamous Intraepithelial Lesion

In the Bethesda System high-grade squamous intraepithelial lesion (HGSIL) encompasses the cellular changes previously known as moderate dysplasia (CIN 2), and severe or marked dysplasia and carcinoma in situ (CIN 3). High-grade SIL is characterized on the smears by the presence of immature cells of the parabasal type, with an increased N/C ratio, containing enlarged, somewhat irregular, hyperchromatic nuclei (Plates 8.4 and 8.5). The chromatin is either granular or reticular, or displays irregular chromatin bands and chromocenters (Plate 8.6). Nucleoli are small or absent. The nuclear membrane is often unevenly stained and its outline may be jagged (Plates 8.7 and 8.8). The cytoplasm is dense and cyanophilic, rarely eosinophilic. These cells can be found isolated or, more often, forming small groups or Indian files (Plate 8.9). The pattern is usually quite uniform, the degree of anisokaryosis is slight (Plate 8.10), and the background in absence of coexistent inflammation is clean. High-grade SIL should be differentiated from squamous metaplasia (see Chapter Five), in which the parabasal cells have a preserved N/C ratio and the chromatin structure, as well as the nuclear membrane outline, are uniform and regular.

Histologic Aspects of HGSIL

High-grade squamous intraepithelial lesions encompass the changes previously known as moderate dysplasia, severe dysplasia, and carcinoma in situ, or CIN 2 and CIN 3. The older concept held that squamous intraepithelial lesions could be classified in accordance to the level of differentiation (ie, if the upper two thirds of the epithelium were differentiated, it was a mild dysplasia; if only the upper third was differentiated, it was a moderate dysplasia; and if there was no differentiation, then it was called a severe dysplasia, or carcinoma in situ). However, this concept was very theoretical. In most cases of pure SIL, there is little or no differentiation. What was perceived as differentiation was, in most cases, the manifestation of HPV infection seen in the upper epithelial layers—what I call the vertical association. The lesion identified previously as "mild dysplasia" or CIN 1, and now as low-grade SIL (Bethesda System) corresponds in most cases to a simple HPV infection. The term "flat condyloma" was explicit enough and could still be used in conjunction with low-grade SIL, although it is preferable to indicate simply "presence of HPV infection."

In HGSIL, the squamous lining is poorly differentiated, although the uppermost layers may be flattened or may demonstrate changes due to HPV infection (koilocytosis and dyskeratosis). The N/C ratio is increased, the scarce cytoplasm is cyanophilic, and the nuclei are hyperchromatic and irregular, sometimes with marked anisokaryosis. The chromatin may be reticular or granular, or display irregular chromatin bands and chromocenters. Small nucleoli can sometimes be seen. The cell borders are often indistinct (Plates

8.11 and 8.12). Mitotic figures, some atypical, can be seen at various levels in the epithelium (Plate 8.13).

Most frequently HGSIL is found in the transformation zone. The basal membrane can be parallel to the surface, or it may bud towards the stroma. The lesion may extend into the glandular spaces, replacing the columnar epithelium. Such extension should not be confused with stromal invasion.

HGSIL must be differentiated from immature metaplasia, in which the N/C ratio is preserved, the cells are of the parabasal type, and the nuclei often contain nucleoli and are uniform and regular with a bland chromatin pattern. In immature metaplasia the cell borders are usually clearly visible.

Repair can also be confused with HGSIL. In repair the cells are large with abundant cytoplasm; the nuclei are regular and often contain macronucleoli. Mitotic figures are common, but not atypical (see Chapter Five).

The association of SIL with HPV infection is described in Chapter Six.

Plate 8.1
Cell spread illustrating squamous cell changes of undetermined significance. These are large intermediate cells; one of them contains two enlarged nuclei surrounded by a faint halo.

Plate 8.2
Enlarged intermediate squamous cells with large, hyperchromatic, slightly irregular nuclei.

Plate 8.3
The nuclei of these intermediate cells are enlarged and hyperchromatic. There is some anisokaryosis. These cells, as well as those depicted in Plates 8.1 and 8.2 can be grouped under the Bethesda category of low-grade squamous intraepithelial lesion (LGSIL).

Plate 8.4
Cellular pattern of high-grade squamous intraepithelial lesion (HGSIL). These parabasal-type cells have enlarged hyperchromatic nuclei. Some of the nuclei contain prominent chromatin bands. Anisokaryosis is slight.

Plate 8.1

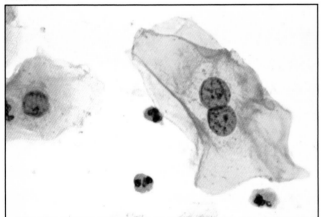

Plate 8.2

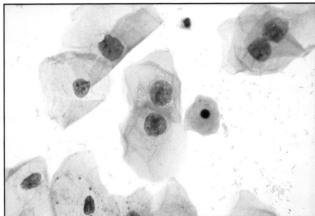

Plate 8.3

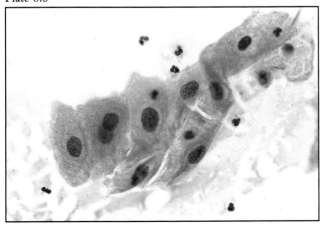

Plate 8.4

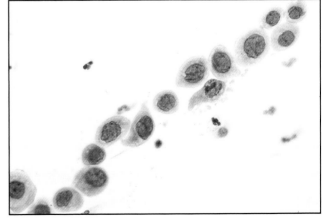

Plate 8.5

Cellular pattern of HGSIL. The N/C ratio is high and there is a moderate degree of anisokaryosis. The hyperchromatic nuclei display a coarse chromatin pattern. There are no nucleoli.

Plate 8.6

Cellular pattern of HGSIL. There is marked anisokaryosis. The chromatin pattern is coarse.

Plate 8.7

Cellular pattern of HGSIL. An Indian file arrangement of the cells. The nuclear membrane is irregular.

Plate 8.5

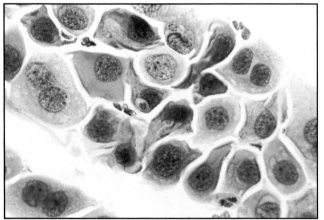

Plate 8.6

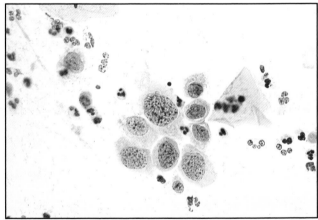

Plate 8.7

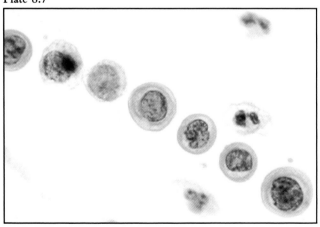

Plate 8.8

Cellular pattern of HGSIL. There is a high N/C ratio, anisokaryosis, an irregular nuclear membrane and a coarse chromatin pattern.

Plate 8.9

Cellular pattern of HGSIL. The cellular changes are marked: anisokaryosis is prominent, the N/C ratio is high, the chromatin is clumped into irregular bands and chromocenters, and the nuclear membrane is very uneven.

Plate 8.10

Cellular pattern of HGSIL. These cells have a very high N/C ratio, with hyperchromatic nuclei, coarse chromatin, and uneven nuclear membranes. Nucleoli are not usually visible in HGSIL. The background is clean.

Plate 8.8

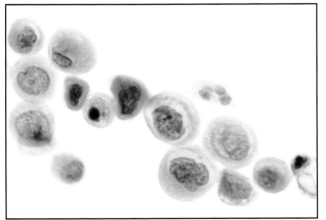

Plate 8.9

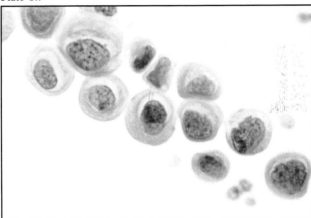

Plate 8.10

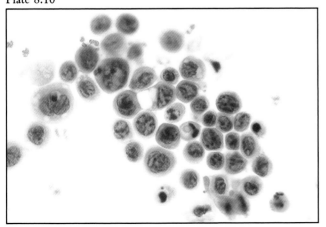

Plate 8.11

Tissue section from a case of HGSIL. There is lack of maturation, loss of polarity, anisokaryosis, and hyperchromasia. One mitotic figure can be seen in the upper middle layers of the lesion.

Plate 8.12

Tissue section from a case of HGSIL. The loss of polarity is quite evident here. In addition, there is anisokaryosis, lack of maturation, and hyperchromasia.

Plate 8.13

Tissue section from a case of HGSIL illustrating numerous mitotic figures at various levels of the lesion.

Plate 8.11

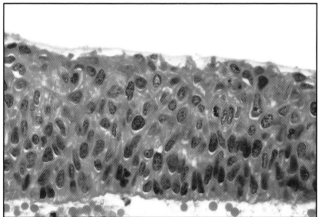

Plate 8.12

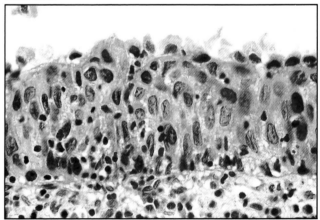

Plate 8.13

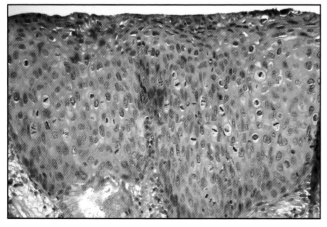

References

(Not all of the following are cited in the text.)

1. Armstrong B, Holman D: Increasing mortality from cancer of the cervix in young Australian women. *Med J Aust* 1:460, 1981.

2. Boon ME, Deng Z, Baowen G, Ryd W: Koilocyte frequency in positive cervical smears as indicator of sexual promiscuity. *Lancet* iii:205, 1986.

3. Brescia RJ, Jenson B, Lancaster WD, Kurman RJ: The role of human papillomaviruses in the pathogenesis and histologic classification of precancerous lesions of the cervix. *Human Pathol* 17:552–559, 1986.

4. Carmichael JA, Clarice DH, Moher D, Ohlike ID, Karchmar EJ: Cervical carcinoma in women aged 34 and younger. *Am J Obstet Gynecol* 154:264–269, 1986.

5. Chu J, White E: Decreasing incidence of invasive cervical cancer in young women. *Amer J Obstet Gynecol* 157:1105–1107, 1987.

6. Coppleson M, Elliott P, Reid BL: Puzzling changes in cervical cancer in young women (Editorial). *Med J Australia* 146:405–406, 1987.

7. Draper DJ, Cook GA: Changing patterns of cervical cancer rates. *Brit Med J* 287:510–512, 1983.

8. Ebeling K, Nischan P, Schindler C: Use of oral contraceptives and risk of invasive cervical cancer in previously screened women. *Int J Cancer* 39:427–430, 1987.

9. Elliott PM, Tattersall MHN, Coppleson M, Russell P, Wong F, Coates AS, Solomon HJ, Bannatyne PM, Atkinson KH, Murray JC: Changing character of cervical cancer in young women. *Brit Med J* 298:288–290, 1989.

10. Green GH: Rising cervical cancer mortality in young New Zealand women. *N Zealand Med J* 89:89, 1979.

11. McMichael AJ, Hiller JE: Pills, partners and preventive prospects: in-situ cancer of the cervix. *Med J Australia* 150:114–116, 1989.

12. Meisels A, Fortin R, Roy M: Condylomatous lesions of the cervix. II. Cytologic, colposcopic and histopathologic study. *Acta Cytol* 21:379–390, 1977.

13. Meisels A, Fortin R: Condylomatous lesions of the cervix and vagina. I. Cytologic patterns. *Acta Cytol* 20:505–509, 1976.

14. Meisels A, Roy M, Fortier M, Morin C, Casas-Cordero M, Shah KV, Turgeon H: Human papillomavirus infection of the cervix: The atypical condyloma. *Acta Cytol* 25:7–16, 1981.

15. Pilotti S, Rilke F, Alasio L, Fontanelli R: Histologic evidence for an association of cervical intraepithelial neoplasia with human papillomavirus infection. *Diagn Gynecol Obstet* 4:357–362, 1982.

16. Pilotti S, Rilke F, De Palo G, Della Torre G, Alasio L: Condylomata of the uterine cervix and koilocytosis of cervical intraepithelial neoplasia. *J Clin Pathol* 34:532–541, 1981.

17. Reid R, Crum CP, Herschman BR, Fu YS, Braun L, Shah KV, Agronow SJ, Stanhope CR: Genital warts and cervical cancer. III. Subclinical Papillomaviral infection and cervical neoplasia are linked by a spectrum of continuous morphologic and biologic change. *Cancer* 53:943–953, 1984.

18. Reid R, Fu YS, Herschman BR, Crum CP, Braun L, Shah KV, Agronow SJ, Stanhope CR: Genital warts and cervical cancer. VI.

The relationship between aneuploid and polyploid cervical lesions. *Am J Obstet Gynecol* 150:189–199, 1984.

19. Rotkin ID: Relation of adolescent coitus to cervical cancer risk. *JAMA* 179:486–491, 1962.

20. Sadeghi B, Hsich EW, Gunn SW: Prevalence of cervical intraepithelial neoplasia in sexually active teenagers and young adults. *Am J Obstet Gynecol* 148:726–729, 1984.

21. Selvaggi SM: Cytologic detection of condylomas and cervical intraepithelial neoplasia of the uterine cervix with histologic correlation. *Cancer* 58:2076–2081, 1986.

22. Sterrett GF, Alessandri LM, Pixley E, Kulski JK: Assessment of precancerous lesions of the uterine cervix for evidence of human papillomavirus infection: a histological and immunohistochemical study. *Pathology* 19:84–90, 1987.

23. Suprun HZ, Schwartz J, Spira H: Cervical intraepithelial neoplasia and associated condylomatous lesions. A preliminary report on 4,764 women from Northern Israel. *Acta Cytol* 29:334–340, 1985.

24. Zhang Z-f, Parkin DM, Yu S-Z, Estève J, Yang X-Z: Risk factors for cancer of the cervix in a rural Chinese population. *Int J Cancer* 43:762–767, 1989.

25. Andolsek L, Kovacic J, Kozuh M, Litt B: Influence of oral contraceptives on the incidence of premalignant and malignant lesions of the cervix. *Contraception* 28:505–519, 1983.

26. Bagi P, Worning AM, Nordsten M, Berget A, Badsberg E: The prognostic significance of virus-associated changes in grade 1 cervical intraepithelial neoplasia. *Acta Obstet Gynecol* 66:441–444, 1987.

27. Barrasso R, Ionesco M, Quinzat D, de Brux J: Cancer in situ du col et papillomavirus. Etude de 111 conisations. *Rev Franç Gynécol Ob* 80:1–5, 1985.

28. Briggs RM: Dysplasia and early neoplasia of the uterine cervix: A review. *Obstet Gynecol Surv* 34:70–99, 1979.

29. Brisson J, Roy M, Fortier M, Bouchard C, Meisels A: Condyloma and intraepithelial neoplasia of the uterine cervix: A case-control study. *Am J Epidemiol* 128:337–342, 1988.

30. Brock KE, Berry G, Brinton LA, Kerr C, MacLennan R, Mock PA, Shearman RP: Sexual, reproductive and contraceptive risk factors for carcinoma-in-situ of the uterine cervix in Sydney. *Med J Australia* 150:125–130, 1989.

31. Buckley CH, Butler EB, Fox H: Cervical intraepithelial neoplasia. *J Clin Pathol* 35:1–13, 1982.

32. Butterworth Jr CE, Hatch KD, Gore H, Mueller H, Krumdieck CL: Improvement in cervical dysplasia associated with folic acid therapy in users of oral contraceptives. *Am J Clin Nutr* 35:73–82, 1982.

33. Byrne MA, Moller BR, Taylor-Robinson D, Harris JR, Wickenden C, Malcolm AD, Anderson MC, Coleman DV: The effect of interferon on human papillomaviruses associated with cervical intraepithelial neoplasia. *Brit J Obstet Gynaec* 93:1136–1144, 1986.

34. Campion MJ, McCance DJ, Cuzick J, Singer A: Progressive potential of mild cervical atypia: prospective cytological, colposcopic and virological study. *Lancet* ii(8501):237–240, 1986.

35. Chang AR: A comparison of the ages of patients with cervical smears

showing human papillomavirus, dysplasia and carcinoma in situ changes (Letter). *N Zealand Med J* 99:205–206, 1986.

36. Clarke EA, Hatcher J, McKeown-Eyssen GE, Lickrish GM: Cervical dysplasia: Association with sexual behavior, smoking, and oral contraceptive use. *Am J Obstet Gynecol* 151:612–616, 1985.

37. Cook GA, Draper GJ: Trends in cervical cancer and carcinoma in situ in Great Britain. *Br J Cancer* 50:367–375, 1984.

38. Crum CP, Mitao M, Levine RU, Silverstein S: Cervical papillomaviruses segregate within morphologically distinct precancerous lesions. *J Virol* 54:675–681, 1985.

39. Curtis EM: Changing concepts: Treating preinvasive cervical neoplasia. *J Med Assoc Georgia* 74:28, 1985.

40. Davies B, Rosenthal M, Munoz ADN: Carcinoma in situ and condyloma acuminatum in the cervix. *Diagn Gynecol Obstet* 3:161–166, 1981.

41. de Brux J: Histoire naturelle des lésions précancéreuses du col utérin. *Bull Cancer (Paris)* 66:409, 1979.

42. de Brux J, Ionesco M, Cochard B, Masson MF, Kaeding H: Condylomes, dysplasies et carcinomes intra-epithéliaux du col utérin. *J Gyn Obst Biol Repr* 9:613–620, 1980.

43. Dinh TV, Powell LC, Hannigan EV, Hang HL, Wirt DP, Yandell RB: Simultaneously occurring condylomata acuminata, carcinoma in situ and verrucous carcinoma of the vulva and carcinoma in situ of the cervix in a young woman. A case report. *J Reprod Med* 33:510–513, 1988.

44. Evans AS, Monaghan JM: Spontaneous resolution of cervical warty dysplasia: The relevance of clinical and nuclear DNA features. A prospective study. *Brit J Obstet Gynaec* 92:165–169, 1985.

45. Falcone T, Ferenczy A: Cervical intraepithelial neoplasia and condyloma: An analysis of diagnostic accuracy of post-treatment follow-up methods. *Am J Obstet Gynecol* 154:260–264, 1986.

46. Friedell GH, McKay DG: Adenocarcinoma in situ of the endocervix. *Cancer* 6:887–897, 1953.

47. Fujii T, Crum C, Winkler B, Fu SY, Richart R: Human papillomavirus infection and cervical intraepithelial neoplasia: histopathology and DNA content. *Obstet Gynecol* 63:99–104, 1984.

48. Fu YS, Reagan JW, Richart RM: Definition of precursors. *Gynecol Oncol* 12:220–231, 1981.

49. Ghosh L, Nadimpalli VR, Ronan SG, Robertson AL Jr: The demonstration of papilloma virus in cervical dysplasia and/or neoplasia. *J Surg Oncol* 32:25–29, 1986.

50. Giacomini G: Cyto-histological correlations in the diagnosis of precancerous lesions of the cervix uteri. *Minerva Ginecol* 27:199–204, 1975.

51. Göppinger A, Birmelin G, Ikenberg H, Elmenthaler U, Hilgarth M, Hillemanns HG, Wied GL: Human papillomavirus standardization and DNA cytophotometry in cervical intraepithelial neoplasia. *J Reprod Med* 32:609–613, 1987.

52. Gross G, Wagner D, Hauser-Brauner B, Ikenberg H, Gissmann L: Bowenoid papulosis and carcinoma in situ of the cervix uteri in sex partners. An example of the transmissibility of HPV-16 infection. *Hautarzt* 36:465–469, 1985.

53. Grunebaum AN, Sedlis A, Sillman F, Fruchter R, Stanek A, Boyce J: Association of human papillomavirus infection with cervical intraepithelial neoplasia. *Obstet Gynecol* 62:448–455, 1983.

54. Guijon FB, Paraskevas M, Brunham R: The association of sexually transmitted diseases with cervical intraepithelial neoplasia: a case-control study. *Am J Obstet Gynecol* 151:185–190, 1985.

55. Harris RWC, Brinton LA, Cowdell RH, Skegg DCG, Smith PG, Vessey MP, Doll R: Characteristics of women with dysplasia or carcinoma in situ of the cervix uteri. *Brit J Cancer* 42:359–369, 1980.

56. Hellberg D, Nillson S, Haley NJ, Hoffman D, Wynder E: Smoking and cervical intraepithelial neoplasia: Nicotine and cotinine in serum and cervical mucus in smokers and nonsmokers. *Am J Obstet Gynecol* 158:910–913, 1988.

57. Hiscock E, Reece G: Cytological screening for cervical cancer and human papillomavirus in general practice. *Brit Med J* 297:724–726, 1988.

58. Hopkins MP, Roberts JA, Schmidt RW: Cervical adenocarcinoma in situ. *Obstet Gynecol* 71:842–844, 1988.

59. Jaworski RC, Pacey NF, Greenberg ML, Osborn RA: The histologic diagnosis of adenocarcinoma in situ and related lesions of the cervix. Adenocarcinoma in situ. *Cancer* 61:1171–1181, 1988.

60. Jenkins D, Tay SK, McCance DJ, Campion MJ, Clarkson PK, Singer A: Histological and immunocytochemical study of cervical intraepithelial neoplasia (CIN) with associated HPV-6 and HPV-16 infections. *J Clin Pathol* 39:1177–1180, 1986.

61. Kadish AS, Burk RD, Kress Y, Calderin S, Romney SL: Human papillomaviruses of different types in precancerous lesions of the uterine cervix. Histologic, immunocytochemical and ultrastructural studies. *Human Pathol* 17:384–392, 1986.

62. Kirkup W, Evans AS, Brough AK, Davis JA, O'Loughlin T, Wilkinson G, Monaghan JM: Cervical intraepithelial neoplasia and "warty" atypia: a study of colposcopic, histologic and cytologic characteristics. *Brit J Obstet Gynaec* 89:571–577, 1982.

63. Koss LG: Dysplasia. A real concept or a misnomer. *Obstet Gynecol* 51:374–379, 1978.

64. Koss LG: Current concepts of intraepithelial neoplasia in the uterine cervix (CIN). *Appl Pathol* 5:7–18, 1987.

65. Lancaster WD, Kurman RJ, Sanz LE, Perry S, Jenson AB: Human papillomavirus: Detection of viral DNA sequences and evidence for molecular heterogeneity in metaplasias and dysplasias of the uterine cervix. *Intervirology* 20:202–212, 1983.

66. La Vecchia C, Franceschi S, Decarli A, Fasoli M, Gentile A, Parazzini F, Regallo M: Sexual factors, venereal disease and their risk of intraepithelial and invasive cervical neoplasia. *Cancer* 58:935–941, 1986.

67. Levine RU, Carrillo EJ, Crum CP: Outpatient management of cervical intraepithelial neoplasia. A summary of 279 cases. *J Reprod Med* 30:351–354, 1985.

68. Levine RU, Crum CP, Herman E, Silver D, Ferenczy A, Richart RM: Cervical papillomavirus infection and intraepithelial neoplasia: A study of male sexual partners. *Obstet Gynecol* 64:16–20, 1984.

69. Lorincz AT, Lancaster WD, Temple GF: Cloning and characteri-

zation of a new human papillomavirus from a woman with dysplasia of the uterine cervix. *J Virol* 58:225–229, 1986.

70. Lovejoy NC: Precancerous lesions of the cervix. Personal risk factors. *Cancer Nursing* 10:2–14, 1987.

71. Lyon JL, Gardner JW, West DW, Stanish WM, Hebertson RM: Smoking and carcinoma in situ of the uterine cervix. *Am J Publ Hlth* 73:558–562, 1983.

72. McCance DJ, Campion MJ, Clarkson PK, Chesters PM, Jenkins D, Singer A: Prevalence of human papillomavirus type 16 DNA sequences in cervical intraepithelial neoplasia and invasive carcinoma of the cervix. *Brit J Obstet Gynaec* 92:1101–1105, 1985.

73. McCance DJ, Walker PG, Dyson JL, Coleman DV, Singer A: Presence of human papillomavirus DNA sequences in cervical intraepithelial neoplasia. *Brit Med J* 287:784–788, 1983.

74. McIndoe WA, McLean MA, Jones RW, Mullins PR: The invasive potential of carcinoma in situ of the cervix. *Obstet Gynecol* 64:451–454, 1984.

75. McMichael AJ, Hiller JE: Pills, partners and preventive prospects: in situ cancer of the cervix. *Med J Australia* 150:114–116, 1989.

76. Meisels A, Begin R, Schneider V: Dysplasia of the uterine cervix. Epidemiological aspects. Role of age at first coitus and use of oral contraceptives. *Cancer* 40:3076–3081, 1977.

77. Melamed MR, Flehinger BJ: Early incidence rates of precancerous cervical lesions in women using contraceptives. *Gynecol Oncol* 1:290–298, 1973.

78. Miglianico L, Reyes M, Poitout P: Cervical intraepithelial neoplasms and flat condylomata. *Ann Pathol* 4:325–328, 1984.

79. Mittal KR, Miller HK, Lowell DM: Koilocytosis preceding squamous cell carcinoma in situ of the cervix. *Am J Clin Pathol* 84:243–245, 1987.

80. Morris HB, Gatter KC, Sykes G, Casemore V, Mason DY: Langerhans cells in cervical epithelium: Effects of wart virus infection and intraepithelial neoplasia. *Brit J Obstet Gynaec* 90:412–420, 1983.

81. Mushika M, Miwa T, Suzuoki Y, Hayashi K, Masaki S, Kaneda T: Detection of proliferative cells in dysplasia, carcinoma in situ, and invasive carcinoma of the uterine cervix by monoclonal antibody against DNA polymerase alpha. *Cancer* 61:1182–1186, 1988.

82. Naib ZM, Nahmias AJ, Josey WE, Kramer JH: Genital herpetic infection. Association with cervical dysplasia and carcinoma. *Cancer* 23:940–945, 1969.

83. Nakajima T, Tsumuraya M, Morinaga S, Teshima S, Shimosato Y, Kishi K, Ohmi K, Sonoda T, Tsunematsu R, Tanemura K, Yamada T, Kasamatsu T: The frequency of papillomavirus infection in cervical precancerous lesions in Japan: An immunoperoxidase study. *Jpn J Cancer Res* 77:891–895, 1986.

84. Naujoks H: Cervical dysplasia: Cytology class III D and CIN I–II. *Pathol Res Pract* 179:401–404, 1985.

85. Nazur MT, Cloud GA: The koilocyte and cervical intraepithelial neoplasia: time-trend analysis of a recent decade. *Am J Obstet Gynecol* 150:354–358, 1984.

86. Nelson JH, Averette HE, Richart RM: Dysplasia, carcinoma in situ, and early invasive cervical carcinoma. *CA* 34:306–327, 1984.

87. Nyeem R, Wilkinson EJ, Grover LJ: Condylomata acuminata of the cervix: Histopathology and association with cervical neoplasia. *Int J Gynecol Pathol* 1:246–257, 1982.

88. Okagaki T, Clark BA, Brooker DC, Williams PP: Koilocytosis in dysplastic and reactive squamous cervical epithelium: An ultrastructural study. *Acta Cytol* 22:95–98, 1978.

89. Okagaki T, Twiggs L, Zachow K, Clark B, Ostrow R, Faras A: Identification of human papillomavirus DNA in cervical and vaginal intraepithelial neoplasia with molecularly cloned virus specific DNA probes. *J Gynecol Pathol* 2:153–159, 1983.

90. Palan PR, Romney SL: Cellular binding proteins for vitamin A in the normal human uterine cervix and in dysplasia. *Cancer Res* 39:3114–3118, 1979.

91. Parent B, Huynk B: Les dysplasies du col utérin. Nouvelle stratégie thérapeutique fondée sur les données virologiques. *J Gynécol Obstét Bio* 15:941–947, 1986.

92. Prakash SS, Reeves WC, Sisson GR, Brenes M, Godoy J, Bacchetti S, de Britton RC, Rawls WE: Herpes simplex virus type 2 and human papillomavirus type 16 in cervicitis, dysplasia and invasive cervical carcinoma. *Int J Cancer* 35:51–57, 1985.

93. Puttemans P, Van Belle Y, de Muylder E: Carbon dioxide laser vaporisation of cervical subclinical papillomavirus infection and intraepithelial neoplasia: short-term effectiveness. *Eur J Obstet Gynecol* 23:167–180, 1986.

94. Reagan JW, Patten SF: Dysplasia: A basic reaction to injury in the uterine cervix. *Ann NY Acad Sci* 97:662–682, 1962.

95. Richart RM: Natural history of cervical intraepithelial neoplasia. *Clin Obstet Gynecol* 10:748–784, 1967.

96. Richart RM: The incidence of cervical and vaginal dysplasia after exposure to DES (Letter). *JAMA* 255:36–37, 1986.

97. Richart RM: Causes and management of cervical intraepithelial neoplasia. *Cancer* 60:1951–1959, 1987.

98. Richart RM, Barron BA: A follow-up study of patients with cervical dysplasia. *Am J Obstet Gynecol* 105:386–393, 1969.

99. Robboy SJ, Noller KL, O'Brien P, Kaufman RH, Townsend D, Barnes AB, Gundersen J, Lawrence WD, Bergstrahl E, et al: Increased incidence of cervical and vaginal dysplasia in 3980 diethylstilbestrol-exposed young women. *JAMA* 252:2979–2983, 1984.

100. Robertson JH, Woodend BE, Crozier EH, Hutchinson J: Risk of cervical cancer associated with mild dyskaryosis. *Br Med J* 297:18–21, 1988.

101. Romney SL, Duttagupta C, Basu J, Palan PR, Karp S, Slagle NS, Swyer A, Wassertheil-Smoller S, Wylie-Rosett J: Plasma vitamin C and uterine cervical dysplasia. *Am J Obstet Gynecol* 151:976–980, 1985.

102. Romney SL, Palan PR, Duttagupta C, Wassertheil-Smoller S, Wylie J, Miller G, Slagle NS, Lucido D: Retinoids and the prevention of cervical dysplasias. *Am J Obstet Gynecol* 141:890–894, 1981.

103. Sadeghi SB, Sadeghi A, Robboy SJ: Prevalence of dysplasia and cancer of the cervix in a nationwide, planned parenthood population. *Cancer* 61:2359–2361, 1988.

104. Saito K, Saito A, Fu YS, Smotkin D, Gupta J, Shah K: Topographic study of cervical condyloma and intraepithelial neoplasia. *Cancer* 59:2064–2070, 1987.

105. Sanz LE, Gurdian J: Human papillomavirus and cervical intraepithelial neoplasia as sexually transmitted diseases. *Semin Adolesc Med* 2:121–124, 1986.

106. Shah KH, Lewis MG, Jenson AB, Kurman RJ, Lancaster WD: Papillomavirus and cervical dysplasia. *Lancet* iii:1190, 1980.

107. Shibata D, Fu YS, Gupta JW, Shah KV, Arnheim N, Martin WJ: Detection of human papillomavirus in normal and dysplastic tissue by the polymerase chain reaction. *Lab Invest* 59:555–559, 1988.

108. Shirasawa H, Tomita Y, Kubota K, Kasai T, Sekiya S, Takamizawa H, Simizu B: Detection of human papillomavirus type 16 DNA and evidence for integration into the cell DNA in cervical dysplasia. *J Gen Virol* 67:2011–2015, 1986.

109. Sillman F, Stanek A, Sedlis A, Rosenthal J, Lanks KW, Buchhagen D, Nicastri A, Boyce J: The relationship between human papillomavirus and lower genital intraepithelial neoplasia in immunosuppressed women. *Am J Obstet Gynecol* 150:300–308, 1984.

110. Singer A, Wilters J, Walker P, Jenkins D, Slavin G, Cowdell H, To A, Husain OAN: Comparison of prevalence of human papillomavirus antigen in biopsies from women with cervical intraepithelial neoplasia. *J Clin Pathol* 38:855–857, 1985.

111. Soutter WP, Wisdom S, Broughs AK, Monaghan JM: Should patients with mild atypia in cervical smear be referred for colposcopy. *Brit J Obstet Gynaec* 93:70–74, 1986.

112. Stern E, Forsythe AB, Youkeles L, Coffelt CF: Steroid contraceptive use and cervical dysplasia: increased risk of progression. *Science* 196:1460–1462, 1977.

113. Sutherland IH, Arulkumaran S, Kitchener HC: Atypical condylomas of the cervix uteri in Singapore women: a histopathological and immunohistochemical study. *N Zealand Med J* 26:151–154, 1986.

114. Syrjänen KJ: Morphologic study of the condylomatous lesions in the dysplastic and neoplastic epithelium of the uterine cervix. *Arch Gynecol* 227:153–161, 1979.

115. Syrjänen KJ: Condylomatous lesions in dysplastic and neoplastic epithelium of the uterine cervix. *Surgery Gynecol Obst* 150:372–376, 1980.

116. Syrjänen KJ: Condylomatous lesions associated with precancerous changes of the uterine cervix. *Neoplasma* 28:497–509, 1981.

117. Syrjänen KJ: Human papillomavirus (HPV) lesions in association with cervical dysplasias and neoplasias. *Obstet Gynecol* 62:617–624, 1983.

118. Syrjänen KJ: Current concepts of human papillomavirus infections in the genital tract and their relationship to intraepithelial neoplasia and squamous cell carcinoma. *Obstet Gynecol Surve* 39:252–265, 1984.

119. Syrjänen KJ, Heinonen U-M, Kauraniemi T: Cytologic evidence of the association of condylomatous lesions with dysplastic and neoplastic changes in the uterine cervix. *Acta Cytol* 25:17–22, 1981.

120. Syrjänen KJ, Syrjänen S: Human papillomavirus (HPV) infections

related to cervical intraepithelial neoplasia (CIN) and squamous cell carcinoma of the uterine cervix. *Ann Clin Res* 17:45–56, 1985.

121. Syrjänen K, Pyrhonen S: Immunoperoxidase demonstration of human papillomavirus (HPV) in dysplastic lesions of the uterine cervix. *Arch Gynecol* 233:52–61, 1982.

122. Syrjänen K, Väyrynen M, Castrén O, Mäntyjärvi R, Pyrhonen S, Yliskoski M: Morphological and immunohistochemical evidence of human papillomavirus (HPV) involvement in the dysplastic lesions of the uterine cervix. *Int J Gynecol Obstet* 21:77–82, 1983.

123. Syrjänen S, Cintorino M, Armellini D, Del Vecchio MT, Leoncini P, Bugnoli M, Pallini V, Silvestri S, Tosi P, Mäntyjärvi R, Syrjänen K: Expression of cytokeratin polypeptides in human papillomavirus (HPV) lesions of the uterine cervix: 1. Relationship to grade of CIN and HPV type. *Int J Gynecol Path* 7:23–38, 1988.

124. Toki T, Oikawa N, Tase T, Wada Y, Yajima A, Suzuki M, Higashiiwai H: Immunoperoxidase demonstration of papillomavirus antigen in dysplasia of the uterine cervix. *Acta Obstet et Gynae* 37:411–415, 1985.

125. Toki T, Oikawa N, Tase T, Vehara S, Wada Y, Yajima A, Ito K, Higashiiwai H, Ito K, Endo N: Cytologic patterns of the cervical dysplasia with papillomavirus antigen. *J Japan Soc Clin Cyt* 24:638–642, 1985.

126. Toki T, Oikawa N, Tase T, Satoh S, Wada Y, Yajima A: Immunohistochemical demonstration of papillomavirus antigen in cervical dysplasia and in vulvar condyloma. *Gynecol Obstet Inves* 22:97–101, 1986.

127. Toki T, Oikawa N, Tase T, Sato S, Wada Y, Yajima A, Higashiiwai H: Immunohistochemical and electronmicroscopic demonstration of human papillomavirus in dysplasia of the uterine cervix. *Tohoku J Exp Med* 149:163–167, 1986.

128. Toki T, Yajima A: "HPV score," a scoring system for histological diagnosis of human papillomavirus infection in dysplasia of the uterine cervix. *Acta Pathologica Jap* 37:449–455, 1987.

129. Trevathan E, Layde P, Webster L: Cigarette smoking and dysplasia and carcinoma in situ of the uterine cervix. *JAMA* 250:499–502, 1983.

130. Villa LL, Franco ELF: Epidemiologic correlates of cervical neoplasia and risk of human papillomavirus infection in asymptomatic women in Brazil. *JNCI* 81:332–430, 1989.

131. Wassertheil-Smoller S, Romney SL, Wylie-Rosett J, Slagle S, Miller G, Lucido D, Duttagupta C, Palan PR: Dietary vitamin C and uterine cervical dysplasia. *Am J Epidemiol* 114:714–724, 1981.

132. Watts KC, Campion MJ, Butler EB, Jenkins D, Singer A, Husain OA: Quantitative deoxyribonucleic acid analysis of patients with mild cervical atypia: A potentially malignant lesion. *Obstet Gynecol* 70:205–207, 1987

133. Watts KC, Husain OA, Campion MJ, Lorriman F, Butler EB, McCance D, Jenkins D, Singer A: Quantitative DNA analysis of low grade cervical intraepithelial neoplasia and human papillomavirus infection by static and flow cytometry. *Brit Med J* 295:1090–1092, 1987.

134. Zaninetti P, Franceschi S, Baccolo M, Bonazzi B, Gottardi G, Serraino D: Characteristics of women under 20 with cervical intraepithelial neoplasia. *Int J Epidem* 15:477–482, 1986.

135. Zuna RE: Association of condylomas with intraepithelial and microinvasive cervical neoplasia: Histopathology of conization and hysterectomy specimens. *Int J Gynecol Pathol* 2:364–372, 1984.

CHAPTER NINE

Invasive Squamous Carcinoma of the Cervix

Taken on a worldwide basis, cancer of the cervix is the second most frequent malignancy in women. Recent estimates of the number of new cases appearing each year worldwide give a figure of 465,600, representing 15% of all cancers diagnosed in women.[28] About 80% of these cases occur in developing countries, where it is the most common of all cancers among women. The rates have been decreasing in most industrialized countries but the relaxation of sexual mores would have produced an increase of epidemic proportions had it not been for cytologic screening programs, which have been available almost everywhere. Even so, there have been reports of increasing rates of cervical cancers in younger populations, particularly under 35 years of age.[7,13,14,20]

The association between sexual activity and cancer of the cervix was first reported by Rigoni-Stern[29] in 1842, who noted that this neoplasia was much more common in prostitutes than in the general population. A century later, in Quebec City, Gagnon,[17] who acted as visiting physician to cloistered nuns, found no cancer of the cervix in his charges. Shortly afterwards, Rotkin,[31] in a series of personal interviews, observed that the most important risk factors were early age at onset of sexual activity and multiplicity of sexual partners. He then postulated that there must exist a transmissible agent that passed from man to woman during the sexual act. This idea was reinforced subsequently with the finding that wives of husbands who reported multiple sexual partners, or whose husbands had carcinoma of the penis, had an increased incidence of cervical cancer.[8,19,24,26,32,33,36,38]

For over two decades, herpes simplex virus II (HSV-2) was held to be the responsible agent. It was observed that women with cancer had an increased rate of positive findings for herpes serum antigens. DNA hybridization revealed that between 10% and 30% of cervical cancers analyzed contained HSV-2 DNA fragments as well as HSV-specific RNA and proteins, in particular the HSV-specific protein ICP10, which could be demonstrated in over 50% of intraepithelial and invasive neoplasia; these HSV fragments were not found in healthy genital tissues from the same patients.[6] Although at one point it was claimed that HSV II fulfilled all of Koch's postulates for the etiologic agent of cancer of the cervix,[2] a direct causal relationship between HSV-2 and genital cancer could not be established because DNA sequences homologous to HSV-2 were not found in a majority of carcinomas of the cervix.[39,40]

Currently there is much interest in the relationship between human papillomavirus and cancer of the genitalia. HPV types 6, 11, and 42 are associated with condyloma acuminatum, a generally benign sexually transmitted disease, while types 16,18,33,35, and others are routinely demonstrated in premalignant and malignant lesions.[4,5,11,18,25] In benign epithelial lesions, HPV DNA is found as an episome, that is, an extrachromosomal circular molecule which reproduces independently; in malignant tumors the HPV DNA sequences are integrated into the host DNA.[12,27] The open reading frames (ORFs) E6 and E7 are never disrupted during integration and seem to play a major role in the neoplastic transformation.[21,22,34] HPV DNA is also found in healthy genital tissues.[9,15,35] It has therefore been postulated that HPV induces neoplastic transformation only with the cooperation of other carcinogens, such as radiation, cigarette smoking, and oncogenic viruses such as HSV (see Chapter Seven).

Oncogenes may also play a role.[10,30] It has been found that c-myc is often amplified and expressed in cervical carcinomas, and this involvement has been described in association with oncogenesis related to both HSV-2 and HPV.[1,3,23,41] At the present time it is thought that HPV may be a necessary factor in genital carcinogenesis, but not sufficient by itself, requiring the presence of a co-carcinogen to produce a malignant tumor.

Classification

Invasive squamous carcinoma of the cervix can be grouped according to its clinical features, or according to the histologic pattern (see Tables 9.1 and 9.2).[16]

The classifications in Table 9.1, however, seem to bear little relation to the outcome of therapy. A more useful system[37] divides invasive squamous carcinoma into the following types:

- *Keratinizing carcinomas* contain abundant keratin, keratin pearls, and intercellular bridges. Nuclei are hyperchromatic or pyknotic, and large, and there are few mitoses (Plate 9.1).
- *Large cell carcinomas* contain uniformly enlarged nuclei with coarse chromatin and prominent nucleoli. There are many mitotic fig-

Table 9.1

Histologic Classification of Invasive Squamous Carcinoma

Grade 1	Well-differentiated carcinoma containing abundant keratin, keratin pearls, and clearly visible intercellular bridges: mitotic figures are fewer than two per high-power microscopic field
Grade 2	Moderately differentiated carcinoma has less apparent keratinization, two to four mitotic figures per high-power field, and anisokaryosis
Grade 3	Poorly differentiated carcinoma with no obvious keratinization, more than four mitotic figures per high-power field, and considerable pleomorphism of cells

lymphocytic cervicitis (see Chapter Five). Small dark cells should always be carefully examined. Unlike lymphocytic cervicitis, in small cell carcinoma there is only one cell type present. The differential diagnosis with small cell malignant lymphoma may be more difficult. In lymphoma the cells are mostly isolated and do not show any molding. In small cell carcinoma clusters of malignant cells do occur, and molding of the nuclei may be seen.

Plate 9.1

Tissue section of a keratinizing invasive squamous carcinoma of the cervix.

Plate 9.2

Tissue section from a large cell invasive squamous carcinoma of the cervix.

Plate 9.3

Tissue section of a small cell invasive squamous carcinoma of the cervix.

Plate 9.4

Low-power view of cervical conization specimen, illustrating a microinvasive squamous carcinoma (depth of penetration, 2.1 mm).

Plate 9.1   Plate 9.2

Plate 9.3   Plate 9.4

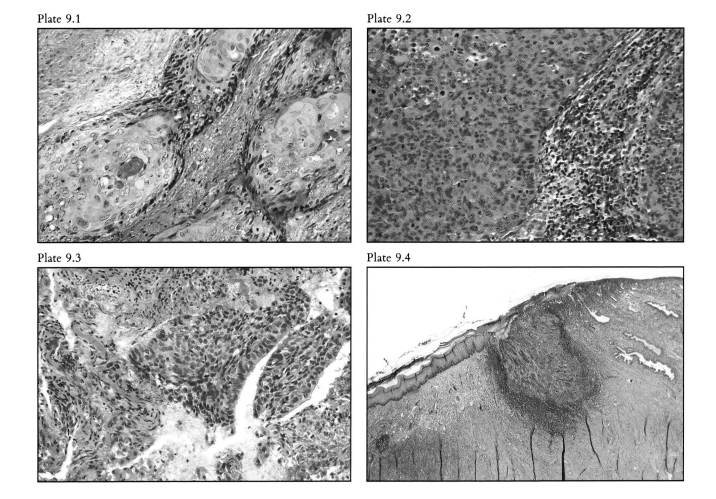

Plate 9.5

High-power view of same lesion as illustrated in Plate 9.4. The stromal reaction, consisting of a lymphocytic cuff surrounding the invasive carcinoma, is clearly visible.

Plate 9.6

Tissue section from a microinvasive squamous carcinoma. Small clusters of malignant cells have separated from the main lesion.

Plate 9.5

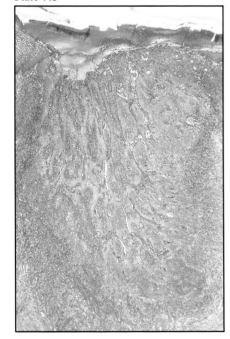

Plate 9.6

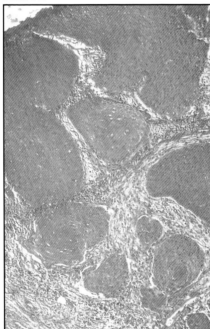

Plate 9.7
High-power view of the lesion illustrated in Plate 9.6. The invasive cells tend to differentiate, become larger, and form small nests, which are often surrounded by a lymphocytic stromal reaction.

Plate 9.8
Cell spread from an early invasive squamous carcinoma. In contrast to HGSIL, anisokaryosis is pronounced and small nucleoli can be seen in some of the nuclei. The background is clean.

Plate 9.9
Cell spread from an early invasive squamous carcinoma. In addition to anisokaryosis, differentiation of some of the malignant cells is shown by the eosinophilic staining of the cytoplasm.

Plate 9.10
Nucleoli are not commonly seen in HGSIL. Their appearance should alert the viewer to the possibility of early invasion. In this cluster, the cells lack distinct boundaries.

Plate 9.7

Plate 9.8

Plate 9.9

Plate 9.10

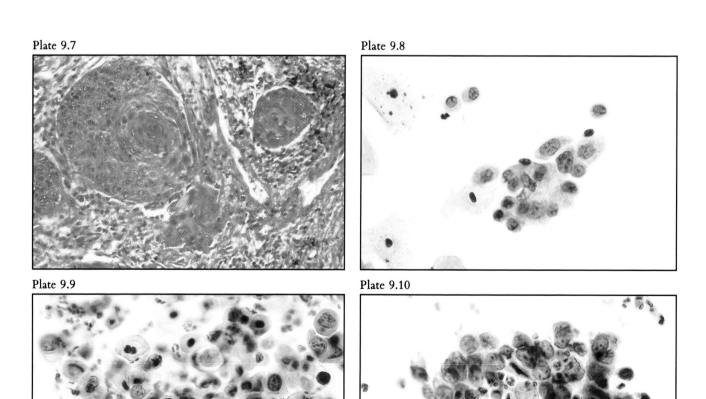

Plate 9.11
The outer limits of the cells are not visible in this cluster from a case of early invasive squamous carcinoma. The arrangement has been called pseudosyncytial.

Plate 9.12
Overlapping of the cells in clusters like this one is another feature that suggests early invasion.

Plate 9.13
Early invasive squamous carcinoma. There is overlapping, lack of distinct cell boundaries, and anisokaryosis. Nucleoli are small, in contrast to the macronucleoli commonly seen in repair (see Plates 5.20 and 5.21 in Chapter Five).

Plate 9.14
Cell spread from an invasive keratinizing squamous carcinoma. The malignant cells are elongated and sometimes eosinophilic, with cigar-shaped pyknotic nuclei. These cells have been called fibroid cells because of their resemblance to fibroblasts.

Plate 9.11

Plate 9.12

Plate 9.13

Plate 9.14

Plate 9.15

Smear from an invasive keratinizing squamous carcinoma. There is marked anisokaryosis. Some of the cells are elongated. The nuclei are hyperchromatic or pyknotic.

Plate 9.16

One keratinized malignant cell showing a tadpole-like shape. The other cells in this field are large, poorly differentiated cancer cells.

Plate 9.17

A single large keratinized cell from an invasive squamous carcinoma. The cytoplasm contains concentric striations. The nucleus is very large, irregular in shape and hyperchromatic.

Plate 9.18

Cell spread from a large cell invasive squamous carcinoma. The cells tend to form irregular clusters. There is marked anisokaryosis. The nuclei are hyperchromatic with coarse chromatin. The nuclear membrane appears irregularly thickened.

Plate 9.15

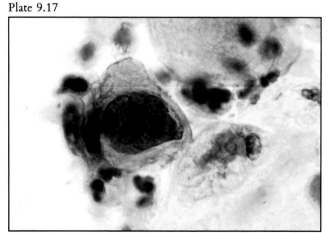

Plate 9.16

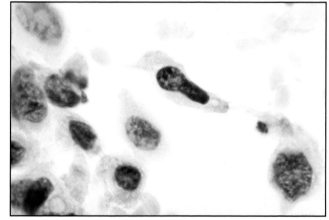

Plate 9.17

Plate 9.18

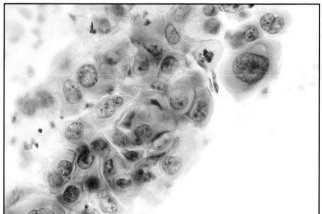

Plate 9.19
A cluster of cells from a large cell invasive squamous carcinoma. The cells tend to overlap and anisokaryosis is considerable. Nuclei contain small nucleoli. A few cells separate from the cluster. The background contains blood.

Plate 9.20
Large cell invasive squamous carcinoma. The nuclei are large and irregular, and contain coarse chromocenters and small nucleoli.

Plate 9.21
Smear obtained from a case of small cell invasive carcinoma. The nuclear/cytoplasmic ratio is increased and the cytoplasm is scarce. The nuclei are darkly stained and anisokaryotic. Compare the size of these cells to those of the large cell carcinoma illustrated above.

Plate 9.22
A cluster of malignant cells from a small cell invasive squamous carcinoma. The variation in size and shape help to distinguish these cells from the small lymphocytes of lymphocytic cervicitis (compare with Plates 5.17–5.19 in Chapter Five).

Plate 9.19

Plate 9.20

Plate 9.21

Plate 9.22

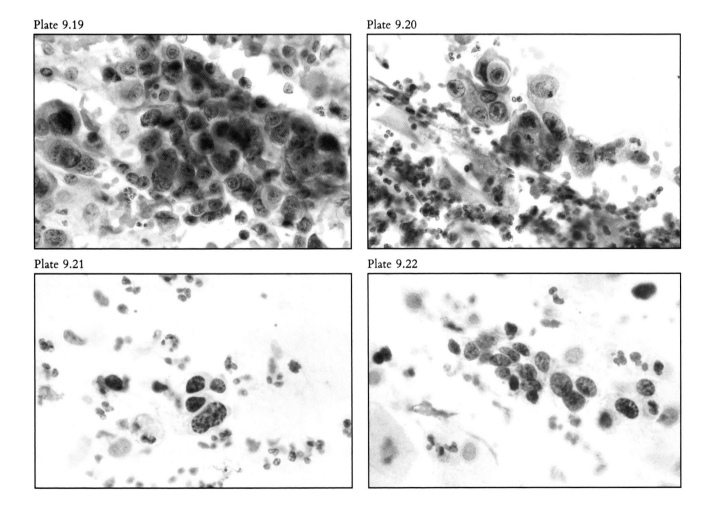

References

1. Adam E, Kaufman RH, Adler-Storthz K, Melnick JL, Dreesman GR: A prospective study of association of herpes simplex virus and human papillomavirus infection with cervical neoplasia in women exposed to diethylstilbestrol in utero. *Int J Cancer* 35:19–26, 1985.

2. Aurelian L, Manak MM, McKinley M, Smith CC, Klacsmann KT, Gupta PK: "The Herpesvirus hypothesis"—Are Koch's postulates satisfied? *Gynecol Oncol* 12:56–87, 1981.

3. Beach R, King CR: The role of HSV and HPV in cervical cancer. *Kansas Medicine* 88:130–131, 1987.

4. Beaudenon S, Kremsdorf D, Croissant O, Jablonska S, Wain-Hobson S, Orth G: A novel type of human papillomavirus associated with genital neoplasias. *Nature* 321:246–249, 1986.

5. Boshart M, Gissmann L, Ikenberg H, Kleinheinz A, Scheurlen W, zur Hausen H: A new type of papillomavirus DNA, its presence in genital cancer biopsies and in cell lines derived from cervical cancer. *Embo J* 3:1151–1157, 1984.

6. Cabral GA, Fry D, Marciano-Cabral F, et al: A herpesvirus antigen in human premalignant and malignant cervical biopsies and explants. *Am J Obstet Gynecol* 145:79, 1983.

7. Campion MJ, Singer A, Clarkson PK, McCance DJ: Increased risk of cervical neoplasia in consorts of men with penile condylomata acuminata. *Lancet* i (8435):943–946, 1985.

8. Carmichael JA, Clarice DH, Moher D, Ohlike ID, Karchmar EJ: Cervical carcinoma in women aged 34 and younger. *Am J Obstet Gynecol* 154:264–269, 1986.

9. de Villiers EM, Wagner D, Schneider A, Wesch H, Miklaw H, Wahrendorf J, Papendick U, zur Hausen H: Human papillomavirus infections in women with and without abnormal cervical cytology. *Lancet* ii:703–705, 1987.

10. Dürst M, Croce CM, Gissmann L, Schwarz E, Huebner K: Papillomavirus sequences integrate near cellular oncogenes in some cervical carcinomas. *Proc Natl Acad Sc* 84:1070–1074, 1987.

11. Dürst M, Gissmann L, Ikenberg H, zur Hausen H: A papillomavirus DNA from a cervical carcinoma and its prevalence in cancer biopsy samples from different geographic regions. *Proc Natl Acad Sci* 80:3812–3815, 1983.

12. Dürst M, Kleinheinz A, Hotz M, Gissmann L: The physical state of human papillomavirus type 16 DNA in benign and malignant genital tumours. *J Gen Virol* 66:1515–1522, 1985.

13. Elliott PM, Tattersall MHN, Coppleson M, Russell P, Wong F, Coates AS, Solomon HJ, Bannatyne PM, Atkinson KH, Murray JC: Changing character of cervical cancer in young women. *Brit M J* 298:288–290, 1989.

14. Fedorkow DM, Robertson DI, Duggan MA, Nation JG, McGregor SE, Stuart GCE: Invasive squamous cell carcinoma of the cervix in women less than 35 years old: Recurrent versus nonrecurrent disease. *Am J Obstet Gynecol* 158:307–311, 1988.

15. Ferenczy A, Mitao M, Nagai M, Silverstein SJ, Crum CP: Latent papillomavirus and recurring genital warts. *New Engl J Med* 313:784–788, 1985.

16. FIGO Cancer Committee: Staging announcement. *Gynecol Oncol* 25:383, 1986.

17. Gagnon F: Contribution to the study of the etiology and prevention of cancer of the cervix of the uterus. *Am J Obstet Gynecol* 60:516–522, 1950.

18. Gissmann L, de Villiers EM, zur Hausen H: Analysis of human genital warts (condylomata acuminata) and other genital tumors for human papillomavirus type 6 DNA. *Int J Cancer* 29:143–146, 1982.

19. Graham S, Priore R, Graham M, Browne R, Burnett W, West D: Genital cancer in wives of penile cancer patients. *Cancer* 44:1870–1874, 1980.

20. Green GH: Rising cervical cancer mortality in young New Zealand women. *N Zealand Med J* 89:89, 1979.

21. Iftner T, Bierfelder S, Csapo Z, Pfister H: Involvement of human papillomavirus type 8 genes E6 and E7 in transformation and replication. *J Virol* 62:3655–3661, 1988.

22. Kanda T, Furuno A, Yoshiike K: Human papillomavirus type 16 open reading frame E7 encodes a transforming gene for rat 3Y1 cells. *J Virol* 62:610–613, 1988.

23. Kaufman RH, Adam E: Herpes simplex virus and human papillomavirus in the development of cervical carcinoma. *Clin Obstet Gynecol* 29:678–692, 1986.

24. Li J, Li FP, Blot WJ, Miller RW, Fraumeni Jr JF: Correlation between cancers of the uterine cervix and penis in China. *J Natl Cancer Inst* 69:1063–1065, 1982.

25. Lorincz AT, Lancaster WD, Temple GF: Cloning and characterization of a new human papillomavirus from a woman with dysplasia of the uterine cervix. *J Virol* 58:225–229, 1986.

26. Martinez I: Relationship of squamous cell carcinoma of the cervix uteri to squamous cell carcinoma of the penis. *Cancer* 24:777–780, 1969.

27. Mincheva A, Gissmann L, zur Hausen H: Chromosomal integration sites of human papillomavirus DNA in three cervical cancer cell lines mapped by in situ hybridization. *Med Microbiol Immuno* 176:245–256, 1987.

28. Parkin DM, Läärä E, Muir CS: Estimates of the worldwide frequency of sixteen major cancers in 1980. *Int J Cancer* 41:184–197, 1988.

29. Rigoni-Stern D: Fatti statistici relativi alle malattie cancerose che servirono di base alle poche cose dette dal dott. *Gior Serv Progr Path* 2:507–517, 1842.

30. Riou G, Barrois M, Tordjman I, Dutronquay V, Orth G: Presence of papillomavirus genomes and amplification of c–myc and c–Ha–ras oncogenes in invasive cancers of the uterine cervix. *C R Acad Sc (Paris)* 299:575–580, 1984.

31. Rotkin ID: A comparison review of key epidemiological studies in cervical cancer related to current searches for transmissible agents. *Cancer Res* 33:1353–1367, 1973.

32. Singer A, Reid BL, Coppleson M: A hypothesis: The role of high-risk male in the etiology of cervical carcinoma. *Am J Obstet Gynecol* 126:110–115, 1976.

33. Smith, PG, Kinlen LJ, White GC, Adelstein AM, Fox AJ: Mortality

of wives of men dying with cancer of the penis. *Br J Cancer* 41:422–428, 1980.

34. Takebe N, Tsunokawa Y, Nozawa S, Terada M, Sugimura T: Conservation of E6 and E7 regions of human papillomavirus types 16 and 18 present in cervical cancers. *Biochem Byophys Res* 143:837–844, 1987.

35. Toon PG, Arrand JR, Wilson LP, Sharp DS: Human papillomavirus infection of the uterine cervix of women without cytological signs of neoplasia. *Brit Med J* 293:1261–1264, 1986.

36. Viñes JJ, Ascunce N: Correlación entre la incidencia del cáncer de cérvix y el cáncer de pene. *Oncología* 9:61–70, 1986.

37. Wentz WB, Reagan JW: Survival in cervical cancer with respect to cell type. *Cancer* 12:384–388, 1959.

38. Zunzunegui MV, ing MC, Coria CF, Charlet J: Male influences on cervical cancer risk. *Am J Epidemiol* 123:302–307, 1986.

39. zur Hausen H: Oncogenic herpes viruses. *Bioch Biophys Acta* 417:25–53, 1975.

40. zur Hausen H: Herpes simplex virus in human genital cancer. *Intern Rev Exp Pathol* 25:307–325, 1983.

41. zur Hausen H: Human genital cancer: Synergism between two virus infection or synergism between a virus infection and initiating events. *Lancet* ii:1370–1372, 1982.

CHAPTER TEN

Adenocarcinoma of the Cervix

Benign Atypia

In the Bethesda System there is a category for atypia of endocervical glandular cells of undetermined significance. In many cases this is a reactive phenomenon, related to chronic endocervicitis or other local conditions. Histologic section shows enlargement of the cells with cytoplasmic eosinophilia[8] (Plate 10.1).

Adenocarcinoma

The frequency of cervical neoplasias that have a glandular component has been evaluated as ranging from 5%[1] to 34%[12] of all cervical cancers. In recent times an absolute increase in the frequency of these lesions has been reported.[44,50] This increase seems to be more than a relative increase compared to squamous carcinomas, which have decreased in frequency. Adenocarcinoma of the cervix appears to be preceded by an in situ phase in most cases, which is predominantly situated within the endocervical canal and may therefore escape detection by colposcopic examination. In at least one third of the patients, adenocarcinoma is associated with a squamous lesion of the cervix.[33,60] The epidemiology is essentially similar to that of squamous neoplasias. The preclinical stage may be protracted.[4] Human papillomavirus, particularly type 18, has been cloned from adenocarcinoma of the cervix[7,10,40,52,59] and its precursors.[54]

Histology

Adenocarcinoma in situ (AIS) is depicted classically[13] as a malignant transformation of the epithelial lining of the endocervical glands. The epithelium usually changes abruptly from benign-appearing to neoplastic. The affected epithelium consists of one or several layers of large cells, containing uneven, hyperchromatic, and enlarged nuclei (Plates 10.2 and 10.3). Mitotic figures are commonly seen, some of which are abnormal. The cytoplasm tends to be eosinophilic and mucin production is reduced or absent. In most cases the necks of the glands are affected. The glands become irregular, with papillary projections in the lumen, infoldings, and cribriform patterns. They may lie back to back.[3,14,15,21,41,55,56]

Jaworski et al[23] described the following subtypes of AIS: an endocervical type characterized by luminal accumulation of mucin-containing cytoplasm, an endometrioid type similar to the endocervical type but without mucin, an intestinal type with neoplastic goblet cells, and miscellaneous types (serous, clear cell, and adenosquamous). In many cases, a squamous intraepithelial lesion is seen in association with AIS (Plate 10.4).

Early invasion is not always easy to recognize[35,45,55] because the stroma is invaded by neoplastic glands, and not by individual cells, as occurs in squamous carcinoma. Invasive adenocarcinoma of the cervix has been classified in subtypes, some of which are the same as in AIS: the most frequently found type is the pure (endocervical) adenocarcinoma, in which the glands are of variable shape and size with budding and branching (Plates 10.5–10.7).[1,5,11,17,26,29,36] Papillary forms occur (Plate 10.8). Mucin is usually present. The epithelium resembles the normal columnar endocervical lining. When this form is particularly well differentiated it may be called "adenoma malignum" (Plate 10.9).[20,25,34,35] In spite of their mild appearance, these tumors often have a poor prognosis.[22,27,48] Adenocarcinoma of endometrial type resembles its counterpart from the uterine cavity.

Less frequent types include the adenoacanthoma, in which there is benign squamous metaplasia integrated within the adenocarcinoma; the adenosquamous carcinoma, in which both the glandular and the squamous components are malignant;[16] the glassy cell carcinoma, in which the cells are large and round with well-defined cellular borders, the cytoplasm has a ground glass appearance and the nucleus is large and contains one or two prominent nucleoli;[24,30,31,37,39,42,43,47,51,53,58,61] the clear cell (mesonephric) adenocarcinoma, characterized by clear cytoplasm and hobnail nuclei;[9,18,19,57] the mucoepidermoid tumor; and the adenoid cystic carcinoma.[32]

Cytology

Endocervical glandular cells may display a gamut of morphologic changes encompassing benign atypias of undetermined significance, patterns suggestive of AIS, and changes consistent with invasive adenocarcinoma.

The benign atypias of undetermined significance consist mostly in enlargement of the nuclei with some degree of anisokaryosis, and presence of nucleoli (Plates 10.10 and 10.11). The endocervical glandular cells are found mostly in clusters or small groupings, without much overlapping. These changes may be reactive (endocervicitis), regenerative, or in some cases, may be precursors to more advanced lesions, like AIS.

In AIS the smears contain numerous endocervical glandular cells forming sheets, strips, or rosettes with sometimes recognizable pseudostratification and loss of polarity. There is little or no overlapping of cells and sometimes a continuous border may be seen on the periphery of the sheets or strips. The nuclei are larger than those of benign endocervical cells, but they remain uniform and somewhat hyperchromatic. Small nucleoli are rarely present (Plates 10.12–10.15). The background is clean.[6,28,38] When there is an associated SIL, the smear may contain predominantly cells from that lesion, and the atypical endocervical cells may be entirely absent, or overlooked.

Early invasion may be suspected when there are isolated cells in addition to the sheets and strips; hyperchromasia, anisokaryosis, and the presence of macronucleoli are also signs pointing towards the possibility of stromal invasion.[2,45]

Cells from invasive adenocarcinomas of the cervix typically form three-dimensional clusters (Plate 10.16). The cells are large, with abundant, often vacuolated cytoplasm. They sometimes conserve their generally columnar shape, which may be best visualized at the periphery of the aggregates (Plate 10.17). In well-differentiated adenocarcinomas, the cells may occur in strips or strands. Nuclei are large, oval, or round, most with some irregularity in their outline. There is anisokaryosis, hyperchromasia, clearing of the chromatin, and loss of polarity (nuclei point in all directions). Macronucleoli are often present, and may be multiple (Plates 10.18–10.22).[4,46,49]

Clear cell carcinomas shed large cells with poorly stained, finely vacuolated cytoplasm. Nuclei are large and often at the center of the cell. The chromatin is granular or reticular with little hyperchromasia. Single round macronucleoli are common. These cells may occur in tight clusters, in sheets, or singly. Since clear cell carcinoma occurs not only on the cervix, but also in the vagina, the endometrium, and the ovary, it is best not to state the origin of the cells.

In adenosquamous carcinoma malignant cells representing both the glandular and the squamous component can be observed. The squamous component is frequently of the large cell type or the keratinizing type. The small cell type is rare. The glassy cell variant can sometimes be recognized by the presence of large malignant cells with an eosinophilic granular cytoplasm and an enlarged nucleus containing a prominent nucleolus.[46,53] Since the squamous component in adenoacanthomas is benign, it is not recognized on cellular samples.

Other rare tumors of the cervix shed malignant cells, which are usually quite difficult to classify. In all such cases, it is in the best interest of all parties to report a finding of malignant cells of undetermined origin.

Plate 10.1

Tissue section of the cervix showing a benign proliferation of endocervical glands. There is pseudostratification of the columnar epithelium, which stains eosinophilic.

Plate 10.2

Tissue section of adenocarcinoma in situ (AIS) of the cervix. An abrupt transition takes place from a normal columnar epithelium to neoplastic, within the gland.

Plate 10.3

Tissue section of AIS. The neoplastic epithelium is eosinophilic, the nuclei are hyperchromatic and crowded, normal polarity has been lost, and mucus secretion has stopped.

Plate 10.4

The lining of the gland shows changes consistent with AIS, with an adjacent area of HGSIL at the surface.

Plate 10.1

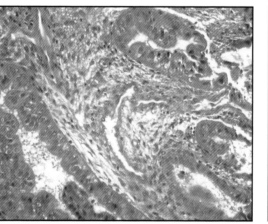

Plate 10.2

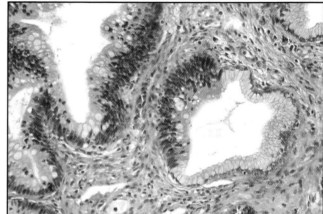

Plate 10.3

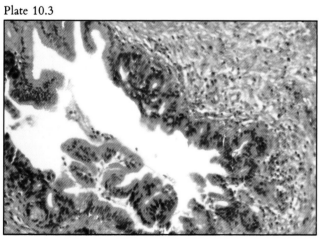

Plate 10.4

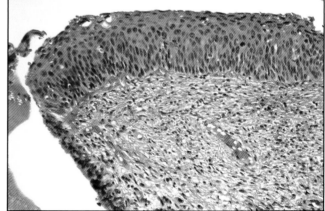

Plate 10.5
Tissue section of an early invasive adenocarcinoma of the cervix. Papillary projections can be seen within the neoplastic glands.

Plate 10.6
Early invasive adenocarcinoma of the cervix. The papillary projections extend from one side of the gland to the other, forming "Roman bridges."

Plate 10.7
Early invasive adenocarcinoma of the cervix. Two normal mucus-secreting glands are seen next to the neoplastic glands.

Plate 10.8
Tissue section of a papillary adenocarcinoma of the cervix.

Plate 10.5
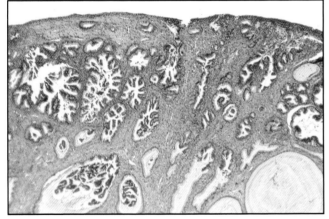

Plate 10.6
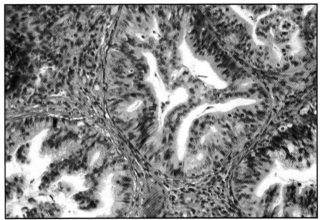

Plate 10.7
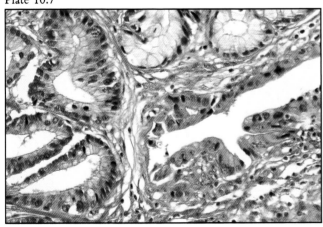

Plate 10.8
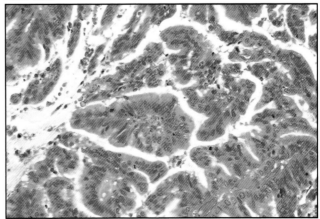

Plate 10.9
Tissue section of a well-differentiated adenocarcinoma of the cervix, the so-called "adenoma malignum."

Plate 10.10
Endocervical sample illustrating atypical glandular cells. There is some clumping together of the cell, with anisokaryosis. Nucleoli are seen in a few nuclei.

Plate 10.11
Atypical endocervical cells, with marked anisokaryosis and prominent nucleoli.

Plate 10.12
Cell pattern of AIS. The endocervical cells are tightly clustered with some overlapping. The nuclei are hyperchromatic.

Plate 10.9

Plate 10.10

Plate 10.11

Plate 10.12

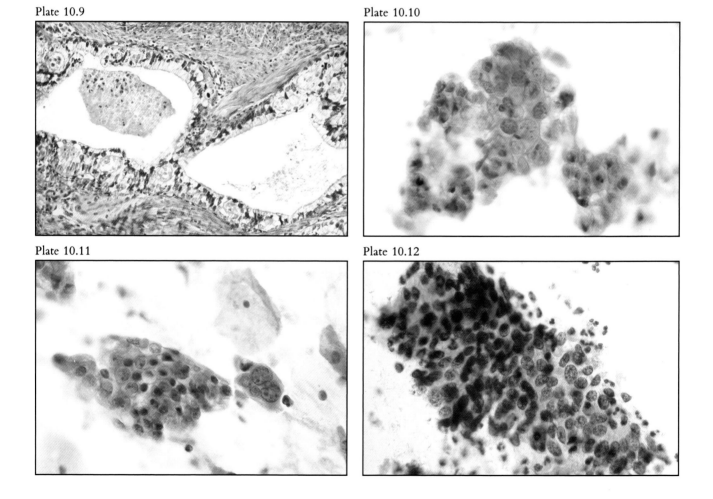

Plate 10.13
Endocervical smear illustrating AIS. There is considerable crowding of the cells, with hyperchromasia. This well-preserved gland formation also shows multistratification.

Plate 10.14
Endocervical smear from a case of AIS. This is the characteristic "strip" formation. The nuclei are large, hyperchromatic, and contain small nucleoli.

Plate 10.15
Endocervical smear from an invasive adenocarcinoma of the cervix. Even in this small group of cells overlapping can be appreciated. Nucleoli are prominent.

Plate 10.16
Cell pattern of invasive adenocarcinoma of the cervix. The cells are tightly clustered. One group forms a papillarylike structure.

Plate 10.13

Plate 10.14

Plate 10.15

Plate 10.16

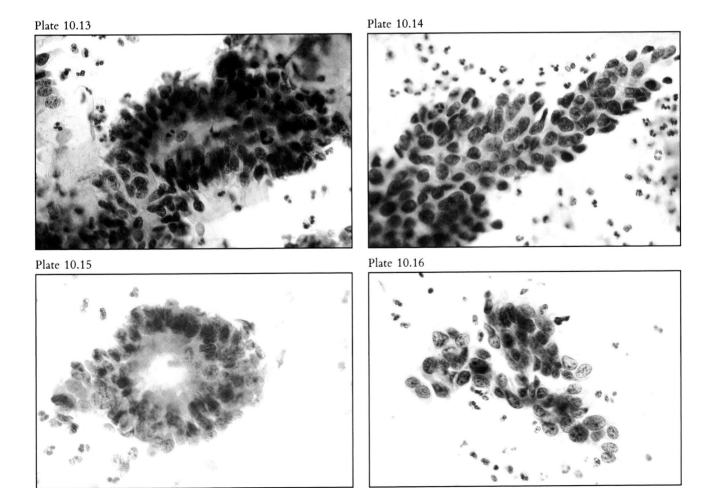

Plate 10.17
Cells from an invasive adenocarcinoma of the cervix. There is marked anisokaryosis, hyperchromasia, and coarsely distributed chromatin within the nuclei. Many cells conserve their columnar shape.

Plate 10.18
A papillary formation from a case of adenocarcinoma of the cervix.

Plate 10.19
Adenocarcinoma of the cervix. These are small vacuolated cells with granulocytic inclusions. The background is bloody.

Plate 10.17

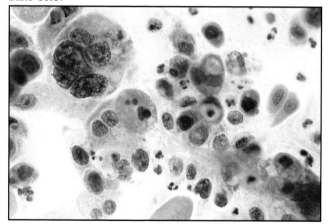

Plate 10.18

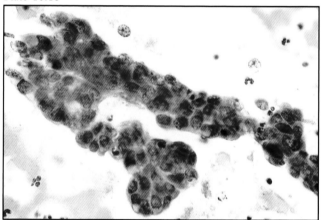

Plate 10.19

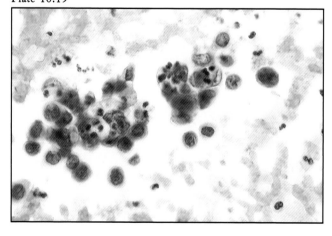

Plate 10.20

Cells from an invasive adenocarcinoma of the cervix. The cytoplasm is eosinophilic. Macronucleoli are visible in some nuclei.

Plate 10.21

Papillary adenocarcinoma of the cervix. The cells form small groups in which the outer cell membranes seem to be continuous from one cell to the other. There is a typical tumor diathesis, consisting of lysed blood and a serous exudate.

Plate 10.22

Cells from a poorly differentiated invasive adenocarcinoma of the cervix. Note the hyperchromasia, the granulocytic inclusions inside cytoplasmic vacuoles, and cell cannibalism.

Plate 10.20

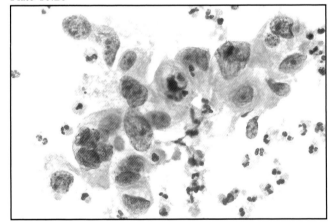

Plate 10.21

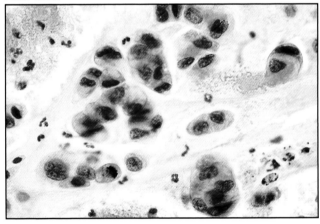

Plate 10.22

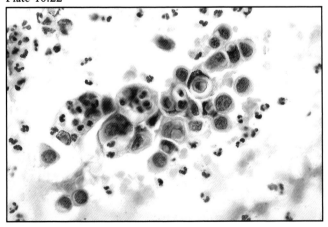

References

1. Abell MR, Gosling JRG: Gland cell carcinoma (adenocarcinoma) of the uterine cervix. *Am J Obstet Gynecol* 83:729–755, 1962.

2. Ayer B, Pacey F, Greenberg M: The cytologic diagnosis of adenocarcinoma in situ of the cervix uteri and related lesions. II. Microinvasive adenocarcinoma. *Acta Cytol* 32:318–324, 1988.

3. Barter RA, Wtares ED: Cyto and histomorphology of cervical adenocarcinoma in situ. *Pathology* 2:33–40, 1970.

4. Boddington MM, Spriggs AI, Cowdell RH: Adenocarcinoma of the uterine cervix: Cytological evidence of a long preclinical evolution. *Brit J Obstet Gynaec* 83:900–903, 1976.

5. Boon ME, Kirk RS, Rietveld-Scheffers PEM: The morphogenesis of adenocarcinoma of the cervix—a complex pathological entity. *Histopathol* 5:565–577, 1981.

6. Bousfield L, Pacey F, Young Q, et al: Expanded cytologic criteria for the diagnosis of adenocarcinoma in situ of the cervix and related lesions. *Acta Cytol* 24:283–296, 1980.

7. Brescia RJ, Jenson AB, Lancaster WD, Kurman RJ: The role of papillomaviruses in the pathogenesis and histologic classification of precancerous lesions of the cervix. *Human Pathol* 17:552–559, 1986.

8. Brown LJR, Wells M: Cervical glandular atypia associated with squamous intraepithelial neoplasia: A premalignant lesion? *J Clin Pathol* 39:22–28, 1986.

9. Buntine DW: Adenocarcinoma of the uterine cervix of probable Wolffian origin. *Pathology* 11:713–718, 1979.

10. Crum CP, Levine RU: Human papillomavirus infection and cervical neoplasia: New perspectives. *Internat J Gynecol Pathol* 3:376–388, 1984.

11. Dallenbach-Hellweg G: On the origin and histological structure of adenocarcinoma of the endocervix in women under 50 years of age. *Pathol Res Pract* 179:38–50, 1984.

12. Davis JR, Moon LB: Increased incidence of adenocarcinoma of uterine cervix. *Obstet Gynecol* 45:79, 1975.

13. Friedell GH, McKay DG: Adenocarcinoma in situ of the endocervix. *Cancer* 6:887–897, 1953.

14. Gloor E, Hurlimann J: Cervical intraepithelial glandular neoplasia (adenocarcinoma in situ and glandular dysplasia). *Cancer* 58:1272–1280, 1986.

15. Gloor E, Ruzicka J: Morphology of adenocarcinoma in situ of the uterine cervix: A study of 14 cases. *Cancer* 49:294–302, 1982.

16. Glücksmann A, Cherry CP: Incidence, histology, and response to radiation of mixed carcinomas (adenoacanthomas) of the uterine cervix. *Cancer* 9:971–979, 1956.

17. Haggard JL, Cotten N, Dougherty CM, Mickal A: Primary adenocarcinoma of the cervix. *Obstet Gynec* 24:183–193, 1964.

18. Hart WR, Norris HJ: Mesonephric adenocarcinomas of the cervix. *Cancer* 29:106–113, 1972.

19. Hasumi K, Ehrmann RL: Clear cell carcinoma of the uterine endocervix with an in situ component. *Cancer* 42:2435–2438, 1978.

20. Hébert H, Hezarkhani M, Abelanet R, Auriol M, Fradet-Gentile A,

Gest J, Guérin P: A propos d'une observation d'adénocarcinome haute-
ment différencié du col utérin. *Sem Hôp Paris* 48:1425–1433, 1972.

21. Hopkins MP, Roberts JA, Schmidt RW: Cervical adenocarcinoma in situ. *Obstet Gynecol* 71:842–844, 1988.

22. Hopkins MP, Schmidt RW, Roberts JA, Morley GW: The prognosis and treatment of stage I adenocarcinoma of the cervix. *Obstet Gynecol* 72:915–921, 1988.

23. Jaworski RC, Pacey NF, Greenberg ML, Osborn RA: The histologic diagnosis of adenocarcinoma in situ and related lesions of the cervix. Adenocarcinoma in situ. *Cancer* 61:1171–1181, 1988.

24. Johnston GA, Azizi F, Reale F, Jones HA: Glassy-cell carcinoma of the cervix: Report of three cases. *J Natl Med Assoc* 74:361–363, 1982.

25. Kaku T, Enjoji M: Extremely well-differentiated adenocarcinoma ("adenoma malignum") of the cervix. *Internat J Gynecol Pathol* 2:28–41, 1983.

26. Korhonen MO: Adenocarcinoma of the uterine cervix: An evaluation of the available diagnostic methods. *Acta Pathol Microbiol Scand* (Suppl) 264:1–52, 1978.

27. Korhonen MO: Adenocarcinoma of the uterine cervix. Prognosis and prognostic significance of histology. *Cancer* 53:1760–1763, 1984.

28. Krumins I, Young Q, Pacey F, et al: The cytologic diagnosis of adenocarcinoma in situ of the cervix uteri. *Acta Cytol* 21:320–329, 1977.

29. Lewis BV, Diaz PRL, Stallworthy JA, Ellis FE: Primary adenocarcinoma of the cervix. *J Obstet Gynaecol Br* 77:277–279, 1970.

30. Littman P, Clement PB, Henriksen B, Wang CC, Robboy SJ, Taft PD, Ulfelder H, Scully RE: Glassy cell carcinoma of the cervix. *Cancer* 37:2238–2246, 1976.

31. Maier RC, Norris HJ: Glassy cell carcinoma of the cervix. *Obstet Gynecol* 60:219–224, 1982.

32. McGee JA, Flowers CE, Tatum BS: Adenoid cystic carcinoma of the cervix. *Obstet Gynecol* 26:356–358, 1965.

33. Maier RC, Norris HJ: Coexistence of cervical intraepithelial neoplasia with primary adenocarcinoma of the endocervix. *Obstet Gynecol* 56:361–364, 1980.

34. McKelvey JL, Goodlin RR: Adenoma malignum of the cervix. *Cancer* 16:549–557, 1963.

35. Michael H, Grawe L, Kraus FT: Minimal deviation endocervical adenocarcinoma: Clinical and histologic features, immunohistochemical staining for carcinoembryonic antigen, and differentiation from confusing benign lesions. *Internat J Gynecol Pathol* 2:261–276, 1984.

36. Mikuta JJ, Celebre JA: Adenocarcinoma of the cervix. *Obstet Gynec* 33:753–756, 1969.

37. Nahhas WA, Abt AB, Mortel R: Stage I glassy cell carcinoma of the cervix with ovarian metastasis. *Gynecol Oncol* 5:87–91, 1977.

38. Nguyen G-K, Jeannot AB: Exfoliative cytology of in situ and microinvasive adenocarcinoma of the uterine cervix. *Acta Cytol* 28:461–467, 1984.

39. Nuñez C, Abdul-Karim FW, Somrak TM: Glassy-cell carcinoma of the uterine cervix: Cytopathologic and histopathologic study of five cases. *Acta Cytol* 29:303–309, 1985.

40. Okagaki T, Tase T, Twiggs LB, Carson LF: Histogenesis of cervical

adenocarcinoma with reference to human papillomavirus 18 as a carcinogen. *J Reprod Med* 34:639–644, 1989.

41. Ostor AG, Pagano R, Davoren RAM, Fortune DW, Chanen W, Rome R: Adenocarcinoma in situ of the cervix. *Internat J Gynecol Pathol* 3:179–190, 1984.

42. Pak HY, Yokota SB, Paladugu RR, Agliozzo CM: Glassy cell carcinoma of the cervix: Cytologic and clinicopathologic analysis. *Cancer* 52:307–312, 1983.

43. Paulsen SM, Hansen KC, Nielsen VT: Glassy-cell carcinoma of the cervix: Case report with a light and electron microscopic study. *Ultrastruct Pathol* 1:377–384, 1980.

44. Peters, RK, Mack TM, Thomas D, Bernstein L, Henderson BE: Increased frequency of adenocarcinoma of the uterine cervix in young women in Los Angeles County. *JNCI* 76:423–428, 1986.

45. Qizilbash AH: In-situ and microinvasive adenocarcinoma of the uterine cervix. A clinical, cytologic and histologic study of 14 cases. *Am J Clin Pathol* 64:155–170, 1975.

46. Reagan JW, Ng ABP: Cellular detection of glandular neoplasms of uterine cervix. In: Compendium on Diagnostic Cytology, Wied GL, Keebler CM, Koss LG, Reagan JW (editors), Tutorials of Cytology, Chicago, 1988.

47. Richard L, Guralnik M, Ferenczy A: Ultrastructure of glassy cell carcinoma of the cervix. *Diagn Gynecol Obstet* 3:31–38, 1981.

48. Saigo PE, Cain JM, Kim WS, Gaynor JJ, Johnson K, Lewis JL Jr: Prognostic factors in adenocarcinoma of the uterine cervix. *Cancer* 57:1584–1593, 1986.

49. Saigo PE, Wolinska WH, Kim WS, Hajdu SI: The role of cytology in the diagnosis and follow-up of patients with cervical adenocarcinoma. *Acta Cytol* 29:785–794, 1985.

50. Schwartz SM, Weiss NS: Increased incidence of adenocarcinoma of the cervix in young women in the United States. *Am J Epidemiol* 124:1045–1047, 1986.

51. Seltzer V, Sall S, Castadot MJ, Muradian-Davidian M, Sedlis A: Glassy cell cervical carcinoma. *Gynecol Oncol* 8:141–151, 1979.

52. Smotkin D, Berek JS, Fu YS, Hacker NF, Major FJ, Wettstein FO: Human papillomavirus deoxyribonucleic acid in adenocarcinoma and adenosquamous carcinoma of the uterine cervix. *Obstet Gynecol* 68:241–244, 1986.

53. Tamimi HK, Ek M, Hesla J, Cain JM, Figge DC, Greer BE: Glassy cell carcinoma of the cervix redefined. *Obstet Gynec* 71:837–841, 1988.

54. Tase T, Okagaki T, Clark BA, Turggs LB, Ostrow RS, Faras AJ: Human papillomavirus DNA in adenocarcinoma in situ, microinvasive adenocarcinoma of the uterine cervix, and coexisting cervical squamous intraepithelial neoplasia. *Int J Gynecol Pathol* 8:8–17, 1989.

55. Teshima S, Shimosato Y, Kishi K, Kasamatsu T, Ohmi K, Uei Y: Early stage adenocarcinoma of the uterine cervix. *Cancer* 56:167–172, 1985.

56. Tobón H, Dave H: Adenocarcinoma in situ of the cervix. Clinicopathologic observations of 11 cases. *Int J Gynecol Pathol* 7:139–151, 1988.

57. Truskett ID, Constable WC: Clear cell adenocarcinoma of the cervix and vaginal vault of mesonephric origin. *Cancer* 21:249–254, 1968.

58. Ulbright TM, Gersell DJ: Glassy cell carcinoma of the uterine cervix: A light and electron microscopic study of five cases. *Cancer* 51:2255–2263, 1983.

59. Wilczynski SP, Walker J, Liao SY, Bergen S, Berman M: Adenocarcinoma of the cervix associated with human papillomavirus. *Cancer* 62:1331–1336, 1988.

60. Wolk BM, Kime W, Albites V: Simultaneous in situ squamous cell carcinoma and microinvasive adenocarcinoma of the cervix. *Int J Gynecol Obstet* 19:69–72, 1981.

61. Zaino RJ, Nahhas WA, Mortel R: Glassy cell carcinoma of the uterine cervix: An ultrastructural study and review. *Arch Pathol Lab Med* 106:250–254, 1982.

CHAPTER ELEVEN

Colposcopy in the Diagnosis and Management of Cervical Intraepithelial Lesions

Céline Bouchard, MD
Michel Fortier, MD

The era of colposcopy was initiated by Hinselmann in 1925 when he proposed the hypothesis that invasive cervical cancer was preceded by preclinical states that could be detected by magnification of cervical epithelium with an optical instrument adapted to the observation of the uterine cervix.[17] His observations led to an exhaustive and cumbersome classification of lesions based on vascularization and whiteness of epithelium revealed after soaking the vagina and cervix with a solution of 5% acetic acid. This new approach to detecting cervical malignancy gained popularity in European countries and proponents used it on all female patients as a screening procedure.

However, cytologically based mass screening programs for cervical pathology were stimulated by Papanicolaou's treatise in 1943. Their quality and efficacy, and the language barrier that prevented wide dissemination of Hinselmann's findings (published in German), were the main reasons that extensive use of Hinselmann's technique was delayed in North American medical practice. In the late sixties, Coppleson[9] in Australia and Stafl[32] in the United States initiated a renewed interest in colposcopy, as a follow-up technique to a finding of abnormal cytology. The simplified and more practical descriptions of cervical anomalies revealed through use of the colposcope were aimed at enabling clinicians to adopt more conservative procedures in their patient management. This new colposcopic approach led to a radical decrease in the rate of major surgical procedures, such as conization and hysterectomy, used to treat cervical intraepithelial neoplasia (CIN). This type of collaboration between researchers and clinicians has completely changed the approach of the medical community to lower genital tract diseases. There is now worldwide acceptance for the use of colposcopy as a clinical tool to evaluate the type, location, and extent of genital disease, to obtain directed biopsies, and to facilitate adequate laser therapy (histology remains the key for selection of management).

Technique

We take endocervical cultures for chlamydia and gonorrhea at a patient's visit. We repeat cytologic analysis only if 3 months have elapsed from the initial referral smear, because the rate of false negatives is too high on the repeat smear.[20]

The colposcope has binocular lenses (Figure 11.1) that magnify 6× to 40× to allow the user to visualize the entire lower genital tract. The best magnification, however, is between 8× and 12×. The speculum is inserted into the vagina in lithotomy position. On the repeat smear a solution of acetic acid (3%–5%) is applied in the vagina and on the cervix with a simple squeeze bottle. Excess liquid is sponged off after 10–20 seconds of cervical soaking. Adequate colposcopic visualization of the cervix must encompass the complete circumference of the transformation zone, which is the cervical area delineated by the endocervical acquired squamocolumnar junction and the so-called exocervical "original" squamocolumnar junction. Colposcopy will identify acetowhite lesions with or without characteristic vascular patterns when present in the transformation zone. Visualization of the original and acquired squamocolumnar junction is mandatory for an adequate colposcopic evaluation. Directed punch biopsy with surgical forceps (Figure 11.2) in the most abnormal spots and endocervical curettage (ECC) (Figure 11.3) will confirm the premalignant or malignant nature of the lesion in question. Cervical biopsies are obtained without anesthesia under colposcopic guidance. Although the specimens sent to the pathologist are small, expert colposcopists can rely on cytologic, histologic, and colposcopic correlation for treatment.

Classification of Lesions

Colposcopic evaluation of lesions is based on the visual aspects of the surface epithelium: color, surface irregularities, vascular patterns, and distribution and extent of abnormalities are used to ascertain the type and severity of disease. The squamous epithelium and columnar epithelium act as a screen for the vessels of the cervical stroma, and modification in the superficial activity is reflected by increased nuclear density, thereby modifying the colposcopic image.

The normal transformation zone is characterized by pinkish surface epithelium with gland openings and yellowish Nabothian cysts. A fine white line delineates the endocervical junction, with grapelike structures representing glandular epithelium (Figure

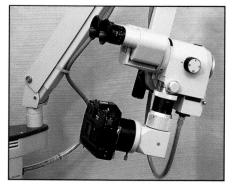

Figure 11.1 Colposcope.

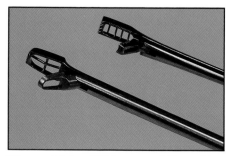

Figure 11.2 Whittner and Kevorkian biopsy forceps.

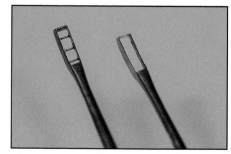

Figure 11.3 Kevorkian endocervical curette.

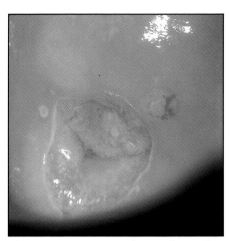

Figure 11.4 Normal transformation zone.

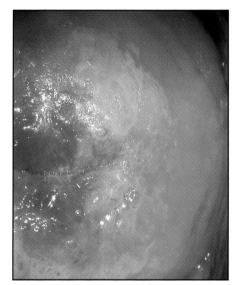

Figure 11.5 Cervical flat condyloma.

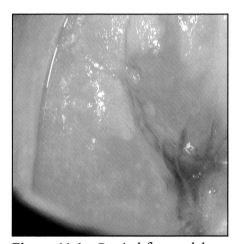

Figure 11.6 Cervical flat condyloma and reverse punctation.

11.4). Expert colposcopists can detect the most abnormal area for sampling for histologic diagnosis. We do not use colposcopic indexes as recommended by some authors[26,27] because we believe that the descriptions of lesions therein are misleading to the novice colposcopist and are useless to the expert.

Adherence to strict triaging of patients without omission of any step of colposcopic protocol (see Triaging and Management, page 197) is necessary for safe management of patients presenting abnormal cytology.

In our department, we stopped using terminology such as dysplasia and carcinoma in situ a few years ago to adopt the grading of CIN as proposed by Barron and Richart.[1,28] We are now changing to the proposed classification of the Bethesda system (see Chapter Two) because new evidence in the field of virology and cervical pathology about a possible link between human papillomaviruses (HPV) and cervical neoplasia[34,41] is establishing that surface lesions are all part of a continuous spectrum.[16,40] Standardization of cytologic, histologic, and colposcopic terminology would eliminate inconsistencies in the literature of various countries and facilitate consensus on clinical management.

This new terminology is clinically oriented and in agreement with histologic description. Colposcopic lesions represent a mixture of acetowhite lesions of various grades. Such lesions may have a vascular pattern of mosaic or abnormal blood vessels, punctation, or hyperkeratosis (Table 11.1). The aim of colposcopy is to rule out invasion by satisfactory visualization of the transformation zone and by appropriate biopsies. Histologic confirmation of the nature of the lesion is mandatory before any form of treatment is undertaken.

Low-Grade Intraepithelial Lesion

Low-grade intraepithelial lesions represent the morphologic expression of HPV infection. Two distinct patterns can be distinguished under the colposcope: the flat condyloma, and the florid condyloma.

Flat Condyloma

The flat condyloma, first described by Meisels et al,[21] is usually located in the transformation zone, rarely in the endocervical canal. Its degree of whiteness varies. Limits are ill-defined, blending into surrounding metaplastic epithelium. Vascularization is usually not visible (Figure 11.5). Sometimes, the lesion presents with sharp borders and fine dots on the surface called reverse punctation,[22] a pathognomonic sign for HPV infection (Figure 11.6).

Small spikes with capillary loops disseminated on the surface of acetowhite lesions (Figure 11.7) in the transformation zone are also typical of HPV lesions but can be an early expression of florid condyloma or an initial form of microconvolution (a high-grade lesion in vertical coexistence with a superficial HPV lesion).[24] Taking biopsies of lesions is essential for adequate diagnosis, no matter what the colposcopic clinical impression.

Table 11.1
Colposcopic Terminology

1. Acetowhite epithelium (modification of epithelium after application of 5% acetic acid solution).
   Grade 1: pale, pinkish appearance of underlying stroma still visible
   Grade 2: whiter epithelium, increased thickness
   Grade 3: very opaque, irregular surface

2. Punctation: set of vascular red dots disseminated in acetowhite lesion. Regularity and coarseness vary with severity of lesion.

3. Mosaic: surface vessels arranged in a mosaic pattern. Density and irregularity of epithelial paving vary with grade of lesion.

4. Hyperkeratosis: white epithelial lesion present before acetic acid application representing surface keratin.

5. Abnormal vessels: abnormal forms of surface vessels described as commas, corkscrews, or spaghettilike. These vessels are signs of invasive disease.

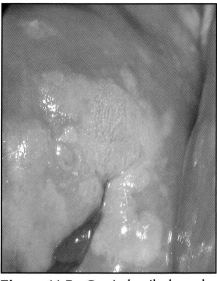

Figure 11.7 Cervical spiked condyloma.

Florid Condyloma

Florid cervical condyloma (Figure 11.8) is occasionally seen in the transformation zone or in the endocervical canal. It is characterized by acetowhite, fingerlike projections, each containing a capillary loop. This lesion is readily seen with the naked eye and is frequently associated with flat acetowhite lesions of low or high grade that are visible with the colposcope (Figure 11.9). Biopsy of surrounding lesions is more important for the expert colposcopist than biopsy of florid lesions since high-grade lesions correlate better with the flat rather than the florid type.

High-Grade Cervical Lesion

The high–grade cervical lesion is located in the transformation zone and is characterized as being of acetowhite Grade 2 or 3 and marked by flat surfaces and sharp geographic contours at the endocervical extremities. Highgrade lesions are thicker than normal metaplastic epithelium.

Vascular patterns, such as punctation or mosaicism, are usually present and are the key to colposcopic diagnostic conclusions (Figure 11.10). Coarseness and irregularity of vascular patterns are signs of severity, while fine and regular patterns can be observed in metaplasia. Heavy and coarse punctation with raising over the surface is often seen in severe forms. With increased severity, mosaicism becomes irregular with coarse and irregular vessels, while epithelial paving appears raised over vascularity.

Biopsy must be directed towards these vascular abnormalities, since abnormal vessels shaped like commas, or spaghettilike or irregular branching in a lesion with an irregular surface frequently reveal microinvasion (Figure 11.11).

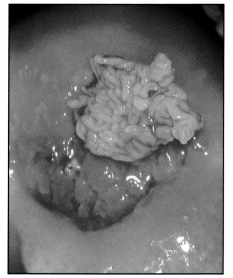

Figure 11.8 Florid cervical condyloma.

High-Grade Lesion with HPV

The high-grade lesion with HPV is colposcopically similar to the one without HPV; minor differences include fine spikes on the surface and variable shades of white. Morin et al[24] recently described a rare lesion of this type: convoluted, acetowhite, well-circumscribed (Figure 11.12). The microconvolutions resembled the surface of the brain and histology demonstrated a typical flat condyloma on the surface with vertical coexistence of high-grade lesion in the lower strata of the epithelium.

On the cervix, this lesion is located in the transformation zone and is sharply distinguished from normal metaplastic epithelium. It is frequently in the neighborhood of either a flat condyloma or a high-grade lesion and can represent a transient form of the disease process in which early gene function and late gene expression of the viral genome are markedly manifested. We have seen convolution spontaneously regress without the disappearance of the acetowhite, high-grade lesion, and transformation of a flat lesion to a convoluted state, in 2 to 3 months of observation.

Triaging and Management

Following colposcopic evaluation, ECC, Schiller's test, and directed punch biopsy, separate patients with abnormal cytology into three major triage groups:

1. Normal colposcopic findings.
2. Abnormal colposcopic findings.
3. Unsatisfactory colposcopic findings.

Normal Colposcopic Findings

With increased transmission of mass media information on sexually transmitted disease (STD), patients are more informed about the possible link between HPV and cervical carcinogenesis. Now aware of the possibility of investigating abnormal Pap tests by colposcopy, they do not want to wait 6 months for a repeat smear when they learn from their practitioner that abnormal cells were detected in their cervico-vaginal routine sampling. Fear of contagious disease and fear of cancer are both very strong motivators in industrialized countries for early colposcopic referral. Many such patients with minimal cytologic atypia, on initial colposcopic evaluation, will demonstrate no lesion, a normal transformation zone, a negative ECC, and a normal Schiller's test.

Those patients with persistent cytologic alterations and normal colposcopic findings should be followed with repeat cytology and repeat colposcopy every 6 months until both return to normal or until a change in triage occurs. Many patients in this group demonstrate koilocytotic cytologic changes corresponding to low-grade intraepithelial lesions, suggesting HPV-infected cells without clin-

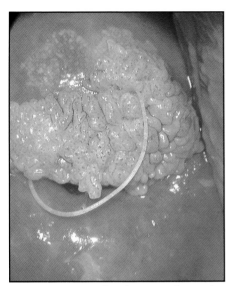

Figure 11.9 Florid cervical condyloma with associated high-grade intraepithelial lesion and string of IUD.

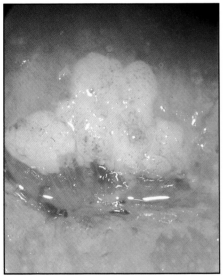

Figure 11.10 High-grade intraepithelial lesion of cervix.

ical evidence of disease. These patients are considered HPV carriers and are at risk of developing subsequently overt HPV lesions or high-grade lesions;[23] close followup of this high-risk group is recommended. Investigation of the male partner is strongly encouraged because detection and treatment of subclinical HPV infection in men may be important for the prevention of genital cancer in women.[30]

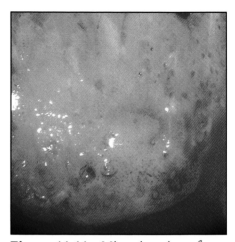

Figure 11.11 Micro invasion of cervix.

Abnormal Colposcopic Findings

Satisfactory colposcopy is obtained by adequate visualization of the entire transformation zone. When invasive disease is ruled out by multiple histologic samplings representative of the most severe areas associated with negative ECC, there is little place for aggressive surgical treatment, such as hysterectomy. Low- and high-grade intraepithelial lesions, associated or not with HPV, should be managed conservatively, by local destructive methods[19] such as cryosurgery, electrocautery, electrodiathermy, or CO_2 laser vaporization.

Controversy surrounds the pertinence of treating low-grade lesions. Some clinicians argue that cervical treatment for this benign lesion, which rarely transforms into malignancy, will not eradicate latent HPV[8] known to exist in proximal tissue and that many lesions regress spontaneously. They advocate observation of these HPV type 6 or type 11 lesions with repeat cytology and colposcopy every 6 months. However, most patients are reluctant to defer treatment of an existing, contagious lesion; reluctance of physicians to repeat colposcopic evaluation and their fears of progression to a more serious state also play a role in the therapeutic decision. Oncogenic HPV types 16 and 18 are occasionally associated with these low-grade lesions[38] and can explain their progression to high-grade lesions.[4,21] Locally destructive methods are simple, well tolerated, and highly effective in eradicating low-grade lesions. Our own approach consists of destroying all colposcopically visible intraepithelial lesions.

We recommend followup every 6 months for the first year, consisting of complete colposcopic assessment. After two negative evaluations, patients are followed by routine cytology every 6 months for 2 years, then yearly thereafter. Abnormal cytology on followup requires a new colposcopic workup.

Cryosurgery

Cryosurgery has been used extensively for the past 30 years for the destruction of intraepithelial cervical lesions, with a mean primary treatment cure rate of 85% to 95% for high-grade lesions.[2,12,29,35] Cellular death is achieved by reducing tissue temperature to a $-20\,^\circ C$ for more than 1 minute. The mechanism of action implies extracellular and intracellular water crystallization with dehydration leading to necrosis.

To be eligible for cryosurgery, patients must fulfill the following criteria:

1. They must have received an adequate colposcopic evaluation and

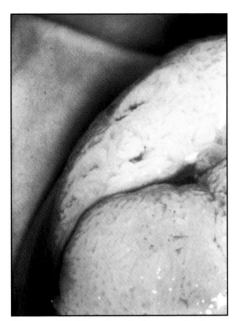

Figure 11.12 Cervical convolutions.

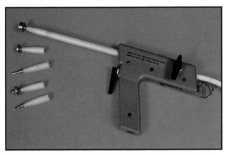

Figure 11.13 Cryogun with interchangeable cryoprobes.

histologic confirmation of the intraepithelial nature of the disease.

2. The entire surface of the lesion should be visible and the lesion confined to the visible portion of the transformation zone.

Although lesions extending far on the ectocervix or onto vaginal fornices may be treated by multiple cryoprobe applications, CO_2 laser vaporization is preferable.

An interchangeable cryoprobe on a cryogun (Figure 11.13) using carbon dioxide (CO_2) or nitrous oxide (N_2O) as a refrigerant is chosen according to the configuration and extension of the lesion (not the grade) and is applied on the cervix. Single[36] and double freeze[11] (freeze, thaw, refreeze) techniques have been used with equally good results. Treatment duration is related to the size of the lesion and is not an important factor for efficacy. Extension of the iceball 7 mm beyond the limits of the lesion is the single most important factor for success.[14] Freezing the endocervical canal is important if the new squamocolumnar junction extends 1 or 2 mm into the canal. This step, in our experience, has not resulted in impaired fertility secondary to cervical stenosis, and followup evaluation is satisfactory in most cases.

As refrigerants, CO_2 or N_2O are equally good. But in our center, after using N_2O for 5 years, we switched to CO_2 after being advised by our anesthetist colleagues that working in areas contaminated by unacceptable amounts of N_2O particles could lead to serious long-term health effects. Air measurements in the colposcopy room after cryosurgery confirmed that the atmosphere was polluted. Therefore, we suggest particular attention be paid to adequate room ventilation when N_2O is used. Measurements should be performed and compared with accepted standards (National Institute for Occupational Safety and Health).

Cervical cryosurgery is a well-tolerated intervention, performed without anesthesia as an outpatient procedure at very low cost. Watery discharge tinged with blood that may persist for 2 to 3 weeks is the most common complaint. Patients are asked to avoid use of tampons and to refrain from intercourse during this period. Serious complications, such as late hemorrhage (after 5–7 days) or infection, are rare and can be prevented by screening and treatment of any concomitant STD at the initial visit. Asymptomatic chlamydial endocervicitis is encountered in 10% of our colposcopy population.

Electrocautery

In Australia, Chanen, Hollyock, and Rome[6,7] have used this method of heat destruction extensively as an outpatient procedure under general anesthesia with a primary cure rate of 95%. Cartier,[5] in France, has proposed complete excision of the transformation zone by use of a diathermic loop allowing complete cervical histologic sampling, achieving at the same time a therapeutic effect. Despite these good results, these electrocautery techniques are not currently much in use in North America.

CO_2 Laser Surgery

With the development of light amplification by stimulated emission of radiation (laser) by Maiman in 1960, a new era of technology emerged, prompting the development of a CO_2 laser instrument (Figure 11.14) that produces parallel beams of light (photons) of a uniform wave length (10.6 μm). At this wave length, light energy is absorbed by water within the cells, thereby causing instant boiling and explosion of the cell walls. The CO_2 laser can vaporize or excise tissue with great precision under colposcopic guidance. The availability of such a precise instrument offers more options in approaching individual lesions.

The laser procedure is done on an outpatient basis without anesthesia in most cases and is rarely associated with serious complications. The most frequent complication reported is late hemorrhage, which usually responds to local measures.

Three types of laser procedures have been described by Wright,[39] selection of which depends on the extent and location of the lesion: the vaporization procedure for a cylindrical dome-shaped defect on an ectocervical lesion, the cylindrical excisional procedure for an endocervical lesion, and the combined procedures for extensive disease.

Results of CO_2 laser surgery are somewhat better than cryosurgery, with primary cure rates of nearly 95% in most series.[33,37,39] The advantage of laser therapy over cryotherapy is its versatility, which permits treatment of both endocervical and ectocervical lesions and scanty post-treatment discharge. It is also the best therapeutic modality for vaginal and vulvar intraepithelial neoplasia.

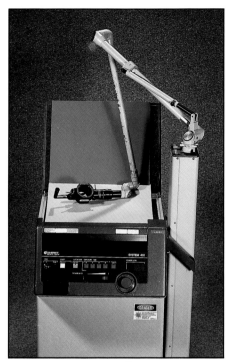

Figure 11.14 CO_2 laser instrument.

Unsatisfactory Colposcopic Findings

When the cytology is abnormal and the transformation zone can not be completely visualized, the colposcopy is unsatisfactory. Invasion must be ruled out to ascertain the nature of the abnormality. Endocervical curettage is performed on all patients and if negative, patients can be closely monitored by repeat cytology, colposcopy, and ECC every 4 months as long as no evidence of malignancy appears on cytologic or histologic analysis. If it does appear, conization is mandatory.

If ECC is positive, diagnostic cervical conization must be performed; this procedure is therapeutic for preinvasive states. Invasion, if revealed by the cone specimen, should be treated according to the stage of disease.

Unsatisfactory colposcopic evaluation represents 10%–15% of total colposcopic exams and is frequently associated with atrophy of the lower genital tract. Correction of atrophy prior to colposcopic evaluation by estrogen replacement for 3 weeks helps to alleviate this condition.

Conization and Hysterectomy

Since Lisfranc reported treating cervical cancer by conization in 1815, this excisional technique has evolved along with knowledge

Table 11.2

Indications for Conization

1. Incomplete colposcopic visualization of transformation zone.
2. Apex of lesion in endocervical canal impossible to assess histologically.
3. Discrepancies in cytologic colposcopic, and histologic reports.
4. Microinvasion on histology.
5. Positive endocervical curettage.
6. Adenocarcinoma of cervix.
7. Persistent disease after repeated conservative therapy.

of cervical pathology and modern technological developments like the laser.

In its early days, conization was performed routinely on all patients presenting with a history of persistent abnormal cytology on smears and was used as a diagnostic tool (hysterectomy being the therapy of choice for intraepithelial disease). With development of colposcopy, the new method for confident evaluation of cervical pathology has resulted in more conservative management, even of patients with abnormal smear cytology, significantly reducing the need for conization.

Studies have consistently shown that the cure and recurrence rates for cervical intraepithelial lesions are the same whether such lesions are treated by hysterectomy or by conservative methods.[15] However, diagnostic conization with the aim of eradicating the lesion is still required for 10%–15% of patients, including those whose lesions have not responded to conservative therapy. Table 11.2 summarizes the indications for this procedure.

Conization is generally indicated when invasive disease has not been completely ruled out by colposcopic workup. Preinvasive disease is cured by this operation, but invasive disease requires more radical therapy. Conization is an out-patient procedure that uses epidural or general anesthesia with the cold knife technique, or preferably, a CO_2 laser. In our center, all cone specimens are obtained using a 30 watt CO_2 laser instrument. The advantages of laser are: the precision of the colposcopic guidance, the bloodless field, the quality of the pathologic specimen, and, in most cases, good healing, resulting in adequate visualization of the squamocolumnar junction on followup. In addition, fertility is not impaired.

The specimen obtained by laser excision is cylindrical rather than cone shaped and the volume of cervical tissue excised by this method is less than that obtained by the cold knife technique. Most specimens include the cervical canal and measure 10–15 mm in length with a mean diameter of 6 mm. Distal positive margins are best treated by laser vaporization at the same session. Positive proximal margins on histology are found in 5% to 10% of cases; therefore, close followup of patients is mandatory. In our experience, most patients with positive endocervical margins will remain free of disease on repeat cytology, colposcopy, and ECC. This can be explained by endocervical reaction to regeneration or by laser vaporization of the cervical bed for hemostatic purposes after excision. Cylindrical endocervical laser excision has a low complication rate. Late hemorrhage, infection, and cervical stenosis can occur but are rare in our experience.

Hysterectomy is not considered the definitive treatment anymore for intraepithelial lesions of the cervix. This radical approach is justified for associated gynecologic conditions, such as fibroids, symptomatic menorrhagia, or genital prolapse, that require a definitive treatment. Persistent intraepithelial lesions after conization in a patient who does not wish to maintain fertility is another indication. Followup of patients by annual cytology after hysterectomy is important because some are at risk for developing vaginal intraepithelial lesions.[3]

Abnormal Cytology and Pregnancy

Abnormal cytology during pregnancy requires colposcopic evaluation as soon as it is detected. Physiologic cervical alterations in pregnant women have been studied by Coppleson and Reid[10] and Singer.[31] With increased hormonal production, eversion of glandular epithelium from the endocervical canal occurs, facilitating colposcopic visualization of the entire transformation zone.

Colposcopic protocol for diagnosis remains the same as for the nonpregnant patient.[13,18] Endocervical curettage is omitted for obvious reasons; treatment of premalignant disease differs in the last 2 months of pregnancy. Unsatisfactory colposcopy with malignant cells on cytology or suspicion of stromal invasion upon colposcopy or histology requires conization, regardless of the stage of pregnancy. Treatment of frank invasion, however, varies according to the stage of disease and the stage of the pregnancy. Microinvasion on the cone specimen does not require termination of pregnancy or caesarean section. Colposcopic revaluation should be repeated every 8 weeks.

References

1. Barron BA, Richart RM: A statistical model of the natural history of cervical carcinoma based on a prospective study of 557 cases. *J Natl Cancer Inst* 41:1343–1353, 1968.

2. Bryson SCP, Lenehan P, Lickrish GM: The treatment of grade 3 cervical intraepithelial neoplasia with cryosurgery: An 11-year experience. *Am J Obstet Gynecol* 151:201–206, 1985.

3. Burghardt E, Holzer E: Treatment of carcinoma in situ; Evaluation of 1609 cases. *Obstet Gynecol* 55:539–545, 1980.

4. Campion MJ, McCance DJ, Cezick J, et al: Progressive potential of mild cervical atypia: Prospective cytological and virological study. *Lancet* 2:237–240, 1986.

5. Cartier R: Colposcopie pratique. S. Karger ed., Suisse, 1977.

6. Chanen W, Hollyock VE: Colposcopy and electrocoagulation diathermy for cervical dysplasia and carcinoma in situ. *Obstet Gynecol* 37:623–628, 1971.

7. Chanen W, Rome RM: Electrocoagulation diathermy for cervical dysplasia and carcinoma in situ: A 15-year survey. *Obstet Gynecol* 61:673–679, 1983.

8. Colgan TJ, Percy ME, Suri M, Shier RM, Andrews DF, Lickrish GM: Human papillomavirus infection of morphologically normal cervical epithelium adjacent to squamous dysplasia and invasive carcinoma. *Hum Pathol* 20:316–319, 1989.

9. Coppleson M: The use of colposcopy in the early detection of carcinoma of the cervix. *Med J Aust* 46:64, 1959.

10. Coppleson M, Reid B: A colposcopic study of the cervix during pregnancy and the puerperium. *J Obstet Gynaecol Br Cmwl* 73:575–585, 1966.

11. Creasman WT, Clarke-Pearson DL, Weed JC Jr: Results of outpatient

therapy of cervical intraepithelial neoplasia. *Gynecol Oncol* 12:s306–s316, 1981.

12. Creasman WT, Wheed JC Jr, Curry SL, Johnston WW, Parker RI: Efficacy of cryosurgical treatment of severe cervical intraepithelial neoplasia. *Obstet Gynecol* 41:501–506, 1973.

13. De Petrillo AD, Townsend DE, Morrow CP, et al: Colposcopic evaluation of the abnormal Papanicolaou test in pregnancy. *Am J Obstet Gynecol* 121:441–445, 1975.

14. Ferenczy A: Comparison of cryo- and carbon dioxide laser therapy for cervical intraepithelial neoplasia. *Obstet Gynecol* 66:793–798, 1985.

15. Fraser R: Hysterectomy for cervical intraepithelial neoplasia. p. 197–200. In: Basic and advanced colposcopy. Wright VC, Lickrish GM, eds. Biomedical Communications, 1989.

16. Gissmann L: Linking HPV to cancer. *Clin. Obstet Gynecol* 32:141–147, 1989.

17. Hinselmann H: Verbesserung der inspektionsmoglichkeit von vulva, vagina und portio. *Munch Med Wochenschr*, 77:1733, 1925.

18. Kohan S, Beckman EM, Bigelow B, Klein SA, Douglas, GL: The role of colposcopy in the management of cervical intraepithelial neoplasia during pregnancy and postpartum. *J Reprod Med* 25:279–284, 1980.

19. Luesley D, Cullimore J: The treatment of cervical intraepithelial neoplasia. *Cancer Surv* 7:529–545, 1988.

20. Meisels A: Are two smears better than one? *Acta Cytol* 34:459–480, 1990.

21. Meisels A, Fortin R, Roy M: Condylomatous lesions of the cervix. II. Cytologic, colposcopic and histopathologic study. *Acta Cytol* 21:379–390, 1977.

22. Meisels A, Roy M, Fortier M, Morin C: Condylomatous lesions of the cervix. Morphologic and colposcopic diagnosis. *Am J Diagn Gynecol Obstet* 1:109–116, 1979.

23. Mitchell H, Drake M, Medley G: Prospective evaluation of risk of cervical cancer after cytologic evidence of human papillomaviral infection. *Lancet* 1:573–575, 1986.

24. Morin C, Bouchard C, Fortier M, Levesque R, Meisels A: A colposcopical lesion of the uterine cervix frequently associated with papillomavirus type 16 as detected by in situ and southern blot hybridization: A cytohistological correlation study. *Int J Cancer* 41:531–536, 1988.

25. Nasiell K, Nasiell M, Valcavinkova V: Behavior of moderate cervical dysplasia during long term follow-up. *Obstet Gynecol* 61:609–614, 1983.

26. Reid R, Campion MJ: HPV-associated lesions of the cervix: Biology and colposcopic features. *Clin Obstet Gynecol* 32:157–179, 1989.

27. Reid R, Stanhope CR, Herschman BR, Crum CP, Agronov SJ: Genital warts and cervical cancer. IV. A colposcopic index for differentiating subclinical papillomaviral infection from cervical intraepithelial neoplasia. *Am J Obstet Gynecol* 149:815–823, 1984.

28. Richart RM: Cervical intraepithelial neoplasia. *Pathol Annual* 8:301–328, 1973.

29. Richart RM, Townsend DE, Crisp W, De Petrillo A, Ferenczy A,

Johnson G, Lickrish GM, Roy M, Villa Santa U: An analysis of long term follow-up results in patients with cervical intraepithelial neoplasia treated by cryotherapy. *Am J Obstet Gynecol* 137:823–826, 1980.

30. Schneider A, Kirchmayr R, De Villiers EM, Gissmann L: Subclinical human papillomaviruses infections in male sexual partners of female carriers. *J Urol* 140:1431–1434, 1988.

31. Singer A: The cervical epithelium during pregnancy and the puerperium. In: Jordan JA, Singer A, eds. The cervix. London: W.B. Saunders, 1976.

32. Stafl A: The clinical diagnosis of early cervical cancer. *Obstet Gynecol Survey* 24:976, 1969.

33. Stafl A, Wilkinson EJ, Mattingly RF: Laser treatment of cervical and vaginal neoplasia. *Am J Obstet Gynecol* 128:128–136, 1977.

34. Syrjanen KJ: Current concepts of human papillomavirus infections in the genital tract and their relationship to intraepithelial neoplasia and squamous cell carcinoma. *Obstet Gynecol Survey* 39:252–265, 1984.

35. Tredway DR, Townsend DE, Hovland DN, Upton RT: Colposcopy and cryosurgery in cervical intraepithelial neoplasia. *Am J Obstet Gynecol* 114:1020–1024, 1972.

36. Townsend DE: Cryosurgery for cervical intraepithelial neoplasia. *Obstet Gynecol Survey* 34:838–840, 1979.

37. Townsend DE, Richart RM: Cryotherapy and carbon dioxide laser management of cervical intraepithelial neoplasia. A controlled comparison. *Obstet Gynecol* 61:75–78, 1983.

38. Willett G, Kurman R, Reid R, et al: Correlation of cervical condylomas and intraepithelial neoplasia with human papillomavirus types. *Int J Gynecol Pathol* 7:350, 1986.

39. Wright VC, Davies E, Riopelle MA: Laser surgery for cervical intraepithelial neoplasia: Principles and results. *Am J Obstet Gynecol* 145:181–184, 1983.

40. zur Hausen H: Human papillomaviruses and their possible role in squamous cell carcinomas. *Curr Top Microbiol Immunol* 78:1, 1977.

41. zur Hausen H: Papillomaviruses in human cancer. *Cancer* 59:1692–1696, 1987.

CHAPTER TWELVE

Quality Assurance in Cervical Cytology

The "Pap" smear has achieved its greatest success in the prevention of carcinoma of the cervix through its use in mass screening programs. In spite of the relaxation of sexual mores, which could have produced a notable increase in the incidence of carcinoma of the cervix, there has in fact been a notable decrease in all areas where systematic screening programs are in effect. It is therefore appropriate to discuss here briefly what such screening programs require in order to achieve the expected results.

The effectiveness of mass screening programs depends foremost on the availability of well-trained cytotechnologists and competent cytopathologists. Still, the laboratory must meet certain standards pertaining to: the adequacy of the space available, the quality of the instrumentation (microscopes, etc), the quality of the samples and of the staining technique, the workload of cytotechnologists and cytopathologists, and the quality assurance program. The area must also have adequate facilities for treatment and followup of patients in whom early lesions are detected.

According to the Bethesda System, the Papanicolaou smear is a medical consultation. This means that smears must be ordered by members of the medical profession, and that the specimen collection is performed by the physician, or by duly authorized members of allied health care personnel. The laboratory should provide written instructions concerning collection techniques, and when the specimen is inadequate, steps must be taken to correct faulty collection or fixation techniques. All cytopreparatory techniques and microscopic examinations should be performed on the premises of the laboratory (not at home, and not in a clinician's office).

The training of cytotechnologists has changed considerably since the time when they were trained "on the bench." Today they generally need 2 or 3 years of college with emphasis on the biological sciences before being admitted into the training program, which consists of formal lectures covering all areas of cytopathology, and considerable practical work at the microscope. The duration of the course is usually 1 year. In Canada the students have to spend another year in practical work before they can sit for the national examination, which gives them the right to practice their profession.

Pathologists also need special training in cytology. In many residency training programs, a 3-month period is dedicated to cytology. Considering the scope of the field, and the great difference between histologic and cytologic pathology, this short training is sorely inadequate and should be increased to at least 6 months. The pathology resident should be exposed to the complete realm of cytology, with particular emphasis on fine needle aspirations. The pathologist must assume responsibility for every cytology report, including the cases screened by cytotechnologists.

An excellent quality assurance program is mandatory in the cytology laboratory. In addition to insuring that the cytotechnologists and pathologists are well trained, the program should specify the steps that must be taken to avoid errors, to the extent that is possible. The work space should be clean, adequately ventilated, and properly lighted (Figure 12.1). Each cytotechnologist should have an adjustable chair to avoid fatigue, a good quality and properly maintained binocular microscope with at least one $10\times$ and one $40\times$ objective lens, and $12.5\times$ oculars. The table, microscope, and chair should be adjusted for maximum comfort. The cytopreparatory area should be separated from the microscopic work area and proper precautions should be taken in the handling of fresh (unfixed) specimens. Great care must be exercised to avoid errors in identifying and labelling smears. Staining and other techniques should be standardized and verified regularly.[6]

One of the most controversial questions is the workload of the cytotechnologist: how many slides should be screened by one person per hour, per day, per week, per year? There is no clear-cut answer. The workload should be adjusted to the individual's capacity and experience. Does the cytotechnologist have other duties, in addition to screening, eg, cytopreparation, record keeping, maintenance of computer files? Each situation will differ; however, a general consensus has emerged in the sense that the *maximum* number of slides screened by one cytotechnologist in one year should not exceed 12,000 gynecologic cases, or about 55 cases in any 24-hour period, although a recent group of experts set the maximum at 21,600 gynecologic slides per year, or about 90 slides per 24 hours.[4] Since many laboratories receive more than one slide per case, these recommendations are actually not so different.

Cytoscreening is a very demanding task, requiring complete concentration and attention to minute morphologic detail during many hours at the microscope. An excessive workload produces tension and failing concentration, with consequent errors. Recent articles in the lay media in the United States (including a Pulitzer Prize winning series in the *Wall Street Journal*, November 2, 1987) have criticized the excessive workload of cytotechnologists (more than 40,000 slides per year in some cases) and pathologists in certain large laboratories, which allegedly has been the cause of serious oversights (false-negative reports). Legislation was promptly enacted to remedy this situation.

On the other hand, the total volume of cases examined should be sufficient to expose the cytotechnologist and the pathologist to the full range of lesions that can be readily diagnosed on a smear. The number of smears processed by a small laboratory may be too limited for staff there to remain proficient at reliably recognizing different lesion types. It has been suggested[15] that a cytology laboratory should report on at least 15,000 cases per year in order to remain efficient.

Complete laboratory records must be kept. Cytology slides and copies of reports should be kept for a minimum of 5 years in benign cases, and for at least 20 years if there is evidence of any significant lesion (Figure 12.2).

In the course of a program of quality assurance, a number of slides have to be reviewed or even rescreened. The original screener should refer all slides showing a significant abnormality to a senior screener (Figure 12.3), and to the pathologist in charge (Figure 12.4). Previous benign smears should be reviewed when the current smear indicates the presence of a significant lesion, so that earlier false negative results can be detected. The pathologist in charge should review all current and previous smears of patients in which the clinician has described a suspicious cervical lesion. Finally, a few slides of each batch prepared should be reviewed to evaluate the quality of the collection, fixation and cytopreparatory techniques.

The practice of rescreening about 10% of negative smears, originally recommended by the International Academy of Cytology, has not proven its value in detecting false-negative results and increases considerably the workload of senior cytotechnologists. Rescreening a much smaller random sample of slides examined by each screener in the laboratory does have a significant value in furthering attention to detail and prevention of errors.

It has been suggested that seeding known significant cases into the screening routine may help in evaluating the accuracy of cytotechnologists. This practice has not proven its value because such slides are easily recognized by the screeners. Also, the logistics of keeping the seeded cases out of the normal laboratory files can be quite complicated.

Peer review is another possible tool of quality assurance. Both normal and abnormal smears are exchanged between cooperating laboratories and any differences in diagnosis are then discussed and clarified. In some areas the laboratory licensing bodies have initiated similar programs, in which a number of normal and abnormal slides are sent to each laboratory and the results are used to determine

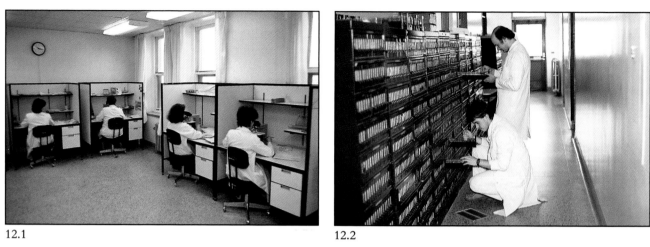

12.1

12.2

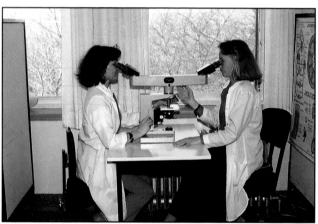

12.3

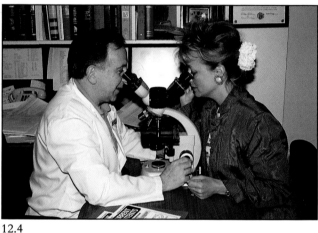

12.4

Figures 12.1–4 (12.1) The work place of cytotechnologists should be well ventilated and lighted. The cubicles installed in our laboratory provide some privacy. Chairs must be adjustable for the most comfortable position.   (12.2) Glass slides must be conserved for a minimum of 5 years for normal cases and for at least 20 years for smears with significant abnormalities. Previous benign slides are retrieved for quality assurance comparisons whenever a current smear presents significant cellular changes.   (12.3) Senior cytotechnologists review slides with other cytotechnologists for quality assurance, but also for continuing education.   (12.4) The pathologist has the final responsibility for the cytologic report. All slides with significant cellular changes, and those obtained from patients with clinically suspicious lesions, are reviewed by the pathologist.

the areas of weakness of any given laboratory, so that specific corrective measures can be initiated.

Proficiency testing has become mandatory in some areas (eg, New York State and Ontario). It has often been regulated by mailing a number of slides several times a year to each laboratory, which in turn must issue a report exactly as if the slides were received from the usual sources: they are screened by cytotechnologists and reviewed by senior cytotechnologists and/or pathologists according to normal procedure. Results are then computed against the diagnoses established by an expert committee.[16] If the laboratory's reports are considered dangerously off-course, remedial action is taken. If the laboratory fails to improve its performance, it may lose its license. The drawback to this system is that it lacks control on how the smears are examined within the laboratory. They may not

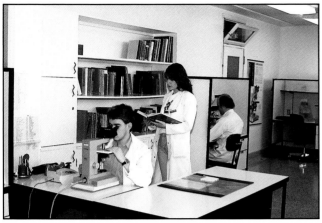

12.5

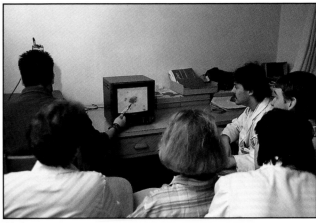

12.6

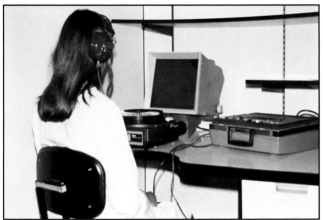

12.7

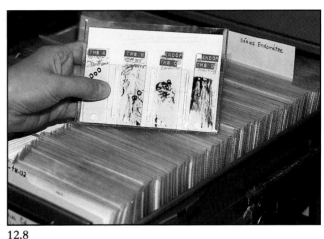

12.8

Figures 12.5–8 Books and specialized journals are as necessary as good microscopes and should be available on the premises for immediate consultation.   (12.6) Continuing education is the responsibility of the pathologist. Regularly scheduled educational sessions help to keep the cytotechnologists and pathologists informed of the latest developments in the ever changing field of diagnostic cytopathology.   (12.7) Audiovisual equipment is a useful tool for continuing education.   (12.8) A collection of study sets of well-identified glass slides should be made available.

be dealt with in a routine manner, but rather be submitted only to senior staff and pathologists for evaluation so as to increase the chance of reaching the right diagnosis.

Proficiency testing can also be done in the laboratory by a visiting team. Slides are presented to each cytotechnologist, who marks any suspicious or malignant cells and refers the case to the pathologist. If no such cells are found, the cytotechnologist reports the case as benign. The passing grade is 90%.[4] If the laboratory fails, it is retested, and if it fails again, remedial action is taken.

One problem with external proficiency testing in cervical cytology is that multiple identical smears are not available. The same set must therefore be circulated among all laboratories for testing to achieve comparable results. When dealing with a large number of laboratories, this may become a logistical nightmare. Although time-consuming and expensive, the visiting team approach offers the best guarantee that tested laboratories are performing good quality cervical cytology.

Followup of all patients whose smears reveal the presence of a significant lesion is one of the most important aspects of quality assurance. The laboratory must take adequate steps to obtain information on the final clinical, or, preferably, histologic diagnosis. A complete review of all slides should be performed when the final result disagrees with the cytologic diagnosis.

Continuing education is an important facet of quality assurance. All involved in the practice of cytology should have the opportunity to attend regional, national or international meetings. An adequate library should be available on the premises of the laboratory, which should include textbooks, monographs, and cytology journals (Figure 12.5). Regular educational sessions should be held in the laboratory (Figure 12.6). Audiovisual products (Figure 12.7) and study slide collections (Figure 12.8) are useful for continuing education. Cytotechnologists should be encouraged to participate actively in these programs. Finally, a recent symposium on quality assurance published in Acta Cytologica[1-3,5,7-14,16] should be consulted as it provides important additional reading.

References

1. Ashton PR: American Society of Cytotechnology quality assurance survey data. Summary report. *Acta Cytol* 33:451–454, 1989.

2. Bonfiglio TA: Quality assurance in cytopathology. Recommendations and ongoing quality assurance activities of the American Society of Clinical Pathologists. *Acta Cytol* 33:431–433, 1989.

3. Collins DN, Patacsil DP: Proficiency testing in cytology in New York. Analysis of a 14-year state program. *Acta Cytol* 30:633–642, 1986.

4. Council on Scientific Affairs (AMA): Quality assurance in cervical cytology. *JAMA* 262:1672–1679, 1989.

5. Gardner NM: In-house quality assurance program in a State cytology laboratory. *Acta Cytol* 33:487–488, 1989.

6. Guidelines for quality assurance programs in cytopathology. Canadian Society of Cytology, February 18, 1989.

7. Gupta PK, Erozan YS: Cytopathology laboratory accreditation, with special reference to the American Society of Cytology programs. *Acta Cytol* 33:443–447, 1989.

8. Kraemer BB: Quality assurance activities of the College of American Pathologists. *Acta Cytol* 33:434–438, 1989.

9. Paris AL: Conference on the state of the art in quality control measures for diagnostic cytology laboratories. Background and introduction. *Acta Cytol* 33:423–426, 1989.

10. Parker JE: Education and training for cytopathologists. Its role in quality assurance. *Acta Cytol* 33:448–450, 1989.

11. Penner DW: An overview of the College of American Pathologists' program in surgical pathology and cytopathology. Data summary of diagnostic performance in cervical cytopathology. *Acta Cytol* 33:439–442, 1989.

12. Rube IF: Experience in managing a large-scale rescreening of Papanicolaou smears and the pros and cons of measuring proficiency with visual and written examinations. *Acta Cytol* 33:479–483, 1989.

13. Solomon D: Introduction to the proceedings of the conference on the state of the art in quality control measures for diagnostic cytology laboratories. *Acta Cytol* 33:427–430, 1989.

14. Steiner C: Cervical cancer screening from the public health perspective. *Acta Cytol* 33:471–474, 1989.

15. Task Force of the Deputy Ministers of Health. Cervical cancer screening programs, II. Screening for carcinoma of the cervix. *Can Med Assoc J* 114:1013–1026, 1976.

16. Thompson DW: Canadian experience in cytology proficiency testing. *Acta Cytol* 33:484–486, 1989.

CHAPTER THIRTEEN

The Computerized Cytopathology Laboratory

George L Wied, MD, FIAC
Harvey E Dytch, PMIAC

Computerization of Routine Laboratory Functions

Computerization of the operation of the routine laboratory is a foregone conclusion: it may be expected that, at least in the United States, Canada, Japan, Sweden, and other developed countries, no laboratory will be operated in the 1990s without computerized systems of data entry, data retrieval, and quality assurance.

At the University of Chicago, computerization of record keeping was initiated in 1959. There are over two million patient records in an on-line computer file available for practically instant retrieval of cytologic, histologic, anamnestic, and therapeutic data.[87,88] Originally, we used an IBM system for the file, translated it to a laboratory-owned PDP-10 (Digital Equipment) computer, followed by another translation to a UNISYS mainframe computer, and eventually back to a laboratory-owned microcomputer (a 25 MHz desktop system, with two 650 MB internal disks, and a 150 MB tape drive for data backup, with a custom program (Interactive Consulting Group, Oswego, IL 60643).

When our cytotechnologists examine a cytologic sample, they have a printout of all previous data on any given patient (in our case as far back as 1959) at their microscopes. Long-term experience with the computerized cytopathology and histopathology file and its operation has persuaded us that centralized major hospital or universitywide systems are uneconomical, inefficient, and unable to

Patient Name: Winter, Catherine C.
Unit No: 333356
Address: 1760 East 50th Place
        Chicago, IL 60615, U.S.A.
Referring MD: Dr. Joseph V. Meig
Specimen was taken in: OPD 2
Date taken: 07/01/89
Date received: 07/01/89
Date reported: 07/02/89
Lab No: V-89-54501
Attending cytopathologist(s): Marluce Bibbo, MD
                              Shelly B. Underhill, MD

The specimen is a VCE smear. The specimen was satisfactory. The epithelial cells were not within normal limits. The cytologic sample exhibits the following microbiologic entities: mixed bacteria. The squamous cell material indicates the presence of invasive squamous carcinoma. Since this is a VCE sample, the present atypia appears mostly in the ectocervix. The hormonal evaluation is not possible due to inflammatory reaction. The following further action on this patient is suggested: repeat smear, colposcopy, and histologic verification. The present lesion is a well differentiated, keratinizing squamous carcinoma.

SAMPLE QUALITY: The specimen was satisfactory.

GENERAL CLASSIFICATION: The epithelial cells were not within normal limits.

SUMMARY DIAGNOSIS: The squamous cell material indicates the presence of invasive squamous carcinoma.

RECOMMENDATION: Immediate histologic verification.

                              Shelly B. Underhill, M.D.
                              Marluce Bibbo, M.D.

Figures 13.1–13.3 Sample output from TBS CLASSVEE program: the diagnostic interpretation is entered from menu displays and translated into a written report.

meet the needs of cytology and histopathology laboratories for on-line availability of large amounts of archival data. Microcomputer systems that are laboratory-owned and -operated decentralize the procedure and are the on-line systems of the future. Microcomputers are relatively inexpensive, and simple to program and interrogate for data retrieval. Admittedly, extensive multivariate analyses will take longer to run on a microcomputer than on a mainframe system. However, such analyses are not required on a daily basis and can be run automatically as a batch-processing operation after the business day or even overnight.

Diagnostic data and patient information are entered into a microcomputer system. For gynecologic cytology reports we are using a computerized version of The Bethesda System (TBS)[68] (designed using a data management system, PARADOX3 by Borland International) for ease of customization of input and output of data. The diagnostic entities are displayed on a CRT in menu form from which the system creates natural English language sentences, although the

Patient Name: Smith, Mary L.
Unit No: 123456
Address: 1234 South State Street
         Chicago, IL 60637, U.S.A.
Referring MD: Dr. John X. Miller
Specimen was taken in: Gyn. Office
Date taken: 07/01/89
Date received: 07/01/89
Date reported: 07/02/89
Lab No: V-89-54321
Attending cytopathologist(s): Shelly B. Underhill, MD

The specimen is a VCE smear. The specimen was satisfactory. The epithelial cells were within normal limits. The cytologic sample exhibits the following microbiologic entities: healthy flora. The glandular epithelial cell material shows presence of endometrial cells in a post-menopausal woman. The hormonal evaluation is compatible with age and history.

SAMPLE QUALITY: The specimen was satisfactory.

GENERAL CLASSIFICATION: The epithelial cells were within normal limits.

SUMMARY DIAGNOSIS: The glandular epithelial cell material shows presence of endometrial cells in a post-menopausal woman.

RECOMMENDATION: Perform Cytobrush sample of endocervix or intrauterine aspirate to exclude glandular atypia.

Shelly B. Underhill, M.D.

Figure 13.2

data are entered as codes. Sample outputs follow (Figures 13.1 through 13.3). The last section of the chapter contains an operational explanation of the computerized Bethesda System (called CLASSVEE) that was developed at the University of Chicago.

The laboratory file system should be on-line and should permit cross referencing of data in a multiparameter query system, so that one may also ascertain for statistical or quality assurance purposes which recommended procedure (repeat smear, biopsy, colposcopic examination, etc) was performed and in what time span, and which clinicians responded expeditiously, who did not respond at all, or who reacted unduly slowly. This kind of system is also useful for providing comparative spreadsheet reports to the hospital administration on past, present, and projected future laboratory performance, and for billing. For scientific analyses, determinations may be made to assess intervals of possible progression from a low-grade alteration (slight dysplasia) to an invasive lesion. Cytometric and histometric data may be attached to a given patient record so that prospective and retrospective analyses are relatively easy to perform.

To acquaint the laboratory staff with the use of microcomputers, it is best to first discontinue the use of typewriters and replace them with word processors. We use Microsoft Word (Version 5) for word processing and Lotus 1-2-3 (Versions 2.2 and 3) for spreadsheets. Some of our word processors are connected to laser printers and

Patient Name: Summer, Anne J.
Unit No: 123478
Address: 4321 North Hollywood Avenue
            Chicago, IL 60611, U.S.A.
Referring MD: Dr. Harry Huerthle
Specimen was taken in: NW Ward 23
Date taken: 07/01/89
Date received: 07/01/89
Date reported: 07/02/89
Lab No: V-89-54666
Attending cytopathologist(s): Anthony G. Montag, MD

The specimen is a VCE smear and a Cytobrush sample. Due to less than optimal adequacy of the sample, the following cytologic interpretation may be equivocal. It was less than optimal due to poor fixation or preservation. The epithelial cells were not within normal limits. The cytologic sample exhibits the following microbiologic entities: Trichomonas sp., and mixed bacteria. There are reactive or reparative changes present, apparently due to inflammation. The squamous cell material indicates the presence of slight atypia of undetermined significance. Since this is a VCE sample, the present atypia appears mostly in the vagina, and the ectocervix. The hormonal evaluation is not possible due to inflammatory reaction. The following further action on this patient is suggested: repeat smear after therapy. The present squamoid atypia warrant repeated cell study after trichomoniasis therapy to assess source of cell changes.

SAMPLE QUALITY: The specimen was less than optimal.

GENERAL CLASSIFICATION: The epithelial cells were not within normal limits.

SUMMARY DIAGNOSIS: The squamous cell material indicates the presence of slight atypia of undetermined significance.

RECOMMENDATION: Repeat after trichomoniasis therapy.

Anthony G. Montag, M.D.

Figure 13.3

some to impact printers, so multisheet forms can be printed via a preprogrammed form-feeding system. Interlaboratory communication and communication with the hospital wards, clinics, and hospitals and outreach programs in cities other than Chicago, as well as with our University administrative offices concerning reports and requests, is by laser G3 or G4 FAXphones that print the output on regular paper.

Quantitative and Analytical Cytology Techniques

In 1924, Feulgen and Rossenbach[44] described the stain that subsequently proved to be specific for double-stranded DNA. In the 1930s, Caspersson and his group[30] measured fluorescence intensity and distribution of DNA, RNA, and proteins in individual cells and documented some principal differences between benign and malignant cells. In the 1950s, Mellors,[66,67] at the Sloan Kettering Institute, applied Caspersson's concepts to the study of exfoliated human cells, using the fluorochrome berberin sulphate, and observed measurable differences of fluorescence between benign cells and cancer cells. Niels Atkin was the initiator of studies using cytophotometry on tumors of the female genital tract and of the breast.[3-5]

Modern instruments use either static image analysis systems to measure cell components in smears,[8,9,24,26,60-62,72,85,86,100,101,104] or flow cytometry systems that use a suspension of single cells or cell nuclei.[7-9,10,55] Analytical and quantitative cytology has two basic purposes: (1) to gather information of prognostic and therapeutic value, and (2) to design systems or machines that will identify subvisual cellular criteria or complement the human eye in the performance of tedious and not easily reproducible objectives.

Flow cytometry provides useful information on DNA content only when rigid criteria for the flow cytometer's performance and for interpretation of data are maintained. A cooperative study by five experienced laboratories demonstrated that maintaining such criteria is not a trivial task.[31] Since practically all tumor cell suspensions analyzed by flow cytometry contains both normal and tumor cells, problems are encountered in detecting tetraploid tumors in lesions of the breast, the ovaries, and the colon.[2,10,47] The methodologic difficulties in detecting tetraploidy by flow cytometry may be responsible for the controversy concerning the prognosis of tetraploid lesions. The introduction of paraffin-embedded material by Hedley et al[50] seemed to initiate a new vista for flow cytometry. However, subsequent investigations by several authors, among them Berlinger,[19] Cornelisse et al,[33] Frierson,[47] and Jacobson,[54] demonstrated that paraffin-embedded yields different flow cytometric results from fresh material. Also, rather high coefficients of variation were shown on paraffin-embedded material by deVere,[35] Cornelisse,[33] Quirke,[74] and Wils.[110] Tumors with near-diploid stemlines may be classified as diploid because of the low resolution. This classification may be of critical prognostic importance, since Iversen[52,53] showed on ovarian lesions that some of these near-diploid tumors have the same poor prognosis as aneuploid tumors.

Image cytometry and flow cytometry each offer certain advantages and disadvantages. For many objectives the simultaneous use of both methods is proposed.[60,61,64,65] The two techniques are compared in Table 13.1.

Most of the information gathered on human cancer is retrospective, based on an analysis of archived material, be it aspiration smears or tissue blocks. DNA measurements can be used to divide human cancer into three groups: The first group is tumors wherein the DNA measurements appear to be of significant value. A good example is the epithelial tumors of the bladder, wherein the diploid pattern corresponds to low-grade papillary tumors and the aneuploid DNA pattern to high-grade tumors and to flat carcinoma in situ, which is the source of most invasive bladder cancers. The DNA measurements are of help in discriminating between bladder tumors

Table 13.1
Comparison of Flow Cytometry with Cell Image Analysis

Features	Low-Resolution Flow Cytometry	High-Resolution Cell Image Analysis
Personnel requirements	Special training required	Standard cytotechnology training
Sample preparation	Specially prepared complex single cell suspension	Existing, routine smear
Staining	Specific fluorochromes	Routine (Pap) or stoichiometric
Number of cells required	Tens of thousands, minimum	A few hundred, minimum
Cytometric features		
DNA content	Yes	Yes
Size	Yes	Yes
Shape	No	Yes
Texture	No	Yes
Color	No	Yes
Principal single parameter	Histograms of fluorescence (DNA content)	Histograms of digitized images based on light absorption or emission (DNA, steroid receptors)
Two or more parameter measurements	Synchronous, limited (DNA vs oncogenes)	Synchronous or sequential
Visual control during measurement	None	Yes
Sorting	With sophisticated sorter only (after measurement)	Electronic sorting or selective scanning (selective enrichment)
Re-examination by reviewer of archived examined material	Impossible	Simple
Specimen retention as permanent record	Impossible	Simple
Comparative analyses of the same cells stained with two reactions (eg, Papanicolaou and Feulgen)	Impossible	Simple with motorized stage
Usefulness for histologic samples	Limited	Yes

of intermediate grade, which are about equally divided into diploid and aneuploid groups, with some evidence, mainly provided by Tribukait,[82,83] that DNA patterns may be translated into behavioral differences. Another example is carcinoma of the prostate, wherein Koss et al[63,64] could show in prospective and retrospective studies that tumors in the diploid range of DNA are much less likely to be aggressive than aneuploid tumors. DNA measurements are therefore of benefit in this case. It must be stressed that even in this group of tumors there are exceptions to the rule.[65]

In the second group of human cancers, the value of DNA measurements is contradictory and must be considered unproven as an independent criterion. Carcinomas of the breast, colon, kidney, and endometrium, and other common cancers belong here. Long-term prospective studies are still needed to shed some light on the clinical usefulness of DNA measurements in tumors derived from these sites.

Finally, there is a group of human cancers wherein the DNA measurements are not of prognostic value (chiefly the tumors of the thyroid gland).[48,65]

While, theoretically, DNA ploidy of human cancers should fall into two distinct categories, diploid and aneuploid, in reality there are a great many problems of histogram interpretation.[65] These problems became apparent in a large prospective study of benign colonic mucosa as a baseline study of colonic cancer.[84] While 75% of the histograms disclosed an approximately diploid pattern corresponding to normal lymphocytes, 25% of the histograms displayed significant variations in the position of the diploid peak. High-resolution cell image analysis can be effectively used in the quantization of estrogen and progestogen receptors.[6,27,28,32,45,46]

Quantitative cytology provides the ability to make objective cellular evaluations. DNA measurements are an important parameter, although not the only useful one, in this endeavor. In addition to visual so-called "global descriptors," such as cell size, shape, color, nuclear size, shape, density, etc, there are significant subvisual features. In the near future, a multitude of unresolved fundamental problems will have to be addressed. There need to be agreements on standards for sample preparation and fixation and staining (including purity of dyes, nature of solvents, the pH, temperature of staining baths, image recording, microphotometric quality, data collection and representation, type and numbers of reference cells, the hydrolysis procedure, if any, etc).

The International Academy of Cytology (IAC) established the Task Force on Quantization and Standardization, which attempts to arrive at internationally acceptable standards on many of these fundamental problems. Assuming that such standards can be established, quantitative and analytical cytology may eventually represent *the* technique to arrive at a reproducible and reliable diagnostic interpretation, and finally at the biologic or diagnostic truth.

Automated Screening

The examination of cells is a subjective procedure, dependent on the skill and expertise of the observer as well as the time devoted to reviewing the slide. As such, it is fallible. No accurate, cost-effective automated system exists which provides an objective analysis of the sample like that available from the clinical hematology laboratory.

Historically, the two major approaches to automating cytologic screening have been (1) high-resolution cell image analysis (Cytoanalyzer[81]) and (2) flow through cell analysis (Kamentsky[55]). Flow cytometry to screen for early detection of ectocervical, endocervical, and intrauterine lesions is undoubtedly an inefficient, uneconomical experiment on the wrong anatomic site. It was a failure when it was conceived by Kamentsky,[55] Koenig et al[57] showed, and has continued to be a dismal failure ever since. If either fully automated or interactive diagnostic computerization is ever used and practically applied to screen cytomorphologically for uterine lesions, it will be by high-resolution cell image analysis.

The effort to use the Cytoanalyzer to automate the diagnosis of cervical smears also collapsed a few years later, and Prewitt and

Mendelsohn[71] used the modified Cytoanalyzer, then called CYDAC, for an image analysis system to classify leukocytes. Subsequently, we developed the TICAS system to analyze cells in cervical smears.[90,92,94-104] Among the important design goals of TICAS and similar systems was to standardize visible and subvisual diagnostic cell features.[11-15,20,21,23,25,37,39-41,56,58,59,75,102] The introduction of computerized cell image analysis of the vaginal/cervical cell sample by the TICAS method was followed by many more or less futile attempts to introduce full automation of the gynecologic cell evaluation in Germany, Great Britain, Holland, Japan, Sweden, and the United States.[29,62,73,78-80,89,91,93,95]

The idea was to automate a rather tedious screening job by a device that would not only be more accurate than cytotechnologists, but would fully screen the entire slide and provide reproducible results quickly and in an economic fashion.

Why then are we not developing a fully automated high-resolution scanning system for gynecologic material? Why have so many attempts failed? The answers are relatively straightforward:

1. A fully automated device requires a monolayer of cells, which means that the material has to be put first in suspension and then placed with a rather sophisticated system[7] on a glass slide. This is time-consuming for the clinician and the laboratory. Such a complex front end existed—probably the only one in actual operation—for the Japanese CYBEST[79,80] System of Toshiba. Toshiba discontinued their entire automation effort in 1986.

2. The clinician expects the cytologic reading to provide information regarding vaginal microbiology, degree and type of infection (eg, HPV, trichomoniasis, herpes, etc), site of infection, hormonal classification, and identification of precursors of squamous and glandular cell lesions. The clinician definitely expects more than only "squamous cancer present" or "no squamous tumor cells found." The computerized recognition of an actual malignant squamous tumor cell is a *trivial* computer recognition routine. This has lead some bioengineers to believe that the entire task of fully automating diagnostic cytology is that simple. In fact, no automated system was or is being programed to discern microbiologic entities or effects of HPV infection, or to clearly identify present well-differentiated adenocarcinoma cells or to classify precursors. However, the main goal of a screening system is to *identify the precursors*, and *not* the frankly malignant tumor cells.

3. The sample's quality has to be classified as "adequate," "inadequate," or "less than optimal." In fact, in 1968, the Vickers Company in the UK announced with great pride, in a cytology conference in Cardiff, Wales, the completion of an automated screening instrument that was so ill-conceived that it could not even tell if there were or were not cells in the sample. It was thus an utter medicolegal monstrosity.[93] The human observer can readily distinguish an adequate sample from an inadequate

or less than optimal sample. However, for a fully automated system, making this distinction is very computer-intensive and time-consuming. On the other hand, if a human observer must scan the smear for sample adequacy, the smear can be fully read while its quality is determined, obviating the need for an automated system.

4. Any automated biologic device must, by necessity, set a threshold beyond which a sample is either classified "positive" or "negative," or "alarm" or "no alarm." It is medicolegally and ethically inconceivable that a machine would be intentionally set at a threshold to miss malignant tumor cell populations. However, if the threshold of an automated device is set such that it will never miss any tumor cell population, there will be a relatively large number of "false alarms." False alarms cost computing time and human re-examination time. This increases the actual cost of operation.

5. Some designers of automated systems state that their system is "as good as an average cytotechnologist," citing statistics in the literature and reports about the occasionally poor performance of cytotechnologists. When saying this, these developers forget that none of us *want or plan* to make diagnostic mistakes. Surely, all of us will make a mistake. However, we do not plan to make mistakes. As a matter of fact, we are very unhappy with ourselves or with one of our associates when such errors occur. The argument that "Statistically, cytotechnologists miss one or more out of 20 cancers; therefore, I can set my machine to miss that many cancers also," leads designers to intentionally design ethically and medicolegally unacceptable, automated malpractice systems.

6. Last but not least, a fully automated diagnostic system could well bring about medicolegal problems for both the producer of the system and the laboratory that uses it, were it to be operated as an unsupervised diagnostic system that would itself thus be liable for diagnostic errors.

The Committee on Cytology Automation of the International Academy of Cytology (IAC) has published guidelines for designers of automated systems[51] that are worthy of repetition upon this occasion. The standards are divided into two major groups: (1) mandatory conditions and (2) highly desirable features (see Table 13.2).

To our knowledge, no system has been designed or developed that meets these criteria of a fully automated system[109] and it is highly doubtful that a commercial system satisfying them will be operational in this century. However, it is quite conceivable that an *interactive* system can be successfully developed that leaves diagnostic judgment largely to the professional and medical personnel. Such interactive systems may, on the least sophisticated level, be just high-resolution cell image scanners that identify "alarms" in the smears, mark their coordinates on the slide electronically, and then replay these cells or artifacts to a human observer for visual re-assessment and diagnostic judgment. We designed such a prescreening alarm

Table 13.2
IAC Guidelines for Automated Systems

Mandatory Conditions (*Conditio sine qua non*)

1. The system shall not be designed or constructed to pass as negative any sample that contains malignant tumor cells.

2. The system shall not flag more "false alarms" on normal cells than could be readily handled by visual manual review.

3. The system shall not use up the entire sample or render the sample unusable for classical microscopic review; the pathologist must be able to examine the sample after routine staining.

4. The system shall yield reproducible results on repeated scannings of the same sample (within appropriate confidence limits).

5. The system shall have an internal calibration standard for quality control.

6. The system shall identify the inadequate (or empty) slide.

Highly Desirable Features (Required for Clinical Application)

1. The system should be able to demonstrate clearly the item that led to an "alarm" for subsequent review by a human observer.

2. The system should include dysplastic cells in the alarm group and should not restrict itself to the identification of frankly malignant tumor cells.

3. The system should detect and identify contamination and artifacts as such to avoid unnecessary human review.

4. The preprocessing of the sample required for a given system should be convenient and inexpensive for the clinician and laboratory (worst case: a system requiring specific preprocessing that is more expensive than the entire routine classical workup and evaluation while not offering improved diagnostic quality).

5. Infectious organisms, such as trichomonads and fungi, as well as "footprints," as in herpes inclusions and koilocytosis, should be identified.

6. The system should operate cost effectively.

identification module[92] that was used to scan the slide in relatively low resolution for alarms while it recognized and "discarded" erythrocytes, leukocytes, and normal squamous epithelial cells. Later, a high-resolution program using the same microscope reevaluated the alarm, discarded artifacts,[38] and attempted to classify the remaining cells. This system worked as far as the software and hardware were concerned, but did not comply fully to the above IAC standards and did not operate in an economic fashion.

Automated screening for gynecologic cancer was the daydream of the 1950s and 1960s. No fully automated systems worked economically and with sufficient accuracy to be clinically useful. From the sublime (Toshiba system)[79,80] to the ridiculous (Vickers system),[93] several instruments were proposed, supported, and finally discontinued. Some tests are still going on, but they are essentially using the same old technology of the 1960s and the 1970s. If automation has a place in screening cytologic samples in the foreseeable future, it will be in an interactive mode where the system scans the sample and shows alarms to a human observer for final analysis. The accelerated scanning by modern parallel processing computers and the decrease of the prices of the processors may make an economical, interactive system a reality in years to come.

Diagnostic Consultants: Expert Systems and Artificial Neural Nets

Expert systems are computer programs that imitate the presentation of a human expert in a particular domain. Expert systems consist of a knowledge base of rules, procedures, and facts and a set of mechanisms for operating on the knowledge base.[1,17,18,36,43,70,76] The use of expert systems and artificial neural networks represents new approaches to the design of medical consultants. Both of these techniques fall into the domain of artificial intelligence (AI): expert systems are knowledge-based programs designed to solve "expert" problems, while artificial neural nets are computational analogues to biologic neural systems that have the ability to "learn" by example. Neural-net systems are modeled on the human brain.[42,69,77] Unlike conventional computers, which consist of disparate electronic switching elements, a neural-net computer makes connections among each element or "neuron" to virtually all of the others on the computer chip. When one neuron "fires," it affects most, if not all, of the others. The result is a machine that can recognize patterns, even when some of the information is missing.[16,34,49,105–108,111]

Years ago, expert systems had to be developed with major programming efforts and expenditure of huge sums of money, since most were developed from scratch using AI languages such as LISP or PROLOG, and few commercially available "shells" were available on anything less than a mainframe computer. This is no longer true and one can now find suitable software packages that provide the novice a sufficiently structured system to enter the facts and rules necessary to specify appropriate action in appropriate cases. Much time is often wasted evaluating the expert system tools or shells. There are usually only minor differences between them. It seems more effective to select an expert system tool useful for the problem and do something with it even on a limited scale. A possible problem in the implementation of expert systems in existing laboratory computer systems is the fact that expert system shells are mostly written for microcomputers and workstations, while currently most major laboratory computers are still either minicomputers or even mainframes. This raises the question of how data are to be transferred and how the network is to be connected unless one uses stand-alone expert system hardware and software.

Most expert system application domains involve uncertainty.[34,111] Rule-based expert systems require a mechanism for managing and reasoning with uncertain knowledge. These mechanisms are usually referred to as Uncertainty Management Systems (UMS). Many UMSs have been proposed. Four of the most well-known UMSs are Bayesian inference, the MYCIN certainty factors, the Dempster-Shafer evidential reasoning, and fuzzy logic.[111] These four main UMSs are commercially available in expert system tools and it is up to the user to select the appropriate system for the specific problem at hand. Practically all knowledge outside of pure mathematics involves some degree or level of uncertainty. Uncertainty arises from limited accuracy of measurement, fuzziness, deficient knowledge or lack of knowledge or observability, or sensitivity to initial conditions (SIC). The type of uncertainty most often experienced in applications exists when measurement devices with limited accuracy are used to observe quantitative parameters. Since these measurement devices have limited accuracy and resolution, some degree of uncertainty is inherent in their measurements. Consider the display of measurements of DNA content in nuclei with a histogram showing four bins between 4N and 8N. Although—at least in our microTICAS system—the individual nuclear measurements are stored accurately, the observer of the histogram sees only that a nucleus falls into a particular range of ploidy. Uncertainty due to real or perceived limited measurement accuracy is generally modeled as a random error.

Another important type of uncertainty is fuzziness.[111] Fuzziness relates to the inherent vagueness of specific classifications or descriptors. Most knowledge obtained from human experts is fuzzy. Fuzziness may appear similar to randomness, but it differs significantly. Fuzzy uncertainty is not necessarily created by any random process. In this case the uncertainty arises from the fuzziness of the knowledge itself. Consider the concept of normal (benign) and abnormal (malignant) nuclear/cytoplasmic ratios. It is evident that a squamous epithelial cell with a N/C ratio of 1:30 is a normal mature cell, and that a large squamous cell with a N/C ratio of 1:1 is abnormal, without even considering other nuclear or cytoplasmic parameters. However, many, if not most, cells fall somewhere in between these extremes. Ignorance of one or more cellular parameters often causes uncertainty in other parameters. Uncertainty arises in practically all domains that apply to artificial intelligence technology. In cyto- and histo-pathologic diagnoses and prognoses, the expert system developer must deal with randomness, fuzziness, limited accuracy of measurement, ignorance, and observability that is deficient or lacking. As the knowledge domain increases, properly interpreting the knowledge becomes more challenging.

A UMS is a set of mathematical algorithms or software shells for the management of uncertain knowledge. The UMS provides the ability to store, generate, and reason with uncertain knowledge. Since each UMS is based on a different mathematical formalism and each assumes a dissimilar model of uncertainty, the selection of the appropriate UMS for developing applications in cyto- and histo-pathology is often key to the project's success. Using the wrong UMS may compromise the system's performance, power, robustness, and reliability. The mathematical details of UMS may be formidable, especially to nontechnical users. However, the use of the appropriate UMS is crucial for success in cytology and histopathology applications. A system that ignores basic uncertainties may erroneously provide completely certain definitions and recommendations that may have very fragile performance.

Expert systems should be designed by a domain expert and a knowledge engineer. Domain experts, ie, the cytopathologists, must be able to effectively verbalize their domain knowledge and their reasoning processes. The knowledge engineers must be acquainted with the available tools and have a working competence in artificial intelligence. They should be familiar with up-to-date developments in the field and be thoroughly involved and interested in the domain under development. Expert systems are already assisting in many levels of diagnostic cytology and histopathology, especially in automated approaches. These expert systems can provide consultations much as a human expert would, and can be restricted to rather brief answers, actions, or recommendations. At the University of Chicago, we are using expert systems of various levels of sophistication in a variety of applications:

1. The cytologic and histologic samples from a given patient are compared cytometrically, and the expert system decides for the purpose of quality assurance if the biopsy is representative of the cytologic sample.[22]
2. Previously stored cytometric, histometric, and clinical data from patients are searched for patterns similar to that of a new patient. When such patterns are identified in the data base, the biologic behavior of similar previous lesions is checked, along with therapeutic history, and the clinician is provided with a comparative assessment for the recommendation of therapy and/or probable prognosis.[16]
3. DNA ploidy measurements are assessed by the expert system, taking into account body site and type of material submitted for DNA analysis. The expert system sets prognostic criteria dependent upon this information (as entered by the microscopist); eg, the system will react to hyperdiploidy differently if it occurs on material from the hematopoietic system rather than squamous epithelium. It will also check the available data base for examples of this type of lesion and provide prognostic probabilities.
4. The cytologic sample of a gynecologic patient with an intraepithelial squamous lesion of the ectocervix is cytometrically evaluated and the data entered into a data base. When and if the patient is treated by laser or cryosurgery, the postoperative sample is rescanned 4 to 6 weeks after therapy and the original scannings are compared with the postoperative scannings. The expert system then compares the pre- and postoperative cytometric findings and evaluates whether or not the therapy was successful in returning the ploidy pattern to normal. Future reexaminations are treated in the same manner, so that the expert system provides a mechanism for ongoing quality control and improved likelihood of success of the therapy.
5. The expert system may also be used to assess anamnestic data and compare these data in conjunction with cytometric data to alert the clinician about possible differential diagnoses. Metarules of the expert system may also be constructed to have a different set of rules invoked for a different set of input data; eg, if the anamnesis shows that the patient was born in England and now lives is Brisbane, Australia and exhibits dark nevi, the system flags the greater possibility of the presence of melanotic cells and consults accordingly. Or if a 65-year-old patient is an obese,

diabetic nullipara, then rules are invoked to consider small squamous parabasal cells "normally expected," but to be more alert to glandular cells from the endometrium.

6. Expert systems can also be used to evaluate subjectively obtained criteria on cytologic and/or histologic samples, such as the descriptive histometric clues a pathologist may use in diagnosis of a tissue specimen. Probabilities (based upon previous cases) of various diagnoses for a given specimen may then be evaluated, together with an explanation as to why the expert system recommended a particular diagnosis.

7. In cytometry, expert systems are being used for scene segmentation (ie, delineation of nuclei and cytoplasm), for automated focus of the microscope, and for recommendations regarding optimal staining and fixation for a given case and the selection of appropriate filters if fluorochromes are used.

The list covers only a few of our applications of expert systems that are currently operational or in development. While expert systems are essentially based on rules comprised of "if" and "then" clauses by means of which the user can always trace how the system arrived at a given answer or recommendation, neural networks are nonalgorithmic and acquire knowledge by learning, essentially as does an infant, learning to walk. Artificial neural networks are based rather loosely on the underlying mathematics of the processing in biologic neural systems, and are comprised of a great many very basic processing elements, roughly corresponding to neurons.[49] They are being used extensively in military reconnaissance to discern man-made objects and identify any possible military intentions (eg, sonar pattern recognition, and visual identification and classification of enemy aircraft or ground vehicles). They are also being used for voice and handwriting recognition. At the University of Chicago we have taken the approach of developing hybrid systems incorporating frame-based and rule-based expert systems that are integrated with artificial neural nets, which often operate as intelligent front-end processors to such systems. The use of artificial neural nets to interpret DNA ploidy spectra, essentially as sophisticated pattern recognition software, is one such example. Using trained artificial neural networks to analyze several hundred ploidy spectra from cervical neoplasias,[108] we were able to obtain 20% better diagnostic separation between various classes than that obtained using a discriminant function classifier. The neural network was configured in a fraction of the time it would have taken a knowledge engineer to build an expert system.

The usefulness of embedded artificial intelligence systems such as these will become increasingly evident in the near future as more research centers enter this important field and as expert system shells and neural network software and hardware become available on inexpensive general purpose microcomputers. While no one expects an artificial intelligence revolution, the additional power of AI techniques grafted on to today's microcomputers and workstations will provide a powerful tool, and possibly the competitive edge, in cell image analysis. Their application will not lead to the replacement of cytotechnologists or pathologists, but will increase the objectivity, reproducibility, and accuracy of their work.

The novice in artificial intelligence mechanisms often expects miraculous results that could not be achieved by the best human brain. Probably only those expert systems that have a limited size and a clearly delineated purpose will have clinical utility in the foreseeable future. The future of expert systems and neural networks depends on technologies that support their high speed and massive storage requirements. Innovations in hardware development and the concurrent reductions in expense per information units processed are continuing (by the development of digital processing chips, gallium arsenide chips and optical computing devices, and wafer, analog, and optical storage devices). Such technological innovations should make artificial intelligence mechanisms so ubiquitous, that it may be anticipated that many laboratory operations, such as diagnostic procedures, the handling of data, microscope control, and quality assurance projects, will have some or more artificial intelligence capabilities added. In years to come, expert systems will be part of most laboratory mechanisms without the user necessarily being aware that there is an artificial intelligence component present.

Computerized Reporting of Vaginal/ Ectocervical/Endocervical Cytology Using the Bethesda System

Hardware and Software Requirements for Using the CLASSVEE system

Hardware Requirements
IBM personal computer or 100% IBM-compatible microcomputer with 640 KB of internal RAM memory, a monochrome or color monitor with adapter, compatible printer (eg, a HPLaserJet II or Epson dot matrix printer), preferable with a 10MB (or more MB) hard disk and a 3.5" (90 mm) floppy disk. Optional: (to obtain even faster performance) an AST Rampage Board, Intel Above Board expanded memory card, or other enhanced memory adapter. For networks: see Paradox Network Pack details from Borland International.

Software Requirements
(1) Operating System: DOS 3.1 or higher, (2) Database Management Program: PARADOX3 (Borland International) or runtime version thereof.

Instructions for Using the CLASSVEE Program in PARADOX3

PARADOX3 is relatively easy to learn. Intricate knowledge of PARADOX3 is not essential for operating or editing (eg, translation of the current English language into other languages or changes of text and explanations) the CLASSVEE (CV) program of The Bethesda System (TBS). Changes such as these (alterations of the text, etc) are allowed by the CV program by using "Modify" command—(see page 231). However, if you contemplate making major changes in the source code, you should read up on PARADOX3 before attempting structural changes. In addition to the six volumes supplied with the PARADOX3 license, you may wish to read "USING PARADOX3" by Bruce and Kramer [ISBN 0-88022-362-6], published 1989 by Que Corp, 11711 N College Avenue, Carmel, IN 46032.

CLASSVEE generates cytopathology reports using a set of fairly universal phrases. It is set up to allow easy data entry, modification, and display through the use of several menu bars. The following instructions are presented in an analogous fashion:

When you receive the floppy disk with the CV program, you will note that the disk is write protected. *Do This Safety Measure First*: Copy the floppy disk onto another floppy disk and put the original disk into a safe place. Then use the copy only and create a batch file called CV.BAT in your main or DOS directory using whichever editor you are comfortable with. It must contain the following:

CD PDOX_DIR
C: PDOX_DIR\PDOX## CLASSVEE##

where PDOX_DIR is the name of the directory into which you have copied CV and PDOX## is the command with which you usually start PARADOX. CV may now be started by typing CV at the DOS C> (or C:\ >) prompt. If your computer does not have a hard disk, copy CV onto a copy of your PARADOX disk and substitute the appropriate drive letter (A: or B:) for the C:

From here on, it is assumed that all parts of CV have been copied from the distribution disk into a PARADOX directory. If you need another copy of the instructions: they can be raised on a HPLaserJet (or compatible laser printer) by writing COPY CVMANUA2.DOC PRN or on an Epson dot matrix printer (or compatible) by writing COPY CVMANUAL.DOC PRN. The laser version represents the original.

General Comments on the Operation of TBS with the CLASSVEE Program

Throughout this document, pressing the Enter key will be shown as <Enter>. Dates should be entered in a mm/dd/yy format, as in 12/30/89. At certain prompts within CV, you will see choices given in square brackets, as in [Y]. This is the default answer you will get by simply using <Enter>.

If an operation requires successive choices from the menu bars, they will be given in braces, as in {Modify} {Patient}. You get these choices by pressing the first letter of each choice. Every time the menu bar is displayed, pressing the Esc key (given as {Esc} in the discussion below) will return you to the preceding menu bar. Pressing a letter or number key and the F keys will be depicted as, for example, {Y} and {F2}, respectively.

During a data entry session, you may be presented with several lists of possibilities for various conditions. If the list is inappropriate, press <Enter>. CV will produce another list. For example, if the epithelial cells in a particular specimen are not within normal limits, there may be several reasons, such as microbiologic entities, preparative changes, etc. The first list CV will present deals with the microbiologic entities. If it is not appropriate (eg, the cells are not normal due to preparative changes), press <Enter> at the prompt.

If, for some reason, you get Paradox system–related error messages while CV is running or if it acts weird ("conks out"), exit the program. The behavior indicates that there are version-incompatible libraries on the distribution disk that must be removed. Corrected libraries will be generated by CV as soon as you start it again. Please do the following:

1. At the DOS level (arrow prompt), go to the directory in which CV is stored with the CD command.
2. Erase the following 3 files:

> EDITLIN.LIB
> CVWORD.LIB
> CVPWORD.LIB

3. Start CV up as usual. You should see messages which indicate that libraries are being generated.

I. Main Menu Bar

CreatePhrases EnterPatient Modify Report Delete Quit

This is the main menu of CV. It should be displayed immediately after CV announces itself. If it is not, CV should be recopied from the distribution disk.

CreatePhrases
This choice is used to create the set of universal phrases used in report generation. They should conform to the Bethesda protocol for GYN cytopathology nomenclature. CreatePhrases should be used only if the set of phrases on the distribution disk has been destroyed. CV will generate easily understood error messages that will tell you what is missing at appropriate points during data entry. If a set of phrases is missing, the patient data you have entered up to that point is not lost. Once the phrases have been entered, use {Modify} {Patient} to continue data entry.

EnterPatient

Relevant patient information, such as name, unit number, address, referring doctor, and attending cytopathologist, may be entered at the appropriate prompts. The patient's name must be entered or CV will generate the error message, "Patient name must be supplied." The rest of the preliminary information is optional. Press <Enter> in the appropriate places to bypass the prompts. CV will also ask for dates regarding the patient's specimen. If you use <Enter>, CV will assume the current date. You may then enter a laboratory reference number and the attending cytopathologist from the displayed list. If choice "other" is made, CV will prompt for the doctor's name.

Other information, such as the type of specimen, adequacy of the specimen, and normalcy of the epithelial cells, is entered at the appropriate places. Should the specimen be other than optimal, CV will display a list of possible causes. Choose up to as many as are listed, including "other." The order you type in your choices will be reflected in the generated report. If you choose "other," you will be asked for your unique reason. Limit your response to 3 lines of 75 characters each and end each line with <Enter>.

If the epithelial cells are not within normal limits, responding with N at the "Are the epithelial cells within normal limits? [Y]:" prompt will cause CV to present several lists of possible causes. Proceed through them until you are done and ready to generate the report. If the cells are normal, respond Y or <Enter> to the prompt, "End of Report? [Y]:"

Once all data has been entered, CV will ask if you want the final report printed on the screen (for quality assurance or a quick review) or on the printer.

Modify

By selecting Modify, you will enter a part of CV where you can modify most of the data used by CV to produce a report. These include patient data, the universal phrases, printer type, and cytopathology findings. This choice will produce the menu bar CreatePhrases.

Report

One of the powerful assets of CV is its database. From the information in the database, you can produce many types of reports. For example, the reports can be based on monthly activity or patients with a certain type of cytopathology finding. This choice is discussed further on page 234.

Delete

Be careful when using this choice! It will permanently erase the information associated with a given patient name. The information is not retrievable.

Quit

Exit CV by using {Quit} {Yes}. You will be returned to PARADOX. Exit PARADOX with {Exit} {Yes}.

II. CreatePhrases

CytologyMD Specimens Adequacy General Descriptive Main

You should not have to use this menu bar often, if at all. These choices let you enter the set of phrases that CV will use to create the final cytopathology report based on your input. This section is self-explanatory once you are creating phrases. There is an interlock which will not allow you to enter phrases at this choice if they already exist. A set of phrases "exists" if the list has been established even though individual items may be missing. You should use the Modify selection at the main menu bar.

III. EnterPatient

This choice has been described in section I.

IV. Modify

Explanations CytologyMD Specimen Patient ReportFormat Main

This is the *main editing* menu bar. From it, *you can change almost everything* that CV uses to produce the cytopathology report. This includes patient information, the way the report is printed, the wording, and on which printer the report will appear.

IV.a. Explanations
This choice will produce the following menu bar:

Adequacy General Descriptive Modify

IV.a.1. Adequacy
You may change the set of universal phrases that describe specimen adequacy from this selection. Choosing Adequacy will produce the following menu bar:

Satisfactory LessThanOptimal Unsatisfactory
Explanations

You may alter the phrases that describe specimen adequacy here. There is full prompting for what you want to change and the changes may be made using CV's own full-screen editor. {Explanations} will return you to the previous menu bar.

IV.a.2. General
This selection will allow you to change how the general categorization (epithelial cells normal or not) is phrased. There is full prompting for what you want to change and the changes may be made using CV's own full-screen editor. Answering {N} <Enter> to the "Any more changes? [N]:" prompt will return you to the previous menu bar. CV will save all changes made.

IV.a.3. Descriptive
This selection will produce the following menu bar:

Micros Changes Squamous Cell VCE-Atypia Glandular
Hormonal Action Return

You may alter any of the sets of phrases associated with the above choices. There is full prompting for what you want to change and the changes may be made using CV's own full-screen editor. Answering {N} <Enter> to the "Any more changes? [N]:" prompt will return you to the above menu bar. {Return} will return you to the previous menu bar (shown in IV.a.).

IV.b. CytologyMD
There is full prompting for what you want to change in the list of attending cytopathologists and the changes may be made using CV's own full-screen editor. Answering {N} <Enter> to the "Any more changes? [N]:" prompt will return you to the above menu bar. {Return} will return you to the previous menu bar (shown in IV.a.).

IV.c. Specimen
There is full prompting for desired modifications to the list of cytology specimen types and the changes may be made using CV's own full-screen editor. Answering {N} <Enter> to the "Any more changes? [N]:" prompt will return you to the above menu bar. {Return} will return you to the previous menu bar (shown in IV.a.).

IV.d. Patient
This selection will produce the following menu bar:

Patient Information Attendings Specimen Descriptive
Modify

IV.d.1. Patient
You may retrieve the record of a patient from this choice. The following menu bar will be displayed:

Name UnitNo LabNo DateReported

You will be asked for the year that the patient record is in as well as for the information with which to search for the patient. Using the above menu bar, you can search for records based on patient's name, unit number, laboratory number, or date the results were reported. The dates should be in the mm/dd/yy form, as in 12/30/89. Should two or more patients be found during the retrieval, the matches will be displayed and you will be asked to choose from among them. If no records are found for desired search, CV will report "Patient not found in current year." In all cases, once the search is complete, you will be returned to the menu bar given in IV.d.

IV.d.2. Information
Once a patient's record has been selected for modification, you can alter the patient's basic information, such as name, address, etc., from this choice. Use the up and down arrow keys to move around

the screen and the backspace key to delete letters and make corrections. Press {F2} to keep or {Esc} to quit and not keep changes.

IV.d.3. Attendings
Once a patient's record has been selected for modification, you can alter the list of attending cytopathologists for the patient from this choice. Up to 3 attendings may be used for a given patient. If you choose "Other," CV will ask for the cytopathologist's name. If no changes are to be made, simply use <Enter>.

IV.d.4. Specimen
The specimen type and general categorization may be changed using this choice. If, at the "Modify specimen type [N]:" prompt, you answer {Y} <Enter>, you will be shown the current specimen type and a list of specimen types. Select as many as necessary from the list. Press <Enter> when done. If no changes are desired, simply press <Enter>. You will then be given the opportunity to change specimen adequacy as well as explanations for the adequacy rating, if any.

IV.d.5. Descriptive
This choice will produce the following menu bar:

Micros Changes SquamousCell VCE Glandular
OtherNeo Hormonal Action Exit

As described above, these choices allow you to modify or add to the cytopathology findings for the patient. Where appropriate, the current findings and a list of phrases will be shown. Make your selection from the list. End your modifications with <Enter>. If no changes are desired, simply use <Enter>.

Changes in other neoplasms ({OtherNeo}) may be made using the built-in full-screen editor. CV will take care of calling up the editor for you. {Exit} will return you to the menu bar given in IV.d.

IV.d.6 Modify
This choice will return you to the Modify menu bar given in IV.

IV.e. ReportFormat
At your option, a printer can be selected for your reports. Two printers have been already defined for use within CV. They are HEWLETT-PACKARD-HPLaserJet and Epson dot matrix printers. (Please note that CV doesn't care if you use capital or lower case letters in the names). CV's response will be "default" when you enter a name that it doesn't understand.

Once you enter the printer type, you can set the page size (header, page size, and margins) to whatever you like. CV will catch most settings that don't make sense. As usual, if no changes are needed, simply use <Enter> at the prompt.

IV.f. Main
Returns you to the main menu bar, given in I.

V. Report

Here you select a patient's records and have them printed. Also, you may generate reports of monthly activity in the lab (based on date reported) and you may select a group of patient records with common attributes. The following menu bar is shown for your selection.

Monthly Patient Select Return

V.a. Monthly
Generate a report of activity for a given month.

V.b. Patient
Print a selected patient's record. You may select the patient by name, unit number, lab number, or date reported. The following menu bar is shown for this use:

Name UnitNo LabNo DateReported

V.c. Select
The real flexibility of CV is its ability to retrieve a group of records based on a set of conditions within a given year. These conditions can be any combination of universal selections that a patient may have. You are given the opportunity to include or exclude the selections. If no choices are made for a selection, it will be assumed you want all conditions possible in a selection. These are shown in the following menu bar:

Year CytologyMD Type Adequacy General Descriptive
Execute

V.c.1. Year
Select a year to work with.

V.c.2. CytologyMD
Select records based on attending cytopathologist.

V.c.3. Adequacy
Select records based on sample adequacy and explanations, if any.

V.c.4. General
Select records based on general categorization.

V.c.5. Descriptive
Select records based on descriptive diagnosis using the following menu bar:

Micros Changes Squamous VCE Glandular OtherNeo
Hormonal Action Exit

These choices are self-explanatory by now. {Exit} will return you to the select menu bar (see V.c.).

V.d. Execute

Retrieve records according to selected parameters and produce a report of basic patient information.

Additional information about TBS or about the above computerized CV version may be obtained by writing to:

The International Academy of Cytology Committee on Continuing Education and Quality Assurance
5841 Maryland Avenue, HM # 449
Chicago, IL 60637
Tel: (312) 702-6569 FAX: (312) 955-8873 TELEX: 4972334

Address of authors: George L Wied, M.D., FIAC
Professor of Pathology and Director, Section of Cytopathology
Harvey E Dytch, SB, PMIAC,
Head, AI Research Center
University of Chicago
5841 Maryland Avenue, HM#449, Chicago, IL 60637

Supported by a grant from the National Cancer Institute, No 1-R35-CA-42517.

References

1. Anderson D: Artificial intelligence and intelligent systems. The implications. Chichester, Ellis Horwood, 1989.

2. Armitage NC, Robins RA, Evans DF, Turner RD, Baldwin RW, Hardcastle JD: The influence of tumour cell DNA abnormalities on survival in colorectal cancer. *Br J Surg* 72:828–830, 1985.

3. Atkin NB, Richards BM: Clinical significance of ploidy in carcinoma of cervix. Its relation to prognosis. *Br Med J* 2:1445–1446, 1962.

4. Atkin NB: Modal DNA-value and survival in carcinoma of the breast. *Br Med J* 86:271–272, 1972.

5. Atkin NB: Prognostic significance of modal DNA value and other factors in malignant tumors based on 1465 cases. *Br J Cancer* 40:210–221, 1979.

6. Bacus S, Flowers JL, Press MJ, Bacus JW, McCarty KS Jr: The evaluation of estrogen receptor in primary breast carcinoma by computer-assisted image analysis. *Am J Clin Pathol* 90:233–239, 1988.

7. Bahr GF, Bibbo M, Oehme M, Puls JH, Reale FR, Wied GL: An automated device for the production of cell preparations suitable for automatic assessment. *Acta Cytol* 22:243–249, 1978.

8. Bahr GF: Frontiers of quantitative cytochemistry: A review of recent developments and potentials. *Analyt Quant Cytol* 1:1–19, 1979.

9. Bahr GF, Bartels PH, Wied GL, Koss LG: Automated cytology. *In*: Diagnostic Cytology and Its Histopathologic Bases. Edited by LG Koss. Third edition, Philadelphia, JB Lippincott, 1979, pp 1123–1186.

10. Baildam AD, Zaloudik J, Howell A, Barnes DM, Turnbull L, Swindell R: DNA analysis by flow cytometry, response to endocrine treatment and prognosis in advanced carcinoma of the breast. *Br J Cancer* 55:553–559, 1987.

11. Bartels PH, Bahr GF, Wied GL: Information theoretic approach to cell identification by computer. *In*: Automated Cell Identification

and Cell Sorting. Edited by GL Wied and GF Bahr. New York, Academic Press, 1970, pp 361–384.

12. Bartels PH, Wied GL: Performance testing for automated pre-screening devices in cervical cytology. *J Histochem Cytochem* 22:660–662, 1974.

13. Bartels PH, Koss LG, Wied GL: Automated cell diagnosis in clinical cytology. *In*: Developments in Clinical Cytology. Edited by LG Koss, D Coleman. London, Butterworths, 1980, pp 314–342.

14. Bartels PH, Abmayr W, Bibbo M, Burger G, Soost HJ, Taylor J, Wied GL: Computer recognition of ectocervical cells—Image features. *Analyt Quant Cytol* 3:157–164, 1981.

15. Bartels PH, Wied GL: Automated image analysis in clinical pathology. *Am J Clin Pathol* 75:489–493, 1981.

16. Bartels PH, Graham A, Kuhn W, Paplanus S, Wied GL: Knowledge engineering in quantitative histopathology. *Applied Optics* 26:3330–3337, 1987.

17. Bartels PH, Weber JE: Expert systems in histopathology. I. Introduction and overview. *Analyt Quant Cytol & Histol* 11:1–7, 1989.

18. Bartels PH, Hiessl H: II. Knowledge representation and rule-based systems. *Anal Quant Cytol & Histol* 11:147–153, 1989.

19. Berlinger NT, Malone BN, Kay NE: A comparison of flow cytometric DNA analyses of fresh and fixed squamous cell carcinomas. *Arch Otolaryngol Head Neck Surg* 113:1301–1306, 1987.

20. Bhattacharya PK, Bartels PH, Bahr GF, Wied GL: A test statistic for detecting the presence of abnormal cells in a sample. *Acta Cytol* 15:533–544, 1971.

21. Bhattacharya PK, Bartels PH, Taylor J, Wied GL: A decision procedure for automated cytology. Test statistic for detecting sample abnormality and inadequacy. *Acta Cytol* 17:538–552, 1973.

22. Bibbo M, Alenghat E, Bahr GF, Bartels PH, Dytch HE, Herbst AL, Keebler CM, Pishotta FT, Wied GL: A quality-control procedure on cervical lesions for the comparison of cytology and histology. *J Reprod Med* 28:811–822, 1983.

23. Bibbo M, Bartels PH, Sychra JJ, Wied GL: Chromatin appearance in intermediate cells from patients with uterine cancer. *Acta Cytol* 25:23–28, 1981.

24. Bibbo M, Bartels PH, Dytch HE, Pishotta FT, Wied GL: High-resolution color video cytophotometry. *Cell Biophys* 5:61–70, 1983.

25. Bibbo M, Bartels PH, Dytch HE, Wied GL: Computed cell image information. *In*: Computer-Assisted Image Analysis Cytology. Edited by SD Greenberg. Monographs in Clinical Cytology. Basel, S Karger, 1984, pp 62–101.

26. Bibbo M, Bartels PH, Dytch HE, Wied GL: Ploidy measurements by high-resolution cytometry. *Analyt Quant Cytol & Histol* 7:81–88, 1985.

27. Bibbo M, Bartels PH, Dytch HE, Puls JH, Wied GL: Rapid cytophotometry and its application to diagnostic pathology. *Applied Pathology* 5:33–46, 1987.

28. Bur M, Bibbo M, Dytch HE, Holt JA, Greene GL, Lorincz M, Wied GL, Press M: Computerized image analysis of estrogen receptor quantitation in FNA of breast cancer. A preliminary report. *Lab Invest* 56:9A, 1987.

29. Burger G, Ploem JS, Goerttler K (Eds): Clinical Cytometry and Histometry. London, Academic Press, 1987.

30. Caspersson T, Santesson L: Studies on protein metabolism in the cells of epithelial tumors. *Acta Radiol* (supp) 46:1–105, 1942.

31. Coon JS, et al: Interinstitutional variability in DNA flow cytometric analysis of tumors. The National Cancer Institute's Flow Cytometry Network experience. *Cancer* 61:128, 1988.

32. Cornelisse CJ, Van Driel-Kulker AM: DNA image cytometry on machine selected breast cancer cells and a comparison between flow cytometry and scanning cytophotometry. *Cytometry* 6:471–477, 1985.

33. Cornelisse CJ, van de Velde CJH, Caspers RJC, Molenaar AJ, Hermans Y: DNA ploidy and survival in breast cancer patients. *Cytometry* 8:225–234, 1987.

34. deLaplace PS: Concerning probability: *In*: World of Mathematics. Edited by JR Newman. New York, Simon & Schuster, 1956.

35. de Vere White RW, Deitch AD, West B, Fitzpatrick JM: The predictive value of flow cytometric information in the clinical management of state 0 (Ta) bladder cancer. *J Clin Pathol* 139:279–282, 1988.

36. Diaper D: Knowledge elicitation. Principles, Techniques and Applications. Chichester, Ellis Horwood, 1989.

37. Dytch HE, Bartels PH, Bibbo M, Pishotta FT, Wied FL: Computer graphics in cytodiagnosis. *Analyt Quant Cytol* 4:263–268, 1982.

38. Dytch HE, Bartels PH, Bibbo M, Pishotta FT, Wied GL: The rejection of noncellular artifacts in Papanicolaou-stained slide specimens by an automated high-resolution system. Identification of important cytometric features. *Analyt Quant Cytol* 5:241–250, 1983.

39. Dytch HE, Bibbo M, Bartels PH, Wied GL: Computer graphics in cytologic and pathologic microscopy. Tools for the clinician and researcher. *Analyt Quant Cytol & Histol* 8:81–88, 1986.

40. Dytch, HE, Bibbo M, Puls JH, Bartels PH, Wied GL: Software design for an inexpensive, practical, microcomputer-based DNA cytometry system. *Analyt Quant Cytol & Histol* 8:8–18, 1986.

41. Dytch HE, Bibbo M, Puls JH, Wied GL: A PC-based system for the objective analysis of histologic specimens through quantitative contextual karyometry. *Applied Optics* 26:3270–3279, 1987.

42. Dytch HE, Wied GL: Artificial neural networks applied to cytologic and histologic samples. *Analyt Quant Cytol & Histol* (in press).

43. Dytch HE, Wied GL: Neurocomputing. Artificial neural net as AI tools for quantitative pathology. *In*: Expert Systems in Cytopathology. Edited by JPA Baak. Springer Verlag, 1990.

44. Feulgen R, Rossenbach H: Mikroskopisch-chemischer Nachweis einer Nukleinsaeure vom Typus der Thymonukleinsaeure Praeparate. *Hoppe-Seylers Z Phys Chem* 135:203–248, 1924.

45. Franklin WA, Bibbo M, Doria MI, Dytch HE, Toth J, DeSombre E, Wied GL: Quantitation of estrogen receptor and Ki-67 in breast carcinoma by the microTICAS image analysis system. *Analyt Quant Cytol & Histol* 9:279–286, 1987.

46. Friedlander ML, Hedley DW, Swanson C, Russel P: Prediction of long-term survival by flow cytometric analysis of cellular DNA con-

tent in patients with advanced ovarian cancer. *J Clin Oncol* 6:282–290, 1988.

47. Frierson H: Flow cytometric analysis of ploidy in solid neoplasms. Comparison of fresh tissues with formalin-fixed paraffin-embedded specimens. *Human Pathol* 19:290–294, 1988.

48. Greenebaum E, Koss LG, Elequin F, Silver CE: The diagnostic value of flow cytometric DNA measurements in follicular tumors of the thyroid gland. *Cancer* 56:2011–2018, 1985.

49. Hecht-Nielsen R: Neural analog processing. Proceedings SPIE-Intl Society Optical Engineering 360:180–189, 1982.

50. Hedley DW, Friedlander ML, Taylor IW, Rugg CA, Musgroove EA: Method for analysis of cellular DNA content of paraffin-embedded pathologic material using flow cytometry. *J Histochem Cytochem* 31:1333–1335, 1983.

51. International Academy of Cytology: Specifications for automated cytodiagnostic systems proposed by the IAC. Acta Cytol 28:352, 1984.

52. Iversen OE: Prognostic value of the flow cytometric DNA index in human ovarian carcinoma. *Cancer* 61:334–339, 1988.

53. Iversen OE: Flow cytometric deoxyribonucleic acid index. A prognostic factor in endometrial carcinoma. *Am J Obstet Gynecol* 155:770–776, 1986.

54. Jacobson AB, Thorund E, Fossa SD, et al: DNA flow cytometry in metastases and recurrence of malignant melanomas. A comparison of results from fresh and paraffin embedded material. *Virchows Arch B* 54:273–277, 1988.

55. Kamentsky LA, Melamed MR, Derman H: Spectrophotometer. New instrument for ultrarapid cell analysis. *Science* 150:630–631, 1965.

56. Katzko MW, Pahlplatz MMM, Oud PS, Vooijs PG: Carcinoma in situ specimen classification based on intermediate cell measurements. *Cytometry* 8:9–13, 1987.

57. Koenig SH, Brown RD, Kamentsky LA, Sedlis A, Melamed MR: Efficiency of a rapid cell spectrophotometer in screening for cervical cancer. *Cancer* 21:1019–1026, 1968.

58. Koss LG, Bartels PH, Sychra JJ, Wied GL: Computer analysis of atypical urothelial cells: II. Classification by unsupervised learning algorithms. *Acta Cytol* 21:261–265, 1977.

59. Koss LG: Diagnostic Cytology and its Histopathologic Bases. 3rd ed. Philadelphia, JB Lippincott, 1979.

60. Koss LG: Analytical and quantitative cytology. A historical perspective. *Analyt Quant Cytol* 4:251–256, 1982.

61. Koss LG, Greenebaum E: Measuring DNA in human cancer. *JAMA* 255:3158–3159, 1986.

62. Koss LG: Automated cytology and histology. A historical perspective. *Analyt Quant Cytol* 9:369–374, 1987.

63. Koss LG: The puzzle of prostatic carcinoma. *Mayo Clin Proc* 63:193–197, 1988.

64. Koss LG, Czerniak B, Herz F, Wersto RP: Flow cytometric measurements of DNA and other cell components in human tumors. A critical appraisal. *Human Pathol* 20:528–548, 1989.

65. Koss LG: The future of cytology. The Wachtel Lecture for 1988. *Acta Cytol* 34:1–9, 1990.

66. Mellors RC, Keane JF, Papanicolaou GN: Nucleic acid content of the squamous cancer cell. *Science* 116:264–269, 1952.

67. Mellors RC, Kupfer A, Hollender A: Quantitative cytology and cytopathology. *Cancer* 6:372–384, 1953.

68. National Cancer Institute Workshop on Terminology: The Bethesda System. *JAMA* 262:931–934, 1989.

69. Obermeier, KK: Natural Language Technologies in Artificial Intelligence. New York, John Wiley & Sons, 1989.

70. Pedersen K: Expert Systems Programming. Practical Techniques for Rule-b based systems. New York, John Wiley & Sons, 1989.

71. Prewitt JMS, Mendelsohn ML: The analysis of cell images. *Ann NY Acad Sci* 128:1035–1043, 1966.

72. Puls JH, Bibbo M, Dytch HE, Bartels PH, Wied GL: microTICAS. The design of an inexpensive video-microphotometer computer system for DNA ploidy studies. *Analyt Quant Cytol & Histol* 8:1–7, 1986.

73. Pressman NJ, Wied GL (Eds): The Automation of Cancer Cytology and Cell Image Analysis. Chicago, International Academy of Cytology, 1979.

74. Quirke P, Dixon MF, Clayden AD, et al: Prognostic significance of DNA aneuploidy and cell proliferation in rectal adenocarcinomas. *J Pathol* 151:285–291, 1987.

75. Rosenthal DL, Suffin S: Predictive value of digitized cell images for the prognosis of cervical neoplasia. *In*: Computer-Assisted Image Analysis Cytology. Edited by SD Greenberg. *In*: Monographs in Clinical Cytology. Edited by GL Wied. Ninth volume. Basel, S Karger, 1984, pp 163–180.

76. Smith B, Kelleher G: Reason Maintenance Systems and Their Applications. Chichester, Ellis Horwood, 1988.

77. Soucek B, Soucek M: Neural and Massively Parallel Computers: The Sixth Generation. New York, John Wiley & Sons, 1988.

78. Stenkvist B, Bergstrom R, Eklund G, Fox CH: Papanicolaou smear screening and cervical cancer. *JAMA* 252:1423–1426, 1984.

79. Tanaka N, Ikeda H, Ueno T, Takahashi M, Urabe M, Imasato Y, Watanabe S, Yoneyama T, Genchi H, Matozaki T, Kashida R: Fundamental study for approaching the automation of cytological diagnosis of cancer and a new automated apparatus CYBEST. *Jap J Clin Pathol* (in Japanese) 22:757–768, 1973.

80. Tanaka N, Ikeda H, Ueno T, Watanabe S, Imasato Y, Kashida R: Fundamental study of automated cyto-screening for uterine cancer. New System for automated apparatus (CYBEST) utilizing pattern recognition method. *Acta Cytol* 21:85–89, 1977.

81. Tolles WE: The cytoanalyzer. An example of physics in medical research. *Trans NY Acad Sci* 17:250–256, 1955.

82. Tribukait B: Flow cytometry in surgical pathology and cytology of tumors of the genito-urinary tract. *In*: Advances in Clinical Cytology. Edited by LG Koss, DV Coleman. Vol 2. New York, Masson Publishing, 1984, pp 163–189.

83. Tribukait B: Flow cytometry in assessing the clinical aggressiveness of genito-urinary neoplasms. *World J Urol* 5:108–122, 1987.

84. Wersto RP, Greenebaum E, Deitch D, Kersbergen K, Koss LG: Deoxyribonucleic acid ploidy and cell cycle events in benign colonic epithelium peripheral to carcinoma. *Lab Invest* 58:218–225, 1988.

85. Wied GL, Messina A, Meier P, Rosenthal E: DNA assessment on Feulgen-stained endometrial cells and comparison with fluorometric values. *Lab Invest* 14:1494–1499, 1965.

86. Wied GL, Messina A, Rosenthal E: Comparative DNA measurements on Feulgen-stained cervical epithelial cells. *Acta Cytol* 10:31–37, 1966.

87. Wied GL, Meier P, Clark LM: An electronic data processing program for cytologic screening projects for uterine carcinoma. *Acta Cytol* 8:385–397, 1964.

88. Wied GL, McGrew EA, Rosenthal E: A cytologic registry and computer system for a city-wide cooperative screening project. *Acta Cytol* 11:150–156, 1967.

89. Wied GL (Editor): Introduction to Quantitative Cytochemistry. New York, Academic Press, 1966.

90. Wied GL, Bartels PH, Bahr GF, Oldfield DG: Taxonomic intracellular analytic system (TICAS) for cell identification. *Acta Cytol* 12:180–204, 1968.

91. Wied GL, Bahr GF (Eds): Automated Cell Identification and Cell Sorting. New York, Academic Press, 1970.

92. Wied GL, Bahr GF, Bartels PH: Automated analysis of cell images by TICAS. *In*: Automated Cell Identification and Cell Sorting. Edited by GL Wied and GF Bahr. New York, Academic Press, 1970, pp 195–360.

93. Wied GL: Automated cell screening—a practical reality or a daydream? *In*: Automated Cytology. Edited by DMD Evans. London, E & S Livingstone, Ltd, 1970, pp 43–47.

94. Wied GL, Bahr GF, Bartels PH: The taxonomic intra-cellular analytic system (TICAS) for cell diagnosis. *In*: Automated Cytology. Edited by DMD Evans. London, E & S Livingstone, Ltd, 1970, pp 252–259.

95. Wied GL, Bahr GF (Eds): Introduction to Quantitative Cytochemistry II. New York, Academic Press, 1970.

96. Wied GL: The future of cytodiagnosis (Betrachtungen ueber die Zukunft der Zytodiagnostik). *Fortschr Med* 26:943–946, 1972.

97. Wied GL, Bartels PH: Modern trends in cytologic diagnosis (Zukunftsaspekte der Zelldiagnostik; Referat). *Verh Dtsch Ges Pathol* 57:169–180, 1973.

98. Wied GL, Bahr GF, Bibbo M, Puls JH, Taylor J, Bartels PH: The TICAS-RTCIP real time cell identification processor. *Acta Cytol* 19:286–288, 1975.

99. Wied GL, Bartels PH, Bibbo M, Puls JH, Taylor J, Sychra JJ: Computer recognition of ectocervical cells. Classification of the efficacy of contour and textural features. *Acta Cytol* 21:753–764, 1977.

100. Wied GL, Bibbo M, Bartels PH: Computer analysis of microscopic images: Application in cytopathology. *Path Annual* 16:367–409, 1981.

101. Wied GL, Bartels PH, Dytch HE, Pishotta FT, Bibbo M: Rapid high-resolution cytometry. *Analyt Quant Cytol* 4:257–262, 1982.

102. Wied GL, Bartels PH, Dytch HE, Pishotta FT, Yamauchi K, Bibbo M: Diagnostic marker features in dysplastic cells from the uterine cervix. *Acta Cytol* 26:475–483, 1982.

103. Wied GL, Bartels PH, Bibbo M: Die Begriffswelten der visuellen und automatisierten Zytodiagnostik: wie eng beruehren sie sich? (The Schools of Thought of Visual and Automated Cytologic Diagnoses: How Interrelated Are They?) *Microscopica Acta* 6:179–186, 1983.

104. Wied GL, Bartels PH, Dytch HE, Bibbo M: Rapid DNA evaluation in clinical diagnosis. *Acta Cytol* 1:33–37, 1983.

105. Wied GL, Bartels PH, Weber J, Dytch HE: Expert systems design under uncertainty of human diagnosticians. IEEE-proceedings (8th Annual Conference on Engineering in Medicine and Biology 1986) CH 2368-9, Vol 25, pp 757–760.

106. Wied GL, Weber JE, Dytch HE, Bibbo M, Bartels PH: TICAS-STRATEX, an expert diagnostic system for stratified cervical epithelium. IEEE Proceedings, EMBS-EMSA, Boston, November 1987.

107. Wied GL, Bartels PH, Bibbo M, Dytch HE: Image Analysis and Quantitative Cyto- & Histopathology. Technical Report No. 2, Chicago, International Academy of Cytology, 1988.

108. Wied GL, Bartels PH, Bibbo M, Dytch HE: Image analysis in quantitative cytopathology and histopathology. *Human Pathol* 20:549–571, 1989.

109. Wied GL: Clinical Cytology. Past, Present and Future. *In*: Oncologia, edited by U. Bonck, S. Karger. Basel, Switzerland (in press).

110. Wils J, van Geuns H, Baak J: Proposal for therapeutic approach based on prognostic factors including morphometric and flow cytometric features in stage III–IV ovarian cancer. *Cancer* 61:1920–1925, 1988.

111. Zadeh Laffi A: Fuzzy sets. Information & Control, Volume 8, 1965.

CHAPTER FOURTEEN

The Gynecologic Smear

A large part of the success of gynecologic cytology depends upon the quality of the smear. Even the most astute cytotechnologist or cytopathologist cannot interpret a smear that is not adequately prepared. Guidelines for the correct sampling, spreading, and fixation of the cellular material should be available in the laboratory and submitted to the individuals responsible for collecting smears.

Sampling

The patient should be instructed not to use a vaginal douche or any vaginal medication or lubricant for at least 24 hours before a smear is to be collected. No lubricant should be used for the introduction of the speculum. The sampling should be done before any pelvic examination. Full visualization of the cervix and upper part of the vagina is necessary in order to obtain an adequate specimen. Originally, smears were obtained only from the posterior vaginal fornix because desquamated cells from the endometrial cavity and the cervix gather in this area. Later it was realized that most epithelial lesions of the cervix originate at the squamocolumnar junction. Therefore, the smear from the posterior fornix was replaced by a scraping of the transitional zone of the cervix. Finally, it was found that the endocervical canal can also harbor early epithelial lesions, and that it was necessary to also sample that area.

For best results, three smears should always be obtained, one from each of these sites. In general, the posterior fornix and the

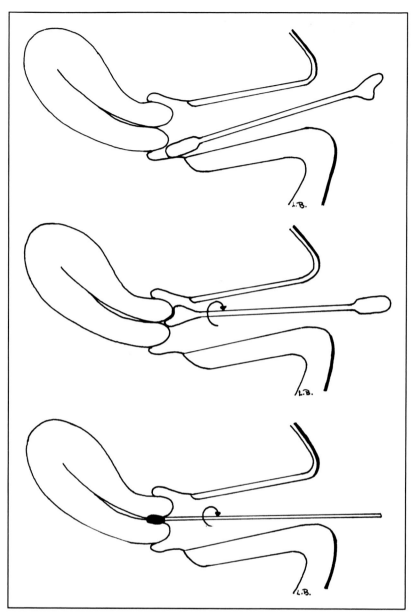

Figure 14.1 Schematic representation of the three samples that are recommended for an adequate sampling of the genital tract.

exocervix are sampled with a wooden or plastic spatula, after removing excess mucus. The endocervical sample is usually obtained with a cotton-tipped applicator, or a commercially available endocervical brush. The resulting three smears can be spread on three glass slides, or, preferably, on a single slide.[1] We prefer this last technique (the V–C–E technique), and have used it successfully for the past 30 years on over 2 million women.

The sampling for the V–C–E technique is performed in the usual manner (Figure 14.1): first a scraping is obtained from the posterior vaginal fornix with a wooden tongue depressor or an Ayre spatula. The material is kept on the instrument. Then a scraping with a second spatula is made from the exocervix, and special care is taken to sample all of the transformation zone. Again, the material is kept on the instrument. Last, the endocervical sample is secured

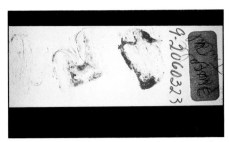

Figure 14.2 A V–C–E smear. The sample next to the label was obtained from the posterior vaginal vault (V), the middle sample by scraping the transformation zone of the cervix (C), and the endocervical (E) sample farthest from the label was obtained with a cotton swab applicator, which is immediately rotated on the glass slide.

with a cotton-tipped applicator. All three samples must be quickly transferred to a slide: the endocervical sample is rolled onto the slide, from one edge to the other near the end farthest from the label, the exocervical sample is spread in the middle area of the slide, and the posterior vaginal vault material is placed nearest to the label (Figure 14.2). This must be done very swiftly to leave no time for drying. As soon as the three samples have been deposited, the glass slide is submerged in 70% ethyl alcohol. A spray fixative may also be used.

The V–C–E smear provides three distinct samples from the genital tract, thus reducing the chances of missing a significant lesion. At the same time it is economical and practical: only one glass slide needs to be stained, screened and stored for each patient. In our experience with nearly 1,000 different sources of gynecologic smears, we have found the V–C–E technique reliable, with a very low rate (1% to 2%) of inadequate smears.

Once the smear has been collected and adequately fixed, it must be sent to the cytopreparatory laboratory as soon as possible, *with the completed requisition form.* The laboratory's first step is to correctly identify the smear and corresponding requisition form by means of a unique access number to avoid confusion. Then the smears are stained, coverslipped and sent to the cytotechnologists for interpretation (Figure 14.3, page 246).

14.1 Modification of Papanicolaou's Stain (EA-65)

Reagents

Hematoxylin (C.I. 75290)
Ethyl alcohol
Aluminum ammonium sulphate
Distilled water
Mercuric oxide
Glacial acetic acid
Phosphotungstic acid
Aqueous light-green staining solution (C.I. 42095)
Eosin Y (C.I. 45380)
Bismark brown staining solution (C.I. 21000)
Ammonium hydroxide
Orange G (C.I. 16230)

Prepared Reagents

1. Harris' hematoxylin solution
   a. Dissolve 15 g hematoxylin in ethyl alcohol at 56 °C (oven or water bath).
   b. Dissolve 300 g aluminum ammonium sulphate in 3,000 mL distilled water by heating over a Bunsen burner with frequent stirring.
   c. Remove from heat.

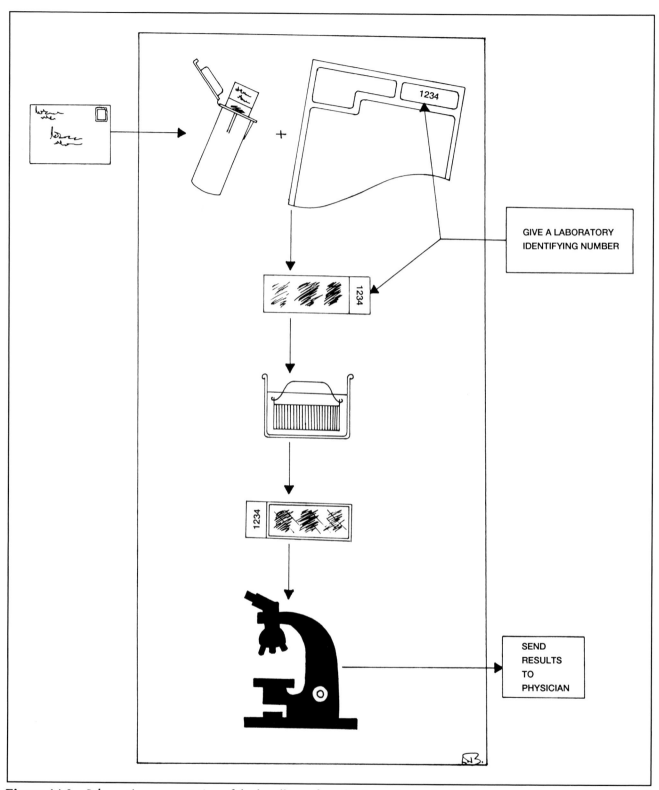

GIVE A LABORATORY
IDENTIFYING NUMBER

1234

SEND
RESULTS
TO
PHYSICIAN

Figure 14.3 Schematic representation of the handling of cytologic specimens in the laboratory. The properly prepared smears arrive in the laboratory by mail, within protective containers. The smears and the requisition form are given an access number. The glass slides are stained and submitted to cytotechnologists for microscopic examination.

d. Add alcoholic hematoxylin solution and bring to boil with frequent stirring.
   e. Turn off Bunsen burner and add 7.5 g mercuric oxide immediately.
   f. After cooling, filter and store in a dark bottle.
   g. Before use, add acetic acid (4 mL for each 100 mL of solution).
2. Orange G (Papanicolaou OG-6) solution
   a. Prepare 10% aqueous solution of orange G with distilled water.
   b. Let stand several days.
   c. Mix 50 mL 10% aqueous solution of orange G, 0.15 g phosphotungstic acid, and 950 mL 95% ethyl alcohol.
   d. Store in a dark bottle. This solution is to be used within 3 months. Filter before use.
3. EA 65
   1. Solution A (Aqueous light green solution)
      a. Prepare 25 mL of 2% aqueous light green solution.
      b. Dilute with 975 mL 95% ethyl alcohol to obtain 0.05% strength solution.
      c. Set aside.
   2. Solution B (Eosin Y)
      a. Mix 5 g eosin Y with 1,000 mL 95% ethyl alcohol.
      b. Set aside.
   3. Solution C (Bismark brown)
      a. Mix Bismark brown with distilled water to obtain 5 mL aqueous solution of 10% strength.
      b. Set aside for a few days.
      c. Mix with 95 mL 95% ethyl alcohol.
      d. Set aside.
   a. Mix 450 mL of solution A, 450 mL of solution B, 100 mL of solution C, and 6 g phosphotungstic acid.
   b. Store in a dark bottle and filter before use. This solution may be prepared every 2 to 3 months.
4. Bluing agent
   a. Mix 394 mL of 70% ethyl alcohol and 6 mL of ammonium hydroxide.

Comments

All dyes used must be certified by the Biological Stain Commission, Rochester, New York. The unequivocal choice of a given dye is obtained by its "color index" (C.I.), which is a catalog system consisting of fixed digits.

Filter all stains and xylene daily with Whatman filter paper No 1 to avoid contamination of smears by cells detached from previous smears. It is best to replace alcohol every day. Maintain an appropriate level of solution in every dish. Discard stain when colored cells start to fade.

14.2 Papanicolaou Staining Technique

Background

Sample the squamous epithelium of the vaginal portion of the cervix, the squamocolumnar junction, and the endocervical epithelium on the same glass slide (V–C–E technique). Fix smear by immersing immediately in 70% alcohol for 15 minutes, or use a commercial spraying fixative. If using a spray, fix smear by holding nozzle about 15 cm from slide and cover with 2 slow sweeps of spray. Allow to dry 5 to 7 minutes.

As a rule of thumb, 1,080 slides can be stained with 800 mL of stain. The slides must be submerged gently by dipping the slides in each solution and then removing them smoothly. Drain slides well between each step. Do not allow cells to dry. Follow the timing of each step exactly.

Reagents

Ethanol
Toluene
Distilled water

Prepared Reagents

1. Harris' hematoxylin solution (see Procedure 14.1.1)
2. Bluing agent (see Procedure 14.1.4)
3. Orange G solution (see Procedure 14.1.2)
4. EA-65 solution (see Procedure 14.1.3)

Procedure

1. Treat smear with 95% ethanol for at least one minute.
2. Dip 10 times in 80% ethanol.
3. Dip 10 times in 70% ethanol.
4. Dip 10 times in 50% ethanol.
5. Rinse by dipping 10 times in distilled water.
6. Stain with Harris' hematoxylin solution for 3 minutes. NOTE: Increase staining time by 30 seconds after staining a lot of 180 slides (First 180 slides: 3 minutes; next 180 slides 3 minutes 30 seconds; next series of 180 slides: 4 minutes; etc).
7. Rinse again by dipping 10 times in distilled water.
8. Rinse again by dipping 10 times in distilled water.
9. Dip 10 times in 50% ethanol.
10. Treat with bluing agent for 1 minute.
11. Dip 10 times in 70% ethanol.
12. Dip 10 times in 80% ethanol.
13. Dip 10 times in 95% ethanol.
14. Stain with Orange G solution for 1 minute.
15. Dip 10 times in 95% ethanol.
16. Dip again 10 times in 95% ethanol.

17. Dip 10 times again in 95% ethanol.
18. Stain with EA-65 for 3 minutes.
19. Dip 10 times in 95% ethanol.
20. Dip again 10 times in 95% ethanol.
21. Dip again 10 times in 95% ethanol.
22. Dip 10 times in 100% ethanol.
23. Dip again 10 times in 100% ethanol.
24. Dip 10 times in 50:50 mixture of ethanol and toluene.
25. Dip 10 times in toluene.
26. Dip again 10 times in toluene.
27. Dip again 10 times in toluene.
28. Coverslip smear with a mounting reagent to which an antioxidant has been added (5 g for 500 mL of mounting reagent) to retard fading of stains.

Staining Reaction

The nuclei are stained by Harris' hematoxylin solution. The keratin takes up yellow stain from Orange G. EA-65 stains the cytoplasm (superficial cells pink and intermediate cells blue-green). Bismark brown, although traditionally included, can be omitted as it provides no staining effect.

Observations	Color	Figure	Chapter
Nuclei	blue	5.2	V
Parabasal cell cytoplasm	deep bluish green	1.12	I
Intermediate cell cytoplasm	bluish green	1.11	I
Superficial cell cytoplasm	pink	1.10	I
Keratinized cell cytoplasm	orange	6.34	VI
Candida albicans	red	4.9	IV
Trichomonas vaginalis	grey-green	4.9	IV

Interpretation

In addition to well-prepared smears with adequate clinical information, cytotechnologists should have access to records of previous cytologic examinations (computer printouts), and when needed, the previous smears of the patient.

All pertinent observations (quality of material submitted, cytologic findings, recommendations, etc) are recorded on the patient's form by the cytotechnologist. Finally, the glass slides are submitted for quality control and/or shown to a senior cytotechnologist or to the pathologist, as appropriate, and finally stored. The form then goes to the data processing unit and is recorded on the computer that prints out the final report to be sent to the patient's doctor (Figure 14.4, see also Chapter 13).

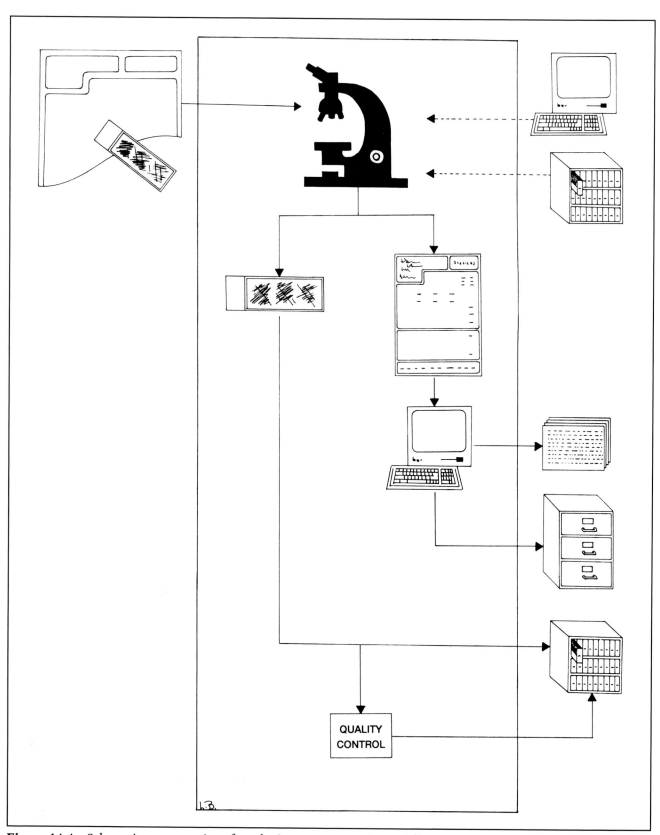

Figure 14.4 Schematic representation of cytologic report preparation and filing. Cytotechnologists have computerized access to previous reports and smears, before and during microscopic examination of the smears. The patient's form is used to register all pertinent findings, which are then entered into the computer for processing. Smears are submitted to quality control or review by senior cytotechnologists or pathologists, and are finally stored for at least 5 years (benign) or 20 years (significant cellular changes).

What is an "Inadequate" Smear?

Recognizing that a smear is suboptimal or frankly inadequate is essential in order to avoid diagnostic errors. The attempt to interpret smears of poor quality is futile and may lead to misinterpretation. It is best to label a smear as inadequate, rather than run the risk of missing an important lesion or of overinterpreting artifactual changes.

Inadequate smears can be the result of faulty sampling, fixation, staining, coverslipping, or a combination of these factors. If the problem lies within the laboratory, remedial action can be taken swiftly and effectively. When the problem is related to sampling and fixation, the person responsible should be contacted, and clear and accurate explanations on how to obtain an adequate sample should be furnished in writing.

Common problems within the laboratory are poor staining with extreme loss of color contrast, the presence of artifacts, and the appearance of "floaters." The use of good quality stains that are regularly replaced, and adherence to proper staining technique will avoid most technical problems in the laboratory. Staining solution should be checked every day to ensure uniform quality. A common and troublesome artifact consists of a golden brown staining of the cytoplasm of intermediate squamous cells. Such cells are called "cornflakes" (Plate 14.1). They have been ascribed to air trapped on the surface of cells when the mounting medium is applied. Floaters are cells detached from the same or another smear that remain suspended in one of the solutions and are picked up during staining. They can usually be recognized because they do not lie on the same plane as the rest of the cells (Plates 14.2 and 14.3).

Other frequent contaminants are spores (Plate 14.4) and other airborne vegetable cells (Plate 14.5), which are deposited on the smears at any time during their preparation. Other contaminants include talcum (Plates 14.6 and 14.7), dust particles (Plate 14.8), fibers from tampons (Plate 14.9), and even flies (Plate 14.10). Hematoidin crystals show up as small rounded cockleburlike formations (Plate 14.11). Inspissated mucus may form spirals, similar to Curshmann's spirals seen in sputum (Plate 14.12).

Faulty sampling may result in smears with scant cellularity (Plate 14.13), or smears that are too thick to be adequately interpreted (Plate 14.14). Gentle spreading of the cell sample is important. If too much force is applied, cells will become elongated and nuclear streaks will appear on the smear (Plate 14.15). If lubricant is used to introduce the vaginal speculum before sampling, the smear will contain an opaque amorphous material that obscures the cellular detail (Plate 14.16).

Incorrect fixation results in loss of cellular staining affinity. Air-dried smears must be rehydrated in the laboratory to avoid drying artifacts. When the smear is fixed with a spray fixative, the nozzle must be held about 15 cm from the glass slide, in order to avoid spreading of the smear, which may make it impossible to interpret (Plate 14.17).

If the sample does not include material from the transformation zone, no elements from that area will be detected on the smear (ie, columnar endocervical cells, metaplastic cells, and/or mucus). Whether the absence of these elements should suffice to label the sample as inadequate remains debatable. Many cases of epithelial abnormalities are detected on smears lacking material from the transformation zone, and conversely, even in the presence of endocervical cells, serious epithelial lesions may not shed diagnostic cells and will therefore be missed.

Smears may be difficult or impossible to interpret because of factors unrelated either to sampling, fixation, or staining. If there is excessive inflammation with or without marked autolysis, numerous granulocytes may entirely obscure the cellular detail (Plate 14.18). Excessive blood (Plate 14.19) as well as large numbers of sperm cells (Plates 14.20 and 14.21) may also impede evaluation of the smear.

References

1. Wied GL, Bahr GF: Vaginal, cervical and endocervical cytologic smears on a single slide. *Obstet Gynecol* 14:361–367, 1959.

Plate 14.1
Artifact: Cornflakes stain golden brown, but should not be confused
with glycogen droplets.

Plate 14.2
A "floater." Such cells lie on a plane above the rest of the smear.
Compare with Plate 14.3 below.

Plate 14.3
This is the plane of the smear over which lies the floater depicted
in Plate 14.2.

Plate 14.4
Contaminant: a spore.

Plate 14.1

Plate 14.2

Plate 14.3

Plate 14.4

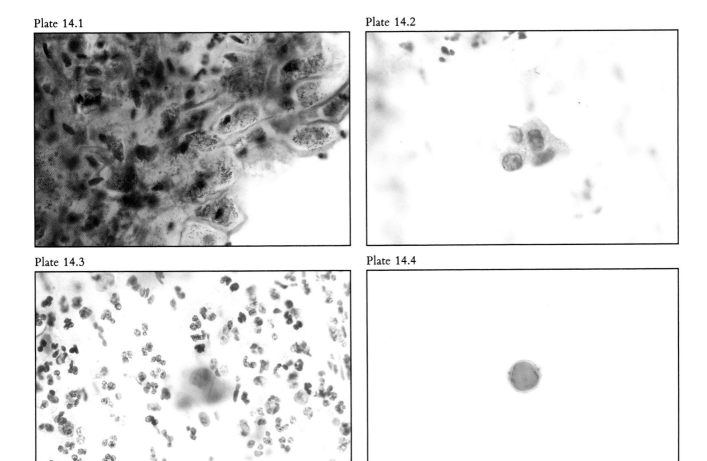

Plate 14.5

Contaminant: a vegetable cell.

Plate 14.6

Contaminant: talcum (see also Plate 14.7).

Plate 14.7

Contaminant: talcum. This is the same area of the smear illustrated in Plate 14.6 under polarized light. Talcum crystals are refringent and display the cross of Malta in their center.

Plate 14.8

Contaminant: a dust particle.

Plate 14.5

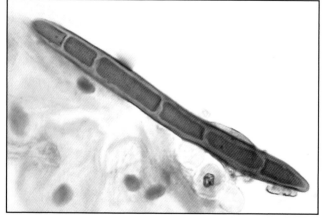

Plate 14.6

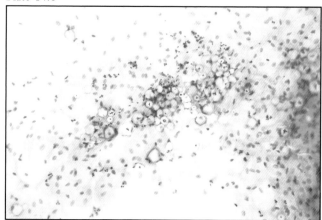

Plate 14.7

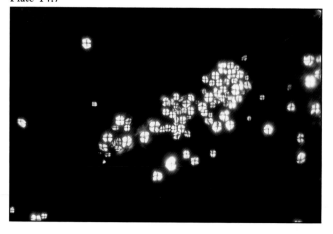

Plate 14.8

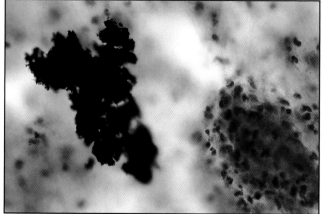

Plate 14.9
Contaminant: a fiber (probably from a tampon).

Plate 14.10
Contaminant: this small fly managed to get mounted on the smear without attracting the attention of the cytopreparatory technologists. Note the squamous cells in the background that provide a sense of scale.

Plate 14.11
Cockleburlike hematoidin crystal.

Plate 14.12
Curschmannlike spiral found on a cervical smear. Represents inspissated mucus.

Plate 14.9

Plate 14.10

Plate 14.11

Plate 14.12

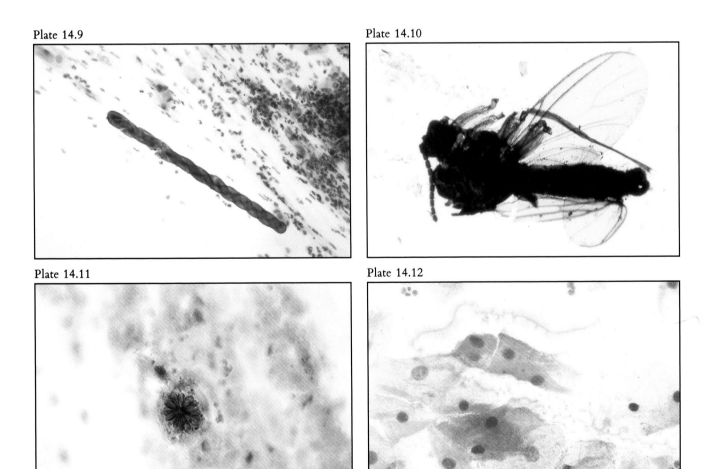

Plate 14.13
Inadequate smear: scant cellularity.

Plate 14.14
Inadequate smear: too thick to be fixed properly, the cell morphology cannot be appreciated.

Plate 14.15
Inadequate smear: streaking due to excessive force of application while spreading the material on the glass slide.

Plate 14.13

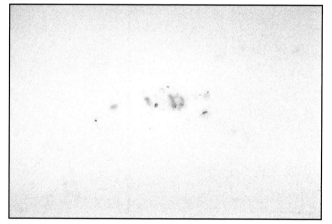

Plate 14.14

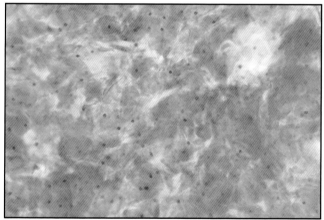

Plate 14.15

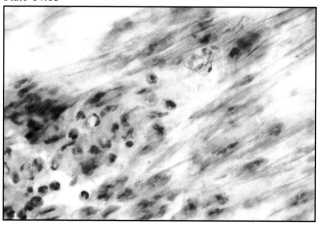

Plate 14.16
Inadequate smear: cellular detail is lost due to heavy overlay of lubricant.

Plate 14.17
Inadequate smear: spray fixative was used too near to the surface of the smear.

Plate 14.18
Inadequate smear: excessive inflammation. The granulocytes completely obscure the cells.

Plate 14.16

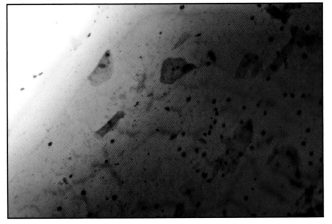

Plate 14.17

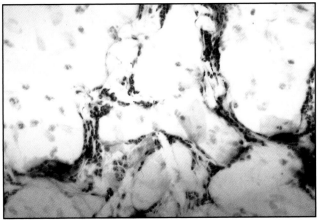

Plate 14.18

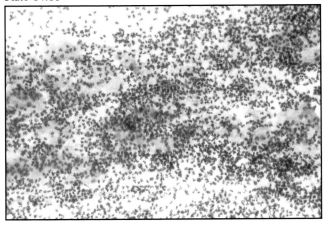

Plate 14.19

Inadequate smear: excessive blood.

Plate 14.20

Inadequate smear: sperm cells cover most of the smear.

Plate 14.21

Inadequate smear: a higher magnification of the smear illustrated in Plate 14.20. The smear consists mostly of sperm cells.

Plate 14.19

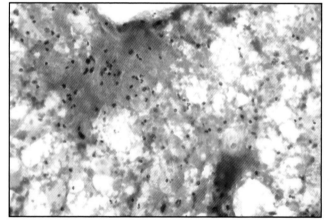

Plate 14.20

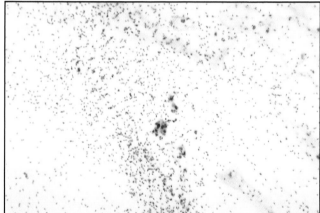

Plate 14.21

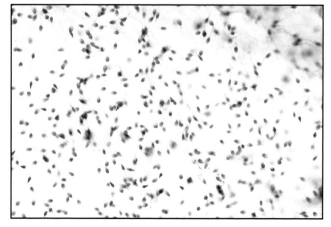

CHAPTER FIFTEEN

Technical Considerations

In 1858, Rudolf Virchow postulated the cell theory, in which the cell was recognized as the basic unit of life. The cell appears as a unit of form, function, and duplication. Fifty years ago morphologic description of cells was the basic approach of cell study. Then cytology and biochemistry were combined to clarify the function of cells, giving birth to biochemical cytology. Later, the electron microscope improved the investigation of the structure of cell organelles down to the level of macromolecules, this was the creation of ultrastructural cytology. The science of immunochemistry was subsequently applied to the relationship between tissue culture, cellular invaders (such as viruses) and the chemical activities of the immunoglobulin molecules, ie, immunocytology. Today we have entered the world of molecular cytology to better understand normal living cells as well as diseased tissue. The cytopathologist and the cytotechnologist must be aware that their fields are not limited to morphologic cytology but that they extend to biochemical, ultrastructural, immunochemical, and molecular cytology. The understanding of normal and abnormal cells requires the use of a battery of different techniques. In the following sections we are going to describe a few techniques complementary to diagnostic cytopathology.

Routine Histology

The development of techniques for the study of tissues (histology) was based on improvements in microscopes, the emergence of dye industries, and the refinement of methods for preparing and observing cells. Histology is defined as the microscopic anatomy of tissue. It is the study of the structure and details of tissues as prepared for and visualized by light microscopy. But it is generally difficult to study living cells and tissues under a conventional light microscope without adequate preparation. The basic techniques of preparing tissues for light microscopy include three main steps:

1. Fixation with chemicals that serve to kill and stabilize structures, prevent self-digestion (autolysis), and preserve lifelike appearance;
2. Embedding in materials that support tissue in order to obtain thin sections that permit light to pass through;
3. Staining with dyes that provide sufficient contrast to differentiate between nucleus and cytoplasm and other cytoplasmic organelles, as well as features of the extracellular environment.

It is beyond this chapter's scope to review theoretical principles of histotechnology. We will describe only those histologic techniques used to prepare the cervical specimens for the many photomicrographs that illustrate this book. For a review of histotechnology (principles and practice) the reader is referred to the paper by Bancroft and Stevens.[1]

15.1 Tissue Fixation
Prepared Reagents

1. Carnoy's fixative
    Ethyl alcohol
    Chloroform
    Glacial acetic acid
    Mix 60 mL ethyl alcohol, 30 mL chloroform, and 10 mL glacial acetic acid. NOTE: This fixative is suitable for Hemalum-Phloxine-Saffron staining, immunohistochemistry, and in situ hybridization.
2. Bouin's fixative
    Saturated aqueous picric acid
    40% formaldehyde
    Glacial acetic acid
    Mix 75 mL saturated aqueous picric acid, 25 mL 40% formaldehyde, and 5 mL glacial acetic acid. NOTE: This fixative is suitable for routine staining and immunohistochemistry.
3. Neutral buffered formalin (10%)
    40% formaldehyde
    Distilled water
    Sodium dihydrogen phosphate (anhydrous)
    Disodium hydrogen phosphate (anhydrous)
    a. Mix 10 mL formaldehyde 40% with 90 mL distilled water.
    b. Add and mix 0.35 g sodium dihydrogen phosphate (anhydrous) and 0.65 g disodium hydrogen phosphate (anhydrous). NOTE: This fixative is appropriate for Hem-

alum-Phloxine-Saffron staining. It is suitable for Hematoxylin-Eosin staining, immunohistochemistry, and in situ hybridization.

Fixation Procedure

Biopsy specimens of the uterine cervix are obtained under colposcopic visualization. The specimen is immediately fixed in Bouin's fluid, Carnoy's fixative, or neutral buffered formalin. We favor Carnoy's fixative because of its versatility: it is suitable for routine hemalum-phloxine-saffron staining, immunohistochemical identification of tissular and viral antigens, and molecular in situ hybridization for the identification of DNA sequences.

Fixation must be done as soon as possible to prevent autolytic and mechanical alterations. Fixation is done at room temperature for a period not exceeding 2 hours. For pieces smaller than 2 mm, 30 minutes is sufficient. Fixation depends on the use of agents that precipitate macromolecules that promote insolubility in order to immobilize tissular constituents in a lifelike state. Carnoy's fixative contains ethanol, which coagulates proteins and breaks hydrogen bonds, thus increasing histochemical reactivity. Ethanol in combination with chloroform and acetic acid give a good fixation for glycogen, which is abundant in cervical specimens. Acetic acid makes an excellent fixative for nucleoproteins by precipitating them. It is a good fixative for nuclei. Therefore, Carnoy's fixative is recommended for Feulgen's reaction and for in situ hybridization (see pp 286–290). The Feulgen's reaction is a cytochemical staining method for the demonstration of DNA in cytologic preparations. This reaction permits the quantitative assessment of the amount of DNA by cytophotometric measurements. Applications and discussion of the Feulgen's reaction in relation to the uterine cervix are reported by Fu et al,[16] Reid et al,[55] Shevchuck and Richart,[65] and Winkler et al.[80]

In order to obtain the best trichrome staining (hemalum-phloxine-saffron), we recommend Bouin's fluid, which is an excellent fixative for the conservation of delicate structures. It can be used for demonstration of glycogen. Fixation of 2–3 hours is sufficient for 2–3 mm pieces. However, Bouin's fluid hydrolyses nucleoproteins and is not recommended for the Feulgen's reaction and for in situ hybridization studies.

15.2 Dehydration, Embedding, and Sectioning
Background

For light microscopy, fixed tissues are usually embedded in paraffin. First, tissues must be dehydrated by soaking them in a series of increasing percentage of ethanol, then soaked in a clearing agent such as toluene (a substance permitting the transition between ethanol and paraffin, ie, a substance that is miscible with both ethanol and paraffin), and finally soaked in melted paraffin.

Prepared Reagents

1. Diluted ethanol
   Dilute absolute ethanol with distilled water in order to obtain the following concentrations: 50%, 70%, 80%, and 95%.
2. Gelatin
   Gelatin
   Absolute ethanol
   Distilled water
   Dissolve 1 g gelatin in 200 mL absolute ethanol. Increase total volume to 1,000 mL with distilled water.

Other Reagents and Equipment

Toluene
Distilled water
Paraffin
Mounting medium (Eukitt)
Automatic tissue changer
Hot paraffin bath
Embedding mold
Microtome and knives
Microscope slides
Coverslips

Dehydration Procedure

The dehydration, clearing, and paraffin soaking schedule is usually performed in an automatic tissue changer. This equipment permits immersion of tissues with constant agitation and the automatic change from one bath to the next one and so on. The immersion schedule is the following:

1. Fixative for 2–3 hours
2. 50% ethanol (dehydration) for 1 hour
3. 70% ethanol (dehydration) for 1 hour
4. 80% ethanol (dehydration) for 1 hour
5. 95% ethanol (dehydration) for 1 hour
6. Absolute ethanol (dehydration) for 1 hour
7. Toluene (clearing) for 1 hour
8. Toluene (clearing) for 1 hour
9. Toluene (clearing) for 1 hour
10. Toluene (clearing) for 1 hour
11. Melted paraffin I for 1 hour
12. Melted paraffin II for 2 hours

Paraffin Embedding and Sectioning Procedure

Tissues are transferred to a mold containing melted paraffin, which cools to become a hard matrix. Thin slices of 4–5 μm in thickness are easily obtained using a microtome. The tissue sections are then mounted on glass slides with 1% gelatin. The sections are allowed to dry in an oven at 37 °C for 2 hours before staining.

15.3 Hemalum-Phloxine-Saffron Stain

Prepared Reagents

1. Bluing agent
     Lithium bicarbonate
     Distilled water
     Mix 40 g of lithium bicarbonate with 4000 mL distilled water.
2. Mayer's hemalum
     Hematoxylin (C.I. 75290)
     Potassium or ammonium alum
     Sodium iodate
     Chloral hydrate
     Citric acid
     Distilled water
     a. Dissolve 1 g hematoxylin, 50 g alum, and 0.2 g sodium iodate in 1,000 mL distilled water.
     b. Add 50 g chloral hydrate and 1 g citric acid. Mix and boil for 5 minutes.
     c. Cool and filter. Keep in a dark bottle.
3. Phloxine
     Phloxine (C.I. 45410)
     Distilled water
     a. Dissolve 4 g of phloxine in 400 mL distilled water.
     b. Filter. Keep in a dark bottle.
4. Saffron
     Saffron (C.I. 75100)
     Absolute ethanol
     a. Dry 2 g of saffron in an oven at 56 °C.
     b. Add 100 mL absolute ethanol and mix well.
     c. Solution may be used the following day. Time improves the staining capacity of saffron.

Other Reagents

Toluene
Absolute ethanol
40% formaldehyde
Tap water

Staining Procedure

1. Treat with toluene for 2 minutes.
2. Treat with toluene for 2 minutes.
3. Dip 10 times in absolute ethanol.
4. Treat with ethanol-formol (9:1) for 10 minutes.
5. Stain with Mayer's hemalum for 5 minutes. NOTE: The staining time for hemalum is 5 minutes the first day. One minute

is added every subsequent day for 5 days, after which the stain is discarded.

6. Rinse in tap water for a few seconds.
7. Differentiate by dipping in bluing agent 10 times.
8. Rinse in tap water for 15–20 minutes.
9. Stain with phloxine for 8–10 minutes. NOTE: Phloxine is replaced every three weeks.
10. Rinse in tap water a few seconds.
11. Dip 10 times in absolute ethanol.
12. Dip 10 times in absolute ethanol.
13. Dip 10 times in absolute ethanol.
14. Stain with saffron for 50 seconds. NOTE: Saffron is replaced every week.
15. Dip 2 times in absolute ethanol.
16. Dip 2 times in absolute ethanol.
17. Dip 2 times in absolute ethanol.
18. Dip 10 times in toluene.
19. Dip 10 times in toluene.
20. Dip 10 times in toluene.
21. Dip 10 times in toluene.
22. Coverslip with a mounting medium.

Staining Reaction

The nuclei are stained dark blue and mucus is stained blue by hemalum. Cell cytoplasm is stained pink by phloxine. Collagen appears yellow-orange (saffron); red blood cells are red and elastic fibers are pink. Plates 10.6 and 6.49 illustrate Hemalum-Phloxine-Saffron staining of sections of the uterine cervix.

15.4 Periodic-Acid-Schiff (PAS) Reaction (for glycogen)

Background

Tissue sections are first oxidized by periodic acid introducing free aldehydes on the polysaccharide chains.[39] These aldehydes groups can react with Schiff's reagent to produce a colored reaction proving the presence of polysaccharides in tissue sections. The Schiff's reagent is a colorless compound obtained by the reaction of basic fuchsin (Pararosanilin, red) and sulphurous acid (H_2SO_4). This reaction is characterized by the loss of the chromophore group localized on the pararosanilin. When aldehyde groups are present in the tissue sections, a red-colored reaction is produced by restoration of the chromophore group.

Prepared Reagents

1. Phosphate buffer (for diastase digestion)
   Sodium phosphate (monobasic)
   Sodium phosphate (dibasic)
   Sodium chloride

Distilled water

Thymol

a. Dissolve 1.97 g sodium phosphate (monobasic), 0.28 g sodium phosphate (dibasic), 8.0 g sodium chloride in 1,000 mL boiling distilled water.

b. Cool and add a few drops of thymol.

c. Keep at 4 °C.

2. Diastase (for digestion of glycogen)

Malt diastase

Phosphate buffer

Dissolve 0.1 g diastase in 100 mL phosphate buffer. NOTE: Prepare diastase daily.

3. Hydrochloric acid (1N HCl)

Concentrated hydrochloric acid (sp g 1.19)

Distilled water

Mix 8.35 mL concentrated HCl with 91.65 mL distilled water.

4. Schiff's reagent

Basic fuchsin (C.I. 42510)

1N HCl

Sodium metabisulfite

Activated charcoal

a. Dissolve 1 g basic fuchsin in 200 mL of boiling water with frequent stirring.

b. Bring the solution to 50 °C and filter.

c. Add 20 mL of 1N HCl to the filtrate.

d. Bring to 25 °C.

e. Add 1 g of sodium metabisulfite.

f. Keep in the dark in a well-stoppered bottle for 24 hours.

g. Add 2 g activated charcoal.

h. Agitate and filter. The filtrate must be colorless and clear.

i. Keep at 4 °C in a dark bottle.

5. 1%-Periodic acid (HIO_4)

Periodic acid

Distilled water

Dissolve 1 g periodic acid in 100 mL distilled water.

6. Sodium (or potassium) metabisulfite

Sodium or potassium metabisulfite

Distilled water

Dissolve 10 g sodium or potassium metabisulfite in 100 mL distilled water.

7. Sulphurous rinse water

10% sodium or potassium metabisulfite

1N HCl

Distilled water

Mix 10 mL 10% sodium or potassium metabisulfite, 10 mL 1N HCl, and 200 mL distilled water.

PAS Staining Procedure

Tissues are fixed in Bouin's fluid, 10% neutral formalin, or Carnoy's fixative (see Procedure 15.1.1–3). It is important to include a second slide used as a negative control. A negative control slide is obtained by a diastase digestion to remove any possible positive reaction. Digestion for 30 minutes is done in the diastase solution heated at 37 °C in a water bath or a laboratory oven. It is also useful to include a positive control slide (a tissue section from the liver which is rich in glycogen). Do not digest the positive control slide. The procedure is as follows:

1. Deparaffinize 2 minutes in toluene.
2. Deparaffinize 2 minutes in toluene.
3. Dip 10 times in absolute ethanol.
4. Treat with ethanol-formol (9:1) for 10 minutes.
5. Rinse in tap water for 5 minutes.
6. Rinse in tap water for 5 minutes.
7. Treat in periodic acid for 5 minutes.
8. Dip 10 times in distilled water.
9. Dip 10 times in distilled water.
10. Dip 10 times in distilled water.
11. Treat in Schiff's reagent for 15 minutes.
12. Rinse in tap water for 15 minutes.
13. Rinse in sulphurous water for 2 minutes.
14. Rinse in sulphurous water for 2 minutes.
15. Rinse in sulphurous water for 2 minutes.
16. Rinse in tap water for 2 minutes.
17. Stain with Mayer's hemalum for 1–5 minutes.
18. Dip 10 times in tap water.
19. Dip 10 times in tap water.
20. Dip 10 times in tap water.
21. Dip 10 times in 70% ethanol.
22. Dip 10 times in 80% ethanol.
23. Dip 10 times in 95% ethanol.
24. Dip 10 times in absolute ethanol.
25. Dip 10 times in toluene.
26. Dip 10 times in toluene.
27. Dip 10 times in toluene.
28. Coverslip with mounting medium.

Staining Reaction

Positive substances stain red. In digested PAS tissues, only mucus stains red and glycogen is digested. In nondigested PAS tissues, mucus and glycogen stain red. Nuclei are blue. Plates 1.8, 6.3, and 6.4 illustrate the results.

Immunohistochemistry

Immunohistochemistry exploits the specific binding property between antibody and antigen to demonstrate a wide range of cellular and infectious components in tissue sections. Antigens are substances (proteins and carbohydrates) that stimulate the immune system of an animal in order to elicit the formation of antibodies. Antibodies (immunoglobulins) are complex protein molecules produced by plasma cells and certain lymphocytes; they combine specifically with inducing antigens.

When an antibody is labelled with a visible fluorescent marker (fluorescein or rhodamine B isothiocyanates) or linked covalently to an enzyme, (peroxidase, alkaline-phosphatase, or glucose-oxidase) capable of reacting in the presence of an appropriate substrate and a suitable chromogen, the labelled antibody becomes a visible probe. Therefore, the labelled antibody-antigen complex is easily visualized and localized within tissue sections by light and electron microscopy (when using enzyme-labelled antibodies) or by immunofluorescence (when using a fluorescent dye as a marker). Because of many disadvantages to immunofluorescent techniques, the use of enzyme markers in immunohistochemistry is becoming more widespread.

Different immunohistochemical techniques are available: the direct technique, the indirect technique, the immunoenzyme bridge technique, the peroxidase-antiperoxidase technique (unlabelled antibody enzyme method), and the avidin-biotin (or streptavidin-biotin) method. It is worth mentioning that these techniques can be performed by computer-assisted robots, which produce cost-effective, simplified, reproducible assays.[5]

Direct Technique

The primary antibody is linked to the marker: horseradish peroxidase for example (see Figure 15.1A). It is the quickest method but also the least sensitive. Another disadvantage is that each primary antibody has to be conjugated with a marker in order to detect different antigens.

Indirect Technique

With the indirect technique the primary antiserum is unlabelled (a rabbit antibody) and used first against a specific antigen (see Figure 15.1B). Then a secondary antibody conjugated with peroxidase is directed against the unlabelled primary antibody (goat anti-rabbit serum). This technique is more sensitive. The versatility of the labelled secondary antiserum permits use of a single conjugated antibody with several primary antibodies directed against different antigens in different tissue sections.

Immunoenzyme Bridge Technique

The antigen is first incubated with unlabelled primary antibody (eg, rabbit antiserum). In the second step, the section is incubated with an unlabelled secondary antibody directed against the primary antibody (eg, a goat anti-rabbit serum). In the third step, the section is incubated with an antihorseradish peroxidase serum (eg, a rabbit immunoglobulin) produced in the same animal species as the primary antibody. Thus the secondary antibody is used as a bridging antibody joining peroxidase to the antigen (see Figure 15.1C).

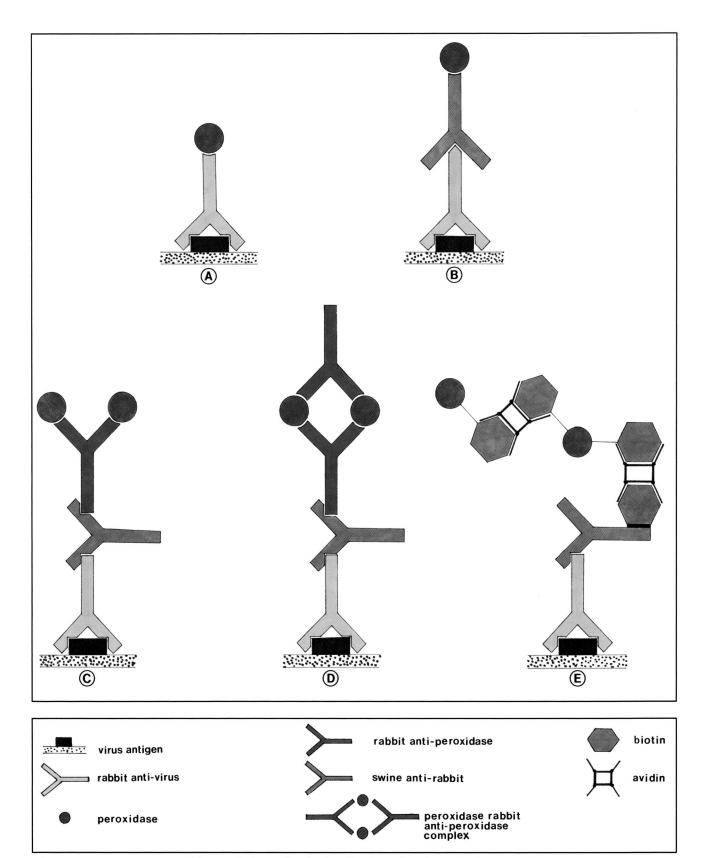

Figure 15.1 Immunoperoxidase techniques for the localization of antigens in tissue sections.

Peroxidase-Antiperoxidase Technique

The principle of the peroxidase-antiperoxidase technique is almost the same as for the immunoenzyme bridge technique except that the third antiserum is replaced by the peroxidase-antiperoxidase (PAP) complex (Sternberger, 1979).[71] This complex is obtained by incubation of the antihorseradish peroxidase antibody with free horseradish peroxidase. The PAP complex and the primary serum must be of the same animal species (eg, rabbit immunoglobulins). The secondary antibody forms a bridge between the primary antibody and the PAP complex (see Figure 15.1D). The intensity of the reaction is amplified with this technique.

Avidin-Biotin Method

This is probably the most popular technique available today. This technique is based on the high-affinity binding between avidin and biotin. The antigen is first incubated with the unlabelled primary antiserum. Subsequently, a biotinylated secondary antibody is directed against the primary antibody. Finally the section is incubated with an avidin-peroxidase (or streptavidin-peroxidase) complex. The avidin binds tightly to the biotinylated antibody at the site of antigen in the tissue section (see Figure 15.1E).

Visualization of Markers at the Antigen Site

Fluorescent markers necessitate the use of a fluorescence microscope in order to visualize the presence of the antigen-labelled complex. In contrast, enzyme markers can be visualized under light microscopy. But they are not visible by themselves, without a previous enzymatic reaction with a substrate and a chromogen. The peroxidase catalyses the transfer of oxygen from the hydrogen peroxide: the substrate. The DAB (diaminobenzidine tetrahydrochloride), the chromogen, acts as a hydrogen donor. An insoluble colored product (gold brown) is then formed at the reaction site. Other chromogens such as AEC (3-amino-9-ethylcarbazole) or the Hanker-Yates reactive (4-chloro-1-naphthol), give respectively a red, alcohol soluble and a blue, alcohol-insoluble precipitate at the reaction site. The use of different chromogens allows the double immunoenzyme staining for the identification of more than one antigen in the same tissue specimen.

Proteolytic Enzyme Digestion

The use of trypsin, pepsin, or pronase can be very useful in enhancing immunoreactivity in paraffin-embedded sections. Variables including temperature, incubation time, and the fixative used must be controlled to obtain maximum reliability with this technique. For instance, tissues fixed in formaldehyde solution benefit greatly from enzyme pre-treatment. However, overdigestion must be omitted because sections may detach from the slide. The use of diluted white glue or poly-L-lysine adhesive may help to prevent the loss of sections.

15.5 Preparation of Tissues for Immunohistochemistry

Background

As a rule, the quality of an immunohistochemical preparation depends upon prompt and proper fixation and processing. There is no perfect fixative for immunohistochemistry. Formalin, Bouin's, and Carnoy's fixatives (see Procedure 15.1) give acceptable results. Formalin is probably the most popular fixative used in many laboratories. But it appears that formalin is not the best-suited fixative for immunohistochemistry. Formalin cross-links proteins around antigenic sites, masking them and preventing optimal antibody binding. In most instances, the antigen can be unmasked using proteolytic enzymes, provided the antigen is resistant to the protease. Bouin's fixative is also effective but not superior to formalin. The alcohol-based fixatives such as Carnoy's fixative assure a superior immunoreactivity to formalin and Bouin's fluid in paraffin-embedded tissues. In our laboratory, we fixed biopsied tissue from the uterine cervix in Carnoy's fluid for 2–3 hours. Tissue processing (dehydration, clearing, and paraffin embedding) can also affect immunoreactivity, mainly if excessive temperatures are used. Paraffin sections not more than 3–5 μm in thickness are recommended. For discussion of dehydration, clearing, and paraffin embedding of biopsied tissue see Procedure 15.2.

Prepared Reagents

1. 2% Hydrochloric acid
   Concentrated hydrochloric acid (sp g 1.19)
   Distilled water
   Add 2 mL concentrated HCl to 98 mL distilled water and mix.
2. 1% glue solution
   White glue
   Distilled water
   Mix 1 mL Elmer's Glue All adhesive with 100 mL distilled water.
3. 0.01% Poly-L-lysine
   Poly-L-lysine (Sigma, Cat No P1399)
   Distilled water
   Dissolve 10 mg poly-L-lysine in 100 mL distilled water.

Other Equipment

Hot plate
Laboratory oven
Microscope slides
Paper towel

Slide Preparation Procedure

1. Clean microscope slides by soaking them in 2% HCl for 15 minutes.
2. Rinse slides twice in distilled water for 2 minutes.
3. Leave slides to air-dry in a dust-free environment.
4. Spread evenly a small drop of 1% white glue on warm slides.
5. Float cut sections onto pre-warmed white glue solution.
6. Allow the sections to stretch out and flatten.
7. Blot on paper towel.
8. Let slides dry overnight at 56 °C in an oven to ensure proper attachment.

NOTE: Another, more expensive, way to ensure adhesion of sections is to use a coating of 0.01% poly-L-lysine instead of white glue. Poly-L-lysine coated slides can be stored at 4 °C prior to collection of tissue sections and staining.

15.6 Avidin-Biotin Complex (ABC) Immunoperoxidase Method

Background

Before starting the immunohistochemical reaction, choose carefully a negative and a positive control slide to guarantee the specificity of the reaction. When searching for papillomavirus, choose a positive papillomavirus-infected skin or genital lesion control section; and for keratin, a squamous cell carcinoma or normal human skin section for a positive control.

Prepared Reagents

1. Phosphate buffered saline (PBS; pH 7.6)
    Sodium chloride
    Sodium phosphate (dibasic)
    Sodium phosphate (monobasic)
    Distilled water
    Dissolve 26.28 g sodium chloride, 4 g sodium phosphate (dibasic), and 0.7 g sodium phosphate (monobasic) in 3,000 mL distilled water.
2. Harris' Hematoxylin (see Procedure 14.1.1)
3. Trypsin solution
    Trypsin
    $CaCl_2$
    Phosphate buffered saline
    Dissolve 0.4 g trypsin and 1.6 g $CaCl_2$ in 400 mL PBS.
4. Hydrogen peroxide-DAB solution
    3% Hydrogen peroxide
    Diaminobenzidine tetrahydrochloride (DAB)
    Phosphate buffered saline
    a. Dissolve 0.6 g DAB in 10 mL PBS. NOTE: It is advisable to prepare this solution under a fume hood because DAB is recognized as a chemical carcinogen. This solution must

be prepared no more than 15 minutes before use. Protect this solution from light. Dispose of DAB as recommended by your institution.

   b. Add and mix 0.1 mL 3% hydrogen peroxide.

5. Antibodies

   Antibody for detection of papillomavirus (Dako)

   Antibody for detection of keratin (Dako)

   Phosphate buffered saline

   Dilute antiserum in PBS according to the manufacturer's recommendations. NOTE: Handle antibodies following the manufacturer's recommendations.

Other Reagents and Equipment

ABC kit (Vector Labs). This kit contains the secondary antibody and the basic immunostaining biochemicals for performing the avidin-biotin complex method.

Normal goat serum (contained in the ABC kit). Dilute according to the manufacturer's recommendations.

Biotinylated goat anti-rabbit IgG (contained in the ABC kit). Dilute according to the manufacturer's recommendations.

ABC complex (contained in the ABC kit)

Toluene

Absolute ethanol

40% formaldehyde

Tap water

Bluing agent (see Procedure 14.1.4)

50%, 70%, 80%, and 95% ethanol

Mounting medium

Coverslips

Freezer

Refrigerator

pH meter

Laboratory oven

Light microscope

All necessary equipment normally available in a histology laboratory

Fume hood

Moist chamber for incubation of tissues

Micropipettes (20 μL; 200 μL; 1,000 μL)

ABC Immunostaining Procedure

1. Deparaffinize in toluene for 5 minutes.
2. Deparaffinize in toluene for 10 minutes.
3. Dip 10 times in absolute ethanol.
4. Treat with ethanol-formol (9:1) for 5 minutes.
5. Block endogenous peroxidase activity with 3% hydrogen peroxide for 30 minutes.
6. Wash in tap water for 5 minutes. NOTE: A prolonged session of rinse is necessary to remove the yellow stain of picric acid if tissue was fixed with Bouin's fluid. A shorter rinse in water

is sufficient for tissue fixed in Carnoy's fluid or in neutral buffered formalin.

7. Rinse in PBS for 5 minutes.
8. Incubate (if necessary) in 0.1% trypsin in PBS at 37 °C for 30 minutes. NOTE: This step is not necessary for detection of papillomavirus antigen, go directly to step 10. But trypsination is essential for detection of keratin.
9. Wash in PBS.
10. Cover tissue with 5% normal goat serum in PBS and incubate at room temperature in a moist chamber for 20 minutes.
11. Decant goat serum and wipe around section.
12. Apply on tissue diluted primary antibody (HPV 1:500; keratin 1:300) and incubate at room temperature in a moist chamber for a period of 2 hours.
13. Dip 10 times in PBS.
14. Wash in PBS for 5 minutes.
15. Wipe around sections and apply biotinylated goat anti-rabbit IgG.
16. Incubate at room temperature in a humid chamber for 30 minutes.
17. During this period of time, prepare the avidin-biotin complex by diluting 2 drops of reactive A and 2 drops of reactive B from ABC kit. NOTE: This ABC solution should be made at least 30 minutes prior to use. It is good for three days.
18. Rinse slides in PBS for 5 minutes.
19. Wipe around sections.
20. Apply ABC solution to sections and incubate at room temperature in a closed humid chamber for a period of 60 minutes.
21. Wash in PBS for 5 minutes.
22. Wearing gloves, apply DAB-substrate solution to the slides and monitor the reaction time under light microscope.
23. Stop reaction by dipping in tap water a few seconds.
24. Counterstain in Harris' hematoxylin for 5 minutes.
25. Dip 10 times in tap water.
26. Dip 10 times in tap water.
27. Dip 10 times in tap water.
28. Dip 10 times in 50% ethanol.
29. Treat sections with the bluing agent for 1 minute.
30. Dip 10 times in 70% ethanol.
31. Dip 10 times in 80% ethanol.
32. Dip 10 times in 95% ethanol.
33. Dip 10 times in absolute ethanol.
34. Dip 10 times in toluene.
35. Dip 10 times in toluene.
36. Dip 10 times in toluene.
37. Coverslip with the mounting medium.

Staining Reaction

A positive result is observed when a colored precipitate is formed (according to the chromogen used). Plates 6.65 and 6.66 illustrate the localization of a papillomavirus antigen characterized by a nuclear gold-brown precipitate. The presence of keratin in the cytoplasm of cells of the uterine cervix is evidenced by the gold-brown staining (Plates 6.6 and 6.7).

Electron Microscopy

The electron microscope has allowed the cytologist to morphologically appreciate the real complexity of cells. Subcellular information on the organization of tissues can be achieved. In fact, it is possible to visualize cellular organelles such as the mitochondria, the nuclear envelope, and the plasma membrane, as well as virus particles. The pathologist can also use electron microscopy to confirm the diagnosis of tumors by observation of desmosomes, tonofilaments, myofilaments, endosecretory granules, and other features.

For transmission electron microscopy (TEM), fixed tissues are embedded in a hard resin. This resin supports sections of 50–100 nm or less in thickness, which are obtained using a glass or diamond knife. Thin sections of tissues are mounted on a screenlike metal grid instead of a microscope slide. This preparation is necessary to allow electrons to pass through the specimen and the metal grid spaces. An image is produced on a fluorescent screen. Without staining, there is little differentiation of structures in the electron microscope. The stains (uranyl acetate and lead citrate) contain heavy metal atoms that combine specifically with certain chemical groups in the cell.

Heavy metals are good absorbers of electrons, preventing them from passing through the specimen which produces an image where stained (metal impregnated) structures appear darker than unstained structures (which absorb few or no electrons). The magnified image is recorded on a photographic plate (a negative); and enlargement of the negative on photographic paper produces a permanent record for analysis and interpretation of cellular structures.

Electron microscopy can be done on biopsy materials as well as cells reprocessed from routine cervical smears. Basic techniques for preparing tissues and cells for electron microscopy include the following steps:

1. Fixation of tissues to preserve the cells with a minimum of alteration and to prepare them for subsequent treatments including embedding, staining, and exposure to the electron beam;
2. Embedding in a resin that allows semi- as well as ultrathin sections;
3. Staining the cells with heavy metal atoms that absorb electrons and thus allow differentiation of structures.

15.7 Fixation, Embedding, and Preparation of Tissue Biopsies for EM

NOTE: The components used in electron microscopy are toxic and may cause skin irritation. Therefore work under an exhaust hood.

Prepared Reagents

1. 0.5M Cacodylate buffer
   Sodium cacodylate
   Concentrated hydrochloric acid (sp g 1.19)
   Distilled water
   a. Dissolve 53.5 g sodium cacodylate in 450 mL distilled water.
   b. Adjust pH to 7.3 with concentrated HCl.
   c. Increase total volume to 500 mL with distilled water.
   d. Keep refrigerated.
2. 0.2M Cacodylate buffer
   0.5M Sodium cacodylate buffer
   Distilled water
   a. Mix 40 mL 0.5M sodium cacodylate buffer with 60 mL distilled water.
   b. Keep refrigerated.
3. 0.1M Cacodylate buffer
   0.5M Sodium cacodylate buffer
   Distilled water
   a. Mix 100 mL 0.5M sodium cacodylate buffer with 400 mL distilled water.
   b. Keep refrigerated.
4. 2.5% Glutaraldehyde fixative
   50% glutaraldehyde
   Distilled water
   a. Mix 10 mL 0.5M sodium cacodylate, 2.5 mL 50% glutaraldehyde and 37.5 mL distilled water.
   b. Keep refrigerated.
5. 2% Osmium tetroxide fixative
   Osmium tetroxide
   Distilled water
   a. Dissolve 1 g osmium tetroxide in 50 mL distilled water.
   b. Keep refrigerated in a dark bottle.
6. 1% Osmium tetroxide fixative (working solution)
   2% Osmium tetroxide fixative
   0.2M sodium cacodylate buffer
   a. Mix 5 mL 2% osmium tetroxide and 5 mL 0.2M sodium cacodylate buffer. Prepare daily.
7. Embedding medium
   Epon 812
   DDSA (Dodecenyl succinic anhydride)
   MNA (Methyl nadic anhydride)
   DMP-30 (an accelerator)
   NOTE: The embedding media is prepared with a mixture of epoxy resin (Epon 812 or a substitute), purified anhydride (DDSA and NMA), and an accelerator (DMP-30). Two mixtures (mixture A: Epon + DDSA; and mixture B: Epon + NMA) are prepared. The hardness of blocks will depend upon the ratio of mixtures A and B. Mixture A gives soft blocks, and mixture B alone gives very hard blocks. Blocks of medium hardness are generally prepared using the following ratio: 6 volumes of mixture A to 4 volumes of

mixture B. Before beginning to prepare embedding medium, pay attention to the weight per epoxide equivalent (WPE) of epoxy resin in order to obtain reproducible embedding (see Table 15.1). The final working embedding medium is obtained according to Table 15.2.

Precautions must be taken to avoid water condensation in the embedding media which causes holes in blocks. Keep all solutions and mixtures in well-capped bottles. Mixtures A and B remain usable for months if they are kept refrigerated. But the mixture must be warmed to room temperature before opening bottles to prevent water capture by hygroscopic anhydrides.

Other Reagents and Equipment

Ethanol
Propylene oxide
Flat silicone rubber mold
Beem capsules
Razor blades
Pasteur pipettes
Two laboratory ovens (one at 42 °C and the other at 60 °C)
pH meter
Rotary shaker
Fume hood

Tissue Preparation for EM Microscopy

1. Small tissue biopsies are immediately fixed in cacodylate buffered 2.5% glutaraldehyde in the colposcopy examination room.
2. When the tissue blocks arrive in EM laboratory, they are cut with a clean, sharp razor blade into blocks no larger than 0.5 mm and are then maintained in glutaraldehyde fixative for 2 hours at 4 °C.
   NOTE: All the following steps are performed using a rotary shaker. The specimens remain in the vials in which they were fixed throughout dehydration, clearing, and infiltration. One solution is removed with a Pasteur pipette and replaced by the next one.
3. Rinse 3 times with 0.1M cacodylate buffer for 60 minutes each. If you wish tissues can remain for many days or weeks in this cold buffer before going to step 4.
4. Fix in cacodylate buffered 1% osmium tetroxide for 90 minutes at 4 °C.
5. Rinse 3 times with 0.1M cacodylate buffer for 20 minutes each.
6. Dehydrate in 50% ethanol for 15 minutes.
7. Dehydrate in 70% ethanol for 15 minutes.
8. Dehydrate in 95% ethanol for 15 minutes.
9. Dehydrate in absolute ethanol for 15 minutes.
10. Dehydrate in absolute ethanol for 15 minutes.
11. Dehydrate in absolute ethanol for 15 minutes.
12. Clear in propylene oxide for 10 minutes. NOTE: Propylene oxide is used as a clearing agent because it is miscible to both

Table 15.1

Quantity of Epoxy Resin for Embedding Medium (according to its w.p.e.)

Epon WPE	Weight of DDSA* (Mixture A) (g)	Weight of NMA** (Mixture B) (g)
140	106	89
141	106	88
142	105	88
143	104	87
144–145	103	86
146	102	85
147	101	85
148	101	84
149	100	84
150–151	99	83

*Quantity to be added to 80 g of Epon (Mixture A)

**Quantity to be added to 100 g of Epon (Mixture B)

Table 15.2
Working Embedding Medium

Block Hardness	Mixture A (g)	Mixture B (g)	Accelerator (g)
Soft	7	3	0.14
Medium*	6	4	0.14
Hard	3	7	0.14

*We usually prepare a medium mixture

ethanol and epoxy resin allowing the tissue to be perfectly impregnated by the resin.

13. Clear in propylene oxide for 10 minutes.
14. Clear in propylene oxide for 10 minutes.
15. Infiltrate with a 1:1 mixture of epon (working solution) and propylene oxide overnight.
16. Continue infiltration in Epon (working solution) for 3–4 hours.
17. Embed in flat molds or Beem capsules. Identify each block.
18. Polymerize for 24 hours at 42 °C.
19. Continue polymerization for another 24 hours at 60 °C.

15.8 Ultramicrotomy
Reagents and Equipment

Glass sticks for making glass knives
Diamond knife
Ultramicrotome
Knifemaker
Adhesive tape
Dental wax
Microscope slides
Coverslips
Hot plate
Razor blades
Copper and nickel grids
Fine tweezers
Filter paper
Wire loops

Procedure for Semithin Sections

Preparations of semithin sections (commonly called thick sections) are first obtained in order to establish a correlation between light and electron microscopy. Thick sections are 0.5–1 μm thick. Glass knives are obtained using a knifemaker. A leakproof trough (made of adhesive tape and then sealed with dental wax) is mounted to enable the sections to be floated onto a liquid surface. Sections are collected using a wire loop and transferred to a drop of water on a microscope slide, which is gently warmed to permit the section to stretch out any wrinkles. The evaporation of water allows the sections to adhere to the slide.

NOTE: The main objective in obtaining and observing thick sections is to select the most significant area for EM scrutiny. Recognition of the precise location of a lesion within a tissue section is crucial because the block must be trimmed to obtain a block face suitable for ultrathin sectioning. With a smaller block face, it is easier to cut ultrathin sections.

Procedure for Ultrathin Sections

After selecting the appropriate area in the stained thick section, trim the corresponding block with a single-edged razor blade to reduce the size of the block face without losing the selected area. Because the shape of the block face facilitates sectioning, it should be cut to produce a trapezoidal face.

Ultrathin sections of 60–90 nm are easily obtained with a diamond knife. Sections are floated on water. Through the binocular microscope of the ultramicrotome, the sections show different colors according to their thickness. Sections showing a silver to gold color allow normal electron microscopic observation.

Sections are collected on a copper or nickel grid maintained in a pair of fine tweezers. The grid is blotted dry by touching its edge to a piece of filter paper.

15.9 Staining Sections for EM

Prepared Reagents

1. 1% Methylene blue-1% Azure II
   Methylene blue (C.I. 52015)
   Azure II (C.I. 52010)
   Borax
   Distilled water
   a. Dissolve 1 g methylene blue, 1 g azure II, and 1 g borax in 100 mL distilled water.
   b. Mix well and filter.
   c. Keep refrigerated in a dark bottle.
2. 10N Sodium hydroxide
   Sodium hydroxide pellets (carbonate free)
   Distilled water
   a. Dissolve 40 g sodium hydroxide pellets in 100 mL boiled distilled water. NOTE: CO_2-free water is obtained by boiling.
3. 70% Ethanol
   Absolute ethanol
   Distilled water
   Mix 70 mL absolute ethanol with 30 mL boiled distilled water.
4. 1% Uranyl acetate
   Uranyl acetate
   70% Ethanol
   a. Dissolve 1 g uranyl acetate in 100 mL 70% ethanol. NOTE: This solution must be protected from light and passed through a Millipore filter before use. Store at 4 °C. Take care in handling this toxic, radioactive stain.
5. Lead citrate
   Lead citrate
   10N Sodium hydroxide
   Distilled water
   a. Dissolve 0.03 g lead citrate in 8 mL boiled distilled water.
   b. Add 0.1 mL 10N sodium hydroxide (carbonate free) and mix.
   c. Shake well for dissolution. Store at 4 °C. Pass through a Millipore filter before use.

Other Equipment

Paper filter (Whatman No. 1)
Mounting reagent
Millipore filter (0.025 μm)
Petri dishes
Dental wax
Parafilm sheets
Fine tweezers
Hot plate

Procedure for Staining Semithin Sections

1. Cover sections with a drop of methylene blue-azure II solution.
2. Heat gently on a hot plate (60 °C) for a few seconds.
3. Drain off excess stain.
4. Wash sections with distilled water.
5. Dry gently on a hot plate.
6. Coverslip with the mounting medium.

Procedure for Staining Ultrathin Sections

1. Prepare two Petri dishes. In the first one, place a filter paper in the bottom and moisten with 70% ethanol to prevent precipitation of stain during uranyl acetate staining. In the second Petri dish place a filter paper in the bottom and add 15–20 moist pellets of sodium hydroxide in the outer internal periphery of the dish to prevent the formation of lead carbonate precipitates during lead staining. A piece of dental wax or Parafilm sheet is then placed on top of the filter paper. Stain solutions are placed directly on this support.
2. Float the grid side down individually on a drop of uranyl acetate that has been deposited on the support sheet in a Petri dish. Replace the lid immediately and protect from light. Stain for 10 minutes.
3. Holding the grid in tweezers, rinse it by dipping repeatedly through the surface of 70% ethanol.
4. Repeat step 3 using boiled distilled water (CO_2-free water).
5. Blot the grid on filter paper.
6. Transfer the grid to the second Petri dish containing a drop of lead citrate. Replace the lid immediately. Stain for 5 minutes.
7. Wash the grid twice in CO_2-free water as in step 3.
8. Blot the grid on a filter paper.
9. Store the grid on clean filter paper in a Petri dish.

15.10 Reprocessing Papanicolaou-Stained Smears for EM

Reagents and Equipment

Toluene
Absolute ethanol

Osmium tetroxide (see Procedure 15.7.6)
Cacodylate buffer (see Procedure 15.7.1–3)
Distilled water
Harris' hematoxylin (see Procedure 14.1.1)
Propylene oxide
Epon 812
DDSA
NMA
DMP-30
Liquid nitrogen
Microscope slides
Rubber embedding molds
Elastic bands
Diamond pencil

Procedure

1. Localize the cells on the smear by light microscopy.
2. Photomicrograph the cell under investigation in order to facilitate identification in step 26.
3. Circle cell locations under the slide with a diamond pencil.
4. Immerse slides in toluene for a period of 24 hours (up to 1 week for old smears) to remove the coverslip.
5. Rehydrate cells in absolute ethanol for 3 minutes.
6. Rehydrate cells in 95% ethanol for 3 minutes.
7. Rehydrate cells in 80% ethanol for 3 minutes.
8. Rehydrate cells in 70% ethanol for 3 minutes.
9. Rehydrate cells in 50% ethanol for 3 minutes.
10. Rehydrate cells in distilled water for 3 minutes.
11. Osmicate in 1% osmium tetroxide in cacodylate buffer for 15 minutes.
12. Rinse in distilled water a few minutes.
13. Stain with Harris' hematoxylin for 2 minutes.
14. Rinse in tap water for 3 minutes.
15. Dehydrate in 50% ethanol for 3 minutes.
16. Dehydrate in 70% ethanol for 3 minutes.
17. Dehydrate in 95% ethanol for 3 minutes.
18. Dehydrate in absolute ethanol for 3 minutes.
19. Treat the slides in propylene oxide for 5 minutes.
20. Treat the slides in the propylene oxide-epon mixture (1:1) for 60 minutes.
21. Embed in epon as follows:
    a. Cut a flat rubber embedding mold to the same dimension as the microscope slide.
    b. Make a hole in the center of the mold. The dimension of the hole must be large enough to surround the cells you wish to examine.
    c. This perforated mold is placed on the microscope slide which becomes the bottom of the mold.
    d. Fill half the mold with epon and use a clean microscope slide to cover the trough. In this way, a "sandwich" is

formed by the smear, the perforated mold and the cleaned slide. Elastic bands are used to keep the sandwich together.

22. Incubate at 37 °C for 24 hours.
23. Incubate at 60 °C for another 24 hours.
24. When epon is polymerized, circle cells you wish to study directly on polymerized epon: the new circle will face the circle made under the slide in step 3.
25. Remove resin block from the glass slide by immersion in liquid nitrogen for 10 seconds.
26. After identifying cells using a microscope and comparing them with the photomicrograph, the block is trimmed, and processed as previously described in routine technique for electron microscopy, ultramicrotomy (see Procedure 15.8), and EM staining (see Procedure 15.9).

15.11 Cytochemical Demonstration of Glycogen in EM

Background

Seligman et al (1965)[64] introduced thiocarbohydrazide (TCH) to replace the classical Schiff-reagent in demonstrating polysaccharides in biologic specimens. TCH was made visible in the electron microscope by treatment by osmium tetroxide (OsO_4) after treatment with periodic-acid. In 1967, Thiery[73] used silver proteinate instead of OsO_4 to visualize TCH. We describe here the procedure used in our laboratory to demonstrate glycogen in specimen of the uterine cervix.

15.11A Tissue Preparation
Prepared Reagents (see Procedure 15.7)

2.5% Glutaraldehyde solution
Cacodylate buffer
1% Osmium tetroxide
50%, 70%, 95%, and absolute ethanol
Embedding medium (see Procedure 15.7.7)

Procedure

1. Fix tissues in 2.5% glutaraldehyde for 2 hours at 4 °C.
2. Wash in 0.1M cacodylate buffer for 1 hour.
3. Wash in 0.1M cacodylate buffer for 1 hour.
4. Wash in 0.1M cacodylate buffer for 1 hour.
5. Fix in 1% osmium tetroxide for 90 minutes.
6. Wash in 0.1M cacodylate buffer for 10 minutes.
7. Wash in 0.1M cacodylate buffer for 10 minutes.
8. Wash in 0.1M cacodylate buffer for 10 minutes.
9. Dehydrate in 50% ethanol for 15 minutes.
10. Dehydrate in 70% ethanol for 15 minutes.

11. Dehydrate in 95% ethanol for 15 minutes.
12. Dehydrate in absolute ethanol for 15 minutes.
13. Dehydrate in absolute ethanol for 15 minutes.
14. Dehydrate in absolute ethanol for 15 minutes.
15. Clear in propylene oxide for 10 minutes.
16. Clear in propylene oxide for 10 minutes.
17. Clear in propylene oxide for 10 minutes.
18. Infiltrate with a 1:1 mixture of epon (working solution) and propylene oxide overnight.
19. Continue infiltration in epon alone (working solution) for 3–4 hours.
20. Embed in flat molds or Beem capsules with epon (working solution).
21. Polymerize for 24 hours at 42 °C.
22. Continue polymerization for another 24 hours at 60 °C. Blocks are now ready for ultramicrotomy (see Procedure 15.8).

15.11B Staining

Prepared Reagents

1. 1% Periodic acid (see Procedure 15.4.5).
   Prepare 20%, 10%, 5%, 2.5%, and 1% acetic acid solution
2. 0.2% Thiocarbohydrazide (TCH)
   Dissolve 100 mg thiocarbohydrazide in 50 mL 20% acetic acid. Filter before use. Keep at 4 °C for 1 week.
3. 1% aqueous silver proteinate
   NOTE: This solution is prepared in very clean glassware with a magnetic stirrer in a dark room (red filter permitted).
   Silver proteinate
   Distilled water
   a. Dissolve 1 g silver proteinate in 100 mL distilled water.
   b. Keep in the dark at 4 °C a few weeks. Filter immediately before use.

Procedure

NOTE: Sections are floated on the different solutions in staining wells at room temperature. Include a control section and omit the first step. This permits you to control the specificity of the staining reaction by preventing the polysaccharide moiety of the tissue to react with the TCH.
The sequence of staining is as follows:

1. Float sections on periodic acid for 20 minutes.
2. Rinse in distilled water for 5 minutes.
3. Rinse in distilled water for 5 minutes.
4. Rinse in distilled water for 5 minutes.
5. Treat in TCH for 24 hours.
6. Wash in 10% acetic acid for 1 minute.
7. Wash in 10% acetic acid for 1 minute.
8. Wash in 10% acetic acid for 20 minutes.
9. Wash in 10% acetic acid for 20 minutes.
10. Wash in 10% acetic acid for 20 minutes.

11. Wash in 5% acetic acid for 20 minutes.
12. Wash in 2.5% acetic acid for 20 minutes.
13. Wash in 1% acetic acid for 20 minutes.
14. Wash in distilled water for 1 minute.
15. Wash in distilled water for 1 minute.
16. Wash in distilled water for 20 minutes.
17. Wash in distilled water for 20 minutes.
18. Wash in distilled water for 20 minutes.
19. Float sections on 1% aqueous silver proteinate in a dark room for 30 minutes.
20. Rinse in distilled water (2–3 changes) until no trace of silver proteinate solution is left on the water surface.

Staining Reaction

Positive sections show large area of darkly stained (black) granules corresponding to glycogen. Positive dense areas are clearly differentiated from other structures (nucleus, mitochondria, etc), which are very slightly visible. The periodic acid-TCH-silver proteinate staining is particularly useful to demonstrate the reduced glycogen in koilocytes. In normal cervical epithelium (Figure 1.3), a large area of glycogen is surrounding the nuclei. In koilocytes (Figures 6.1 and 6.2) a small, patchy, positive area indicates that the quantity of glycogen is metabolically diminished possibly as a result of HPV infection.

DNA Studies

Genetic information is stored in the nucleic acids: deoxyribonucleic acid (DNA) and ribonucleic acid (RNA). RNA and DNA consist of a single (for RNA) or double intertwined (for DNA) chain of four different nucleotides. Nucleotides have three parts: a phosphate group, a sugar, and an organic base. The names of the bases are: adenine (A), guanine (G), cytosine (C), thymine (T) (found only in DNA), and uracil (U) (found only in RNA). In the double chain (or duplex structure) of DNA, the bases on opposite strands are held together by hydrogen bonds in such a way that adenine is always paired with thymine; and that guanine is always paired with cytosine. RNA molecules exist predominantly as single-stranded molecules, but it can also adopt the configuration of a double-stranded molecule where cytosine is paired with guanine and adenine with uracil. This base-pair complementarity of DNA and RNA is the basis for the technique of nucleic acid hybridization.

Because the sequence of bases in DNA and RNA is unique for each organism and for each gene in an organism, there is nearly no probability of finding the same sequence of 20 successive nucleotides in two different genes or two different organisms. Therefore the genetic information present in the chromosome(s) of living cells or viral particles can be identified with a near absolute specificity by hybridization with a complementary nucleic acid probe that is labelled by incorporation of a radioactive or biotinylated nucleotide into the molecule.

In living cells, DNA is maintained as a duplex structure except when it replicates. Upon replication, the two strands unwind and separate from each other to synthesize new strands of DNA. Under experimental conditions, it is possible to separate (to melt, to dissociate, to denature) the two nucleotide chains (strands) from one another to form single-stranded DNA molecules. Dissociation occurs after heating DNA in the presence of a low-salt solution or by raising the pH. Under reverse conditions, ie, if the temperature is lowered and the concentration of salt is raised, or if the pH is lowered, complementary single strands reassociate or anneal to form stable duplexes or hybrids. This experimental reassociation is termed molecular hybridization. Under appropriate conditions DNA-DNA, RNA-RNA, and RNA-DNA hybrids can be formed.

The stability of the hybrids is expressed as a function of their melting temperature (Tm), which is the point at which half of the duplexes have dissociated. Double-stranded DNA molecules dissociate at temperatures above their own melting temperature. The optimal rate of reassociation of single-stranded DNA molecules to form hybrids occurs at 25 °C below their Tm. At this temperature (Tm-25 °C), hybridization is said to occur in standard conditions of stringency. Variations in temperature increase or decrease the stringency of the hybridization reaction. The melting temperature of a double-stranded DNA molecule is a function of the G+C content, the concentration of monovalent cation, and reaction temperature, which is reduced by organic denaturants such as formamide. McConaughty et al (1969)[37] have presented the following equation to calculate the Tm of any DNA:

$$Tm = 81.5 + 16.6 \, (\log M) + 0.41 \, (\%CG) - 0.72$$
$$(\% \text{ Formamide) where M is the molarity of}$$
$$\text{monovalent cation.}$$

Under high-stringency conditions (eg, Tm −20 °C) only the most stable duplexes are formed. In other words, under these conditions, a viral DNA probe will detect a virus harboring a strongly homologous base-pair matching. Under relaxed or low-stringency conditions (eg, Tm −40 °C), the formation of hybrids with lower stability is possible. This means that a target virus could be detected with a viral probe showing a reduced degree of base-pair homology. It is therefore the stringency of the reaction which determines the specificity of the hybridization reaction.

In the following sections, we are going to review different techniques for the molecular detection of papillomavirus sequences: In situ hybridization (ISH), filter in situ hybridization (FISH), dot/blot hybridization, southern blot hybridization, and the polymerase chain reaction (PCR).

In Situ Hybridization

The technique of in situ hybridization was originally developed by Gall and Pardue (1969)[17] and John et al (1969).[28] The technique is used for the detection of specific cellular or viral genomes in histologic or cytologic preparations. Radioactive or biotinylated probes can be used. The genomic sequences are visualized as dark grains (for radioactive probes) or a colored precipitate (for biotinylated probes) directly within the cells. This method permits the study of the spatial distribution of specific sequences relative to given lesions.

In this section, we are not going to describe the in situ technique using radiolabelled probes (for more information see Pardue).[53] Detection applications for papillomaviruses using in situ hybridization with radiolabelled probes have been reported widely, most notably by Stoler and Broker (1986),[72] Gupta et al (1985),[23] Gupta et al (1987),[22] Del Mistro et al (1987),[13] McDonnell et al (1987),[38] Nagai et al (1987),[47] Ostrow et al (1987),[51] and still others.[18,21,43,48–50,56,81,83] Radioactively labelled probes, though highly specific and sensitive, have several disadvantages: the relatively high cost, the short half-life of radioisotopes, safety issues for personnel, waste isotope disposal problems, and the rather long exposure time that is necessary for autoradiography using a photographic emulsion: for example, 7 days for ^{35}Sulphur and up to 4 weeks for tritium.

An alternative approach using biotin-labelled probes was developed by Langer-Safer et al (1982),[32] Manuelidis et al (1982),[36] and Singer and Ward (1982).[69] Adaptation of this technique for the detection of viral genomes including parvoviruses, polyomaviruses, herpes simplex viruses, adenoviruses and retroviruses was performed by Brigati et al (1983).[4] Cytomegalovirus infection was investigated with biotinylated DNA probes by Myerson et al (1984).[45,46] Detection and localization of human papillomavirus DNA in human genital condylomas specifically was accomplished by Beckmann et al (1985).[2] Since then many other varieties of research and other descriptive works concerning the detection of human papillomaviruses using biotinylated probes have been subsequently published.

Biotinylated probes are visualized by sequential immunocytochemical reactions using antibiotin antibodies together with an enzyme-labelled second antibody or by the high-affinity reaction that occurs between biotin and avidin or streptavidin (Chaiet and Wolf, 1964),[7] itself conjugated with an enzyme. The enzyme label is generally peroxidase although polyalkaline phosphate has been used (Unger et al, 1986;[76] Lewis et al, 1987[33]). The presence of hybridized biotinylated probe coupled with the streptavidin-peroxidase complex is then detected by addition of a chromogen such as 3',3'-diaminobenzidine (DAB) or aminoethylcarbazole (AEC) and a hydrogen peroxide substrate. The reaction yields a brown precipitate in the presence of DAB, or a red precipitate in the presence of AEC. When using alkaline phosphatase, a dark blue precipitate is obtained at the hybridization site in the presence of nitroblue tetrazolium (chromogen) and 5-bromo-4-chloro-3-indolyl phosphate (BCIP) as substrate. Tissue sections are lightly counterstained with hematoxylin, light green, methyl green, or metanil yellow and subsequently mounted with a coverslip.

15.12 In Situ Hybridization Technique

15.12A General Preparations and Equipment

Carnoy's fixative (see Procedure 15.1.1)
Neutral buffered formalin (see Procedure 15.1.3)
Absolute ethanol
Toluene
Double-distilled water
Paraffin
Mounting medium (Eukitt)
Mayer's hemalum (see Procedure 15.3.2)
2% HCl
1% Glue solution (see Procedure 15.5.2)
0.01% Poly-L-lysine (see Procedure 15.5.3)
Hydrogen peroxide-DAB solution (H_2O_2-DAB solution, see Procedure 15.6.4)
Streptavidin peroxidase conjugate (Dilute accordingly to the manufacturer's recommendations)
Bluing agent (see Procedure 15.3.1)
Automatic tissue changer
Hot paraffin bath
Embedding mold
Microtome and knives
A hot plate
A laboratory oven
Microscope slides
20 × 20 mm glass coverslips

Prepared Reagents

1. Phosphate buffered saline
   Sodium chloride
   Sodium phosphate (dibasic)
   Sodium phosphate (monobasic)
   Double-distilled water
   Dissolve 7.6 g sodium chloride, 0.99 g sodium phosphate (dibasic), 0.36 g sodium phosphate (monobasic) in 1,000 mL double-distilled water. Sterilize by autoclaving.
2. Proteinase K (1 mg/mL)
   Proteinase K
   Double-distilled water
   Dissolve 1 mg proteinase K in 1 mL double-distilled water. Store at $-20\,°C$.
3. Proteinase K (200 μg/mL)
   Aqueous proteinase K (1 mg/mL)
   PBS
   Mix 200 μL aqueous proteinase K with 800 μL PBS.
4. 4% Paraformaldehyde
   Paraformaldehyde
   PBS
   Dissolve 2 g paraformaldehyde in 50 mL PBS.

5. Deionized formamide

  Formamide (Sigma)

  AG501-X8 ion-exchanged resin (20–50 meshs; BioRad)

  Whatman No. 1 filter paper

  Magnetic stirrer

  a. Mix 5 g resin in 50 mL formamide on a magnetic stirrer for 30 minutes at room temperature.

  b. Filter through a Whatman No. 1 filter paper. Prepare this solution daily.

6. 50% deionized formamide in 0.1% PBS

  Deionized formamide

  PBS

  Double-distilled water

  a. Mix 25 mL deionized formamide, 5 mL PBS, and 20 mL double-distilled water.

7. 50% (w/v) Dextran sulfate

  Sodium dextran sulfate (M.W. 500,000)

  Sterile double-distilled water

  a. Dissolve 50 g dextran sulfate in 100 mL sterile double-distilled water.

  b. Heat to 60 °C to help dissolution. Store at 4 °C.

8. 10N Sodium hydroxide

  Sodium hydroxide pellets

  Double-distilled water

  a. Dissolve 40 g NaOH pellets in 80 mL double-distilled water.

  b. Increase total volume to 100 mL with double-distilled water.

9. 20× SSC

  Sodium chloride (NaCl)

  Sodium citrate (M.W. 294.10)

  10N NaOH

  Double-distilled water

  a. Dissolve 175.3 g NaCl and 88.2 g sodium citrate in 800 mL double-distilled water.

  b. Adjust pH to 7.0 with 10N NaOH.

  c. Increase total volume to 1,000 mL with double-distilled water.

  d. Sterilize by autoclaving.

10. Sheared denatured salmon sperm DNA

  Salmon sperm DNA (Type III, sodium salt; Sigma)

  Double-distilled water

  Magnetic stirrer

  18-gauge hypodermic needle

  a. Dissolve 250 mg salmon sperm DNA in 25 mL double-distilled water.

  b. Stir on magnetic stirrer for at least 4 hours at room temperature.

  c. Shear DNA by passing it 10–12 times through an 18-gauge hypodermic needle.

  d. Boil DNA for 10 minutes.

  e. Store at −20 °C in small aliquots.

11. 10% Triton X-100
    Triton X-100
    Double-distilled water
    Mix 1 mL Triton X-100 with 9 mL double-distilled water.
12. 0.025% Triton X-100 in PBS
    10% Triton X-100
    PBS
    Mix 125 μL 10% Triton X-100 in 100 mL PBS.

15.12B Preparation of Hybridization Probes

Background

The preparation of DNA probes is done by the introduction of a radioactive (^{35}S or tritium) or a nonradioactive marker (biotin) into the sequence of nucleic acid used as a probe. At the end of the reaction, the marker must be visualizable if the target DNA sequences are present in the studied sample. Cloned HPV-DNA types 6, 11, 16, or 18 are viral DNA sequences which can be used as probes when they are biotin-labelled with biotinylated deoxyuridine triphosphate to replace thymidine triphosphate in the nick-translation reaction catalyzed by *E coli* DNA polymerase I (Rigby et al, 1977).[57]

The process of "nick translation" uses DNase I to introduce single-strand nicks in double-stranded DNA. Then the 5' to 3' exonuclease action of *E coli* DNA polymerase I is used to remove DNA sequences from one strand of the double-stranded template starting at the nicks. Finally the missing DNA stretches are replaced (or repaired) by incorporation of labelled deoxyribonucleotides using the 5' to 3' polymerase action of the same enzyme. Unincorporated deoxyribonucleotides are separated from labelled probe after chromatography through a small column of Sephadex G-50. The labelled DNA is excluded from the column and eluted ahead of the unincorporated deoxyribonucleotides. After denaturation of the probe, short single-stranded probe molecules are obtained and ready for the hybridization reaction. The whole procedure is simplified using a commercial "nick translation" kit.

Probes, Reagents and Equipment

Papillomavirus DNA probes
A commercial nick translation kit for labelling of DNA
Biotinylated deoxyuridine triphosphate (Bio-11-dUTP; Enzo Biochem)
Sephadex G-50
A controlled-temperature water bath
Follow the recommendations included in the "nick translation" kit for labelling of 1 μg of DNA. Separate labelled DNA from unincorporated nucleotides by spun-column chromatography.[60]

15.12C Preparation of Hybridization Mixture

Prepared Reagents

Deionized formamide (see Procedure 15.12A.5)
50% dextran sulfate (see Procedure 15.12A.7)
20× SSC (see Procedure 15.12A.9)
Sheared salmon sperm DNA (see Procedure 15.12A.10)
Biotin-labelled probe
For each 100 μL hybridization cocktail, mix
   a. 50 μL deionized formamide
   b. 20 μL 50% dextran sulfate
   c. 10 μL 20× SSC
   d. 16 μL of biotinylated probe
   e. 4 μL of sheared salmon sperm DNA
NOTE: This 100 μL quantity is sufficient for hybridization of 5 tissue samples. This mixture is stable for at least 12 months at 4 °C.

15.12D In Situ Hybridization Procedure

1. Fix tissue biopsies in Carnoy's fixative or in neutral buffered formalin for 2 hours (see Procedure 15.1).
2. Dehydrate and embed tissue biopsies (see Procedure 15.2).
3. Prepare tissue sections on acid-cleaned slides (see Procedure 15.5).
4. Deparaffinize tissue sections in toluene for 5 minutes.
5. Deparaffinize tissue sections in toluene for 5 minutes.
6. Deparaffinize tissue sections in toluene for 5 minutes.
7. Immerse in absolute ethanol for 5 minutes.
8. Immerse in 70% ethanol for 5 minutes.
9. Immerse in phosphate buffered saline (PBS) for 5 minutes.
10. Spot proteinase K over tissue sections.
11. Incubate at 37 °C for 10 minutes.
12. Remove excess enzyme by immersion of slides in PBS for 10 minutes.
13. Postfix tissues in 4% paraformaldehyde. NOTE: This postfixation markedly reduces the loss of cellular DNA during in situ hybridization (Haase)[24] and increases the strength of the hybridization signal three- to fivefold (Brigati et al).[4]
14. Dip 10 times in PBS.
15. Immerse tissues in 50% ethanol for 5 minutes.
16. Immerse tissues in 70% ethanol for 5 minutes.
17. Immerse tissues in absolute ethanol for 5 minutes.
18. Air-dry tissue sections.
19. Spot 20 μL of hybridization mixture on dried tissue sections.
20. Coverslip and seal with rubber cement.
21. Place slides in a Petri dish.
22. Float the Petri dish in a 95 °C water bath for 10 minutes. NOTE: In this step, DNA probe and tissular DNA are denatured together as previously described by Beckmann et al.[2]
23. Then float Petri dish in an ice water bath for 10 minutes.

24. Allow tissues to hybridize by placing slides in an oven at 37 °C for 18–24 hours.
25. Carefully remove coverslip.
26. Immerse tissue sections in 50% deionized formamide prepared in 0.1% PBS for 10 minutes.
27. Immerse in 0.025% Triton X-100 for 5 minutes.
28. Immerse in PBS for 5 minutes.
29. Spot the streptavidin-peroxidase conjugate diluted 1:300 in PBS on tissue sections.
30. Incubate at room temperature for 30 minutes.
31. Rinse in PBS for 5 minutes.
32. Rinse in PBS for 5 minutes.
33. Spot the DAB-H_2O_2 solution on tissue sections.
34. Incubate at room temperature for 5–8 minutes.
35. Dip 10 times in distilled water.
36. Counterstain with Mayer's hemalum (see Procedure 15.3.2).
37. Rinse in tap water for a few seconds.
38. Differentiate in bluing agent by dipping 10 times.
39. Rinse in tap water for 10 minutes.
40. Dip 10 times in absolute ethanol.
41. Dip 10 times in absolute ethanol.
42. Dip 10 times in absolute ethanol.
43. Dip 10 times in toluene.
44. Dip 10 times in toluene.
45. Dip 10 times in toluene.
46. Coverslip with the mounting medium.

NOTE: A protocol for automation of in situ hybridization was recently developed by Elizabeth Unger and her collaborators.[77]

Staining Reaction

Nuclei staining golden brown are positive, ie, contain DNA homologous to the corresponding probe (see Plates 6.67 and 6.68).

Comments

In situ hybridization presents many advantages and a few disadvantages. For instance in lesions that contain very few nuclei harboring a large amount of viruses, in situ hybridization is more sensitive than any other technique for viral detection. This technique is particularly useful to detect viral DNA in fixed tissues for retrospective studies. Also in situ hybridization allows identification of specific cell types harboring the viral genome. The use of specific probes under conditions of high stringency allows the recognition of specific types of viruses.

15.13 Filter In Situ Hybridization

Background

This technique was developed by Wagner et al in 1984.[79] It was used widely for the screening of large populations.[10,12,14,26,30,40,62,63]

In this method, exfoliated cells are filtered onto a membrane without DNA extraction. Then cells are lysed and denatured by alkaline treatment, and neutralized. Preferably, hybridization is carried out under stringent conditions. Washing of the filter and autoradiography are performed as usual.

15.13A Cell Collection

PBS (see Procedure 15.12A.1)
Centrifuge
Eppendorf tubes
50 mL conical tubes
Vortex

a. Collect cellular samples with spatula or swab.
b. Place spatula or swab in 50 mL conical tube containing 10 mL PBS.
c. Vortex specimen to remove material from spatula and swab.
d. Remove and discard spatula and swab.
e. Centrifuge specimens at 3,000 rpm for 20 minutes.
f. Remove supernatant fluid from each tube.
g. Resuspend pellet in 200 μL PBS. This sample may be stored frozen at $-20\,°C$ or $-70\,°C$ in an Eppendorf tube.

15.13B Cell Treatment
Prepared Reagents

1. 5M Sodium chloride
   Sodium chloride (NaCl)
   Double-distilled water
   a. Dissolve 292.2 g NaCl in 800 mL double-distilled water.
   b. Adjust the volume to 1,000 mL double-distilled water.
   c. Aliquot and sterilize by autoclaving.
2. Denaturation solution
   10M NaOH
   5M NaCl
   Double-distilled water
   a. Mix 2.5 mL 10M NaOH, 15 mL 5M NaCl, and 32.5 mL double-distilled water. Keep refrigerated.
3. 1M Tris-HCl (pH 7.4)
   Tris base
   Concentrated hydrochloric acid (HCl)
   Double-distilled water
   a. Dissolve 121.1 g Tris base in 800 mL double-distilled water.
   b. Adjust pH to 7.4 by adding 70 mL HCl.
   c. Increase total volume to 1,000 mL with double-distilled water.
   d. Aliquot and sterilize by autoclaving.
4. Neutralization solution
   1M Tris-HCl (above)
   5M NaCl (above)

a. Mix 25 mL 1M Tris-HCl and 25 mL 5M NaCl. Sterilize by autoclaving.

Other Materials

Nylon membrane (GeneScreen Plus, Nen, Dupont)
Whatman 3MM filter paper

Procedure

1. Prepare duplicate nylon membranes by drawing in pencil a grid of 2 cm squares. Up to 50 specimens can be included on a 14 × 15 cm membrane.
2. Thaw specimens at room temperature.
3. Vortex specimens.
4. Spot an aliquot of 100 μL of each specimen in predetermined square on two different membranes placed on the surface of 3MM filter paper that has been moistened with double-distilled water. NOTE: Each membrane will be hybridized with different HPV probes. Always include a negative and a positive control.
5. Allow specimens to air-dry.
6. Saturate 3 layers of Whatman 3MM paper with the denaturation solution for 15 minutes.
7. Transfer the air-dried membranes to surface of saturated Whatman 3MM paper.
8. Saturate another 3 layers of Whatman 3MM paper with neutralization solution for 15 minutes.
9. Transfer membranes to surface of neutralization-saturated Whatman 3MM paper.
10. Allow membranes to air-dry at room temperature. NOTE: According to supplier recommendations, it may be necessary to bake the membranes to permit the complete adherence of materials. Then the membranes are stored in envelopes until hybridization procedures.

15.13C Preparation of Probes (see Procedure 15.12B)

The probes (cloned papillomavirus DNA) are labelled using a nick translation labelling kit. Instead of using a biotin-labelled nucleotide, we use here a radioactive nucleotide (^{32}P-nucleotide). The specific activity of the probe is determined by liquid scintillation counting. Only probes with a specific activity of at least 1×10^8 dpm/μg are used for hybridization.[34,60]

15.13D Prehybridization Mixture

Prepared Reagents

1. 10% Sodium dodecyl sulfate (SDS)
   Electrophoresis-grade SDS
   Double-distilled water

Concentrated HCl

NOTE: Wear a mask when preparing SDS solution.

  a. Dissolve 100 g SDS in 900 mL double-distilled water.
  b. Heat to 68 °C to assist dissolution.
  c. Adjust pH to 7.2 by adding a few drops of concentrated HCl.
  d. Increase total volume to 1,000 mL with double-distilled water.

2. Prehybridization mixture

Deionized formamide (see Procedure 15.12A.5)
50% Dextran sulfate (see Procedure 15.12A.7)
10% SDS (see above)
Double-distilled water
Sodium chloride (NaCl)
Water bath with automatic agitation

  a. Mix 5 mL deionized formamide, 2 mL dextran sulfate, 1 mL 10%-SDS, and 2 mL double-distilled water.
  b. Incubate in water bath at 42 °C for 15 minutes.
  c. Add 0.58 g NaCl to the tube and mix by inversion.
  d. Incubate at 42 °C for 15–20 minutes.

Procedure

1. Place each membrane in a plastic bag.
2. Pour 10 mL prehybridization mixture into the bag.
3. Squeeze out air bubbles and seal.
4. Incubate in water bath at 42 °C for a minimum of 15 minutes with constant agitation.

15.13E Hybridization Protocol
Prepared Reagents

1. Labeled probe (see Procedure 15.13C)
2. Sheared salmon sperm DNA (see Procedure 15.12A.10)
3. Double-distilled water

For each membrane, mix 100 μL of salmon sperm DNA, radioactive probe corresponding to 1–4 $\times$ 10^5 dpm/mL, and enough double-distilled water to make a total of 1 mL hybridization solution.

Denature the probe and the salmon sperm DNA together by heating in boiling water for 5 minutes.

Procedure

1. Open the bag containing the prehybridization solution with scissor.
2. Add 1 mL denatured hybridization mixture. NOTE: A mixture of probes can be added to the same bag in step 2. For instance in the first bag, containing membrane no. 1, labelled HPV-6 and HPV-11 can be added; in the second bag, containing membrane no. 2, labelled HPV-16 and HPV-18 can be added. The final concentration of probes must be made of 50% of each.

3. Reseal the plastic bag.
4. Incubate overnight with a constant agitation at 42 °C.

15.13F Washing Protocol

Prepared Reagents

1. 20× SSC (see Procedure 15.12A.9)
2. 10% SDS (see Procedure 15.13D.1)
3. Double-distilled water

Washing Solutions

1. 2× SSC (Washing solution 1)
   Mix 100 mL 20× SSC with 900 mL double-distilled water.
2. 2× SSC-1% SDS (Washing solution 2)
   Mix 100 mL 20× SSC, 100 mL 10% SDS, and 800 mL double-distilled water.
3. 0.1× SSC (Washing solution 3)
   Mix 5 mL 20× SSC and 995 mL double-distilled water.

Procedure

1. Remove membrane from hybridization solution.
2. Wash membrane with washing solution 1 at room temperature with constant agitation for a period of 5 minutes.
3. Repeat step 2.
4. Place the membrane in a new plastic bag.
5. Add 200 mL washing solution 2 to the bag.
6. Squeeze out air bubbles and seal the bag.
7. Wash membrane in a water bath at 68 °C with constant agitation for 20 minutes.
8. Open bag and discard used solution.
9. Repeat steps 5, 6, 7, and 8.
10. Repeat steps 5, 6, 7, and 8.
11. Remove membrane from plastic bag.
12. Place membrane in labware plate.
13. Add 200 mL washing solution 3.
14. Rinse for 20 minutes at room temperature with constant agitation.
15. Discard used solution no. 3.
16. Repeat steps 13, 14, and 15.
17. Repeat steps 13, 14, and 15.
18. Place membrane with the DNA face-up on Whatman 3MM paper. NOTE: Allow membrane to air-dry at room temperature but not completely to prevent irreversible binding of the probe to the membrane. This precaution will favor probe removal (dehybridization) and subsequent rehybridization with other probes on the same membrane.

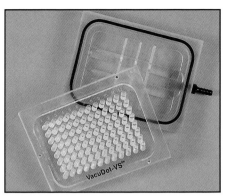

Figure 15.2 Illustration of the VacuDot-VS manifold.

15.13G Autoradiography

Materials

Plastic bags
X-ray film cassette
Intensifying screen
Transparent tape
Kodak X-Omat AR film
Low-temperature freezer ($-70\ °C$)
Darkroom facility

Procedure

1. Place moist membrane in a plastic bag.
2. Open an X-ray film cassette.
3. Place intensifying screen in bottom of cassette.
4. Tape bag containing membrane on top of intensifying screen.
5. In darkroom, place sheet of X-ray film on top of membrane.
6. Place second intensifying screen on top of film.
7. Close X-ray film cassette.
8. Expose at $-70\ °C$ for 1–5 days.
9. Develop and fix film accordingly to supplier's recommendations.
10. If signal intensity is insufficient, place another film in the cassette, and repeat autoradiography for a longer period of time.

Interpretation of Results

In order to achieve a good interpretation of the autoradiographic signal, it is necessary to compare intensity of samples with negative and positive controls. These controls must be processed exactly like the specimens. A specimen will be considered as positive if the signal is above the signal of the negative control. The cells containing viral DNA appear as dark spots on the autoradiograms (Figure 15.2), but differentiation of specific signals from background noise is sometimes difficult.[19]

15.13H Dehybridization

Prepared Reagents

1. 0.4N Sodium hydroxide
   10N Sodium hydroxide
   Double-distilled water
   Mix 40 mL 10N NaOH and 960 mL double-distilled water.
2. 0.1× SSC–0.1% SDS–0.2M Tris-HCl solution
   20× SSC (see Procedure 15.12A.9)
   10% SDS (see Procedure 15.13D.1)
   1M Tris-HCl, pH 7.4 (see Procedure 15.13B.3)
   Double-distilled water

a. Mix 5 mL 20× SSC, 10 mL 10% SDS, and 200 mL 1M Tris-HCl, pH 7.4.

b. Increase total volume to 1,000 mL with double-distilled water. Sterilize by autoclaving.

3. Dehybridization solution

   20× SSC (see Procedure 15.12A.9)

   10% SDS (see Procedure 15.13D.1)

   Double-distilled water

   a. Mix 5 mL 20× SSC and 100 mL of 10% SDS.

   b. Increase total volume to 1,000 mL with double-distilled water.

Dehybridization (Probe Stripping) Protocol

NOTE: Remember that the membrane must not be allowed to air-dry completely after hybridization and washing schedule.

1. Incubate membrane in 100-200 mL 0.4N NaOH at 42 °C for 30 minutes with gentle agitation.
2. Wash membrane with gentle agitation at 42 °C in 100-200 mL of 0.1× SSC–0.1% SDS–0.2M Tris-HCl for 30 minutes.
3. Blot membrane. *Do not* allow to air-dry.
4. Autoradiograph for 24 hours to confirm probe removal.
5. If probe is still bound to the membrane, repeat steps 1, 2, 3, and 4.
6. If no signal is detected, prehybridize and hybridize membrane.

Dot/Blot Hybridization

In dot/blot hybridization,[25] DNA extracted from frozen or fixed tissues is first denatured by heat and/or alkaline treatment and applied to a membrane through a filtration manifold device. There is no restriction digestion of DNA and no electrophoresis steps. Total DNA is concentrated into small area on the membrane. The membrane is then hybridized as described for the filter in situ hybridization procedure. In this section, we are going to describe a dot/blot hybridization using DNA extracted from paraffin embedded tissues. The whole process of DNA preparation from paraffin embedded tissues and dot/blot hybridization is summarized in Figure 15.3.

15.14 DNA Extraction from Paraffin-Embedded Tissues

Prepared Reagents

1. 0.5M EDTA, pH 8.0

   Disodium ethylene diamine tetraacetate · 2H$_2$O (EDTA)

   Double-distilled water

   10M NaOH

   Magnetic stirrer

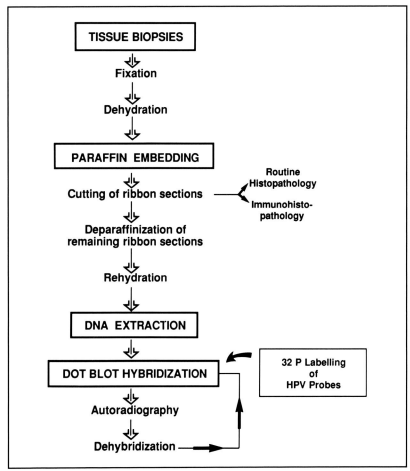

```
                TISSUE BIOPSIES
                      ⇓
                   Fixation
                      ⇓
                  Dehydration
                      ⇓
              PARAFFIN EMBEDDING                      Routine
                      ⇓                              Histopathology
           Cutting of ribbon sections ─────────⟨
                      ⇓                              Immunohisto-
            Deparaffinization of                      pathology
            remaining ribbon sections
                      ⇓
                  Rehydration
                      ⇓
                DNA EXTRACTION
                      ⇓                              32 P Labelling
            DOT BLOT HYBRIDIZATION ←──────┐              of
                      ⇓                    │         HPV Probes
                Autoradiography            │
                      ⇓                    │
            Dehybridization ───────────────┘
```

Figure 15.3 Diagram of the whole protocol for dot/blot hybridization study of DNA extracted from paraffin embedded tissue biopsies.

    a. Add 186.1 g EDTA to 800 mL double-distilled water.

    b. Stir on magnetic stirrer.

    c. Adjust pH to 8.0 with NaOH. NOTE: EDTA will not go into solution until the pH is approaching 8.0 by the addition of NaOH.

    d. Increase total volume to 1,000 ml with double-distilled water. Sterilize by autoclaving.

2. 0.1M EDTA (pH 8.0)

    0.5M EDTA solution (above)

    Double-distilled water

    Mix 200 mL 0.5M EDTA with 800 mL double-distilled water. Sterilize by autoclaving.

3. 1M Tris-HCl (pH 7.5)

    Trizma hydrochloride (Sigma)

    Trizma base (Sigma)

    Double-distilled water

    a. Add 127 g Tris-HCl and 23.6 g Tris-base to a volumetric beaker.

    b. Increase total volume to 1,000 mL with double-distilled water. Sterilize by autoclaving.

4. 0.4M Tris-HCl (pH 7.5)

    1M Tris-HCl, pH 7.5 (above)

    Double-distilled water

    Mix 400 mL 1M Tris-HCl (pH 7.5) with 600 mL double-distilled water. Sterilize by autoclaving.

5. Extraction buffer

    1M Tris-HCl (pH 7.5)

    0.1M EDTA

    10% SDS (see Procedure 15.13D.1)

    Double-distilled water

    Mix 1 mL 1M Tris-HCl, 1 mL 0.1M EDTA, 5 mL 10% SDS, and 93 mL double-distilled water. Sterilize by autoclaving.

6. Proteinase K (5 mg/mL)

    Proteinase K (Boehringer)

    Double-distilled water

    37 °C water bath

    a. Dissolve 25 mg proteinase K in 5 mL double-distilled water.

    b. Preincubate proteinase K solution 1 hour at 37 °C before use. NOTE: If the solution is not intended to be used immediately, keep at −20 °C.

7. 0.1M Tris-HCl (pH 7.9)

    Trizma base (Sigma)

    Trizma hydrochloride (Sigma)

    Double-distilled water

    Dissolve 13.7 g Trizma-HCl and 1.6 g Trizma base in 1,000 mL double-distilled water. Sterilize by autoclaving.

8. Phenol

    Redistilled phenol (molecular grade)

    0.1M Tris-HCl (pH 7.9)

    a. Liquify phenol in water bath at 68 °C. NOTE: Phenol can cause severe burns. Wear safety glasses and gloves when working with phenol.

    b. Mix 66 mL liquified phenol and 34 mL 0.1M Tris-HCl (pH 7.9).

    c. Store in dark bottle at 4 °C. This solution remains stable for at least 1 month.

9. Chloroform-isoamyl alcohol (24:1)

    Chloroform (molecular grade)

    Isoamyl alcohol

    Mix 4 mL isoamyl alcohol and 96 mL chloroform. Store in well-stoppered dark bottle at 4 °C.

10. TE buffer (0.01M Tris-HCl, 0.001M EDTA)

    .1M Tris-HCl (pH 7.9)

    0.1M EDTA

    Double-distilled water

    a. Mix 100 mL 0.1M Tris-HCl (pH 7.9) and 10 mL 0.1M EDTA.

    b. Increase total volume to 1,000 mL with double-distilled water. Sterilize by autoclaving.

Other Reagents and Equipment

Absolute ethanol
70% ethanol
50% ethanol
PBS (see Procedure 15.12A.1)
Anhydrous ethanol
5M NaCl
Carnoy's fixative (see Procedure 15.1.1)
1.5 mL Eppendorf tubes
Pasteur pipettes
Microcentrifuge

DNA Extraction Protocol

1. Use 25 to 35 ribbon sections from routinely embedded tissue blocks for dot/blot hybridization.
2. Remove excess paraffin around tissues with a blade.
3. Deparaffinize and vortex all pieces of tissues in 1.5 mL Eppendorf tubes filled with 1 mL toluene.
4. Microcentrifuge for 5 minutes.
5. Remove toluene.
6. Add 1 mL toluene, and vortex.
7. Microcentrifuge for 5 minutes.
8. Remove toluene (if necessary use a Pasteur pipette to prevent disturbing the tissue pellet).
9. Repeat steps 6, 7, and 8, replacing toluene by 1 mL of each of the following reagents: two absolute ethanol, one 70% ethanol, one 50% ethanol, and finally two washings in PBS.
10. Add 450 μL extraction buffer and 50 μL proteinase K (5 mg/mL).
11. Incubate at 37 °C for 1 hour.
12. Add 450 μL distilled phenol.
13. Vortex for a few seconds.
14. Microcentrifuge for 5 minutes.
15. Remove the lower organic phase with Pasteur pipette.
16. Add 900 μL chloroform-isoamyl alcohol.
17. Vortex for a few seconds.
18. Remove the upper, aqueous phase containing DNA, and transfer it into a clean Eppendorf tube. Discard organic phase.
19. Add 9 μL NaCl and 900 μL anhydrous ethanol to the tube containing extracted DNA.
20. Precipitate DNA at −20 °C overnight.
21. Microcentrifuge precipitated DNA for 15 minutes at 14,000 rpm.
22. Remove ethanol and discard.
23. Resuspend the DNA pellet in 50 μL TE.

15.15 Dot/Blot Technique

Dot/blot procedures described herein are done according to the technique described by the supplier of GeneScreen Plus filter (NEN-Dupont).

Solutions for Denaturation and Neutralization of DNA

1. Denaturation solution (0.25M NaOH)
   Commercial 1M NaOH solution
   Double-distilled water
   a. Mix 25 mL 1M NaOH solution with 75 mL double-distilled water.
2. Neutralization solution
   0.25M NaOH
   20× SSC (see Procedure 15.12A.9)
   Double-distilled water
   a. Mix 50 mL 0.25M NaOH and 625 µL 20× SSC.
   b. Increase total volume to 100 mL with double-distilled water. Sterilize by autoclaving.

Other Materials and Equipment

GeneScreen Plus filter
A filtration manifold device (see Figure 15.2)

Dot/Blot Protocol

In order to ascertain the reproducibility of the technique, HeLa cells (positive to HPV-18) and CaSki cells (positive to HPV-16) are fixed in Carnoy's fixative, embedded in paraffin, sectioned into 5 µm ribbons and studied by the dot/blot protocol. A negative control also must be prepared. It is best to denature and dot cloned HPV-DNAs on each membrane.

1. Soak GeneScreen Plus membrane cut to the dimension of filtration manifold in 0.4M Tris-HCl (pH 7.5) for at least 30 minutes before use in step 5.
2. Denature 50 µL DNA with 50 µL 0.25M NaOH denaturation solution for 10 minutes at room temperature.
3. Chill DNA on ice for 5 minutes.
4. Neutralize with 100 µL neutralization solution.
5. Place soaked filter in manifold and clamp tightly.
6. Add denatured DNA to wells of manifold and permit to settle *without* suction for 30 minutes.
7. Apply light suction for 30 seconds.
8. Remove membrane from manifold.
9. Allow to air-dry at room temperature.

Probe Labelling, Hybridization, and Autoradiography

Probe labelling, hybridization, washing conditions and autoradiography are performed as described in Procedure 15.13C–G. To assess fully the quantity and conservation of DNA extracted from paraffin blocks and snared on filters, the relative amounts of DNA can be compared by hybridization to a ^{32}P-labelled probe that con-

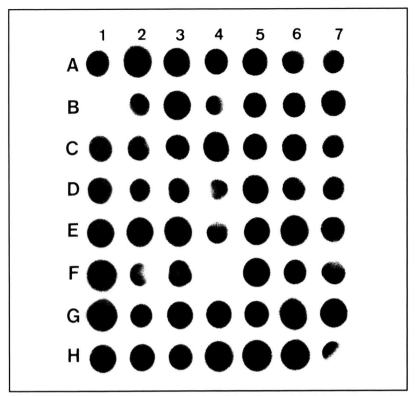

Figure 15.4 Autoradiogram of a dot/blot filter with 56 DNA samples after hybridization with the ALU repeat. Black spots are positive results proving the presence of human DNA. Note that 2 samples (positions A2 and F4) are negative. For a comparison of the same filter hybridized with HPV-16 under stringent conditions, see Figure 6.82.

tains an ALU repeat sequence[61] (Oncor). This probe is extremely sensitive and will detect many similar sequences in the human genome. It is also wise to perform control hybridizations with ^{32}P-pBR322 (HPV probes have been isolated from plasmids containing pBR322) in order to eliminate the possibility of contamination with this sequence.

Interpretation of Results

A black dot on the autoradiogram is considered to be a positive result when the intensity is above the background signal of the negative control. An autoradiograph of a filter with 48 DNA samples after hybridization with the ALU repeat probe is shown in Figure 15.4. The same filter hybridized under high-stringency conditions with HPV-16 is illustrated in Figure 6.16.

Dot/blot hybridization does have limitations:[6,19] a lower sensitivity than Southern blot hybridization, an inability to determine virus subtype, and the necessity of repeated rounds of hybridization with the individual probes to differentiate between related HPV types. However, advantages of the technique are also evident: capacity to screen a large number of specimens; the possibility of retrospective studies of suitable gynecologic materials; the ease of correlative studies between histomorphology, immunohistopathology and HPV-typing on the same biopsy specimen (hence, no need for frozen biopsies); and low cost for each test.

15.16 Southern Blot Hybridization

The hybridization method developed by Southern[70] in 1975 is the most sensitive technique for the detection and characterization of DNA. Total DNA is first extracted from clinical specimens using digestion of cells by a protease, followed by organic extraction with phenol and chloroform, and DNA precipitation with ethanol. Then purified DNA (5–10 μg) is digested with restriction endonucleases producing characteristic fragments of different size. These DNA fragments are separated by agarose gel electrophoresis. The DNA fragments are then denatured in situ by alkali (NaOH), then neutralized, and then transferred by capillary action onto a hybridization membrane. Labelled probes are hybridized under conditions of high or low stringency, with DNA covalently bound to the filter. The filter is washed according to the same conditions of stringency as those used during hybridization. Results are obtained after autoradiography.

15.16A Sampling and Storage of Specimens

Reagents and Equipment

Wooden spatulas
Cotton swabs
50 mL conical centrifuge tube
Phosphate buffered saline (PBS) (see Procedure 15.12A.1)
Vortex
Tabletop clinical centrifuge
1.5 mL Eppendorf tubes
Low-temperature freezer ($-70\ °C$) or at least a $-20\ °C$ freezer

Cell Scrape Specimen Procedure

1. Scrape cervix with a wooden spatula and a cotton swab.
2. Place spatula and swab into a 50 mL conical centrifuge tube containing 25 mL phosphate buffered saline (PBS).
3. Vortex to dislodge cells from spatula and swab.
4. Discard spatula and swab.
5. Centrifuge cells in clinical centrifuge at 1,500 rpm for 15 minutes.
6. Pour off PBS.
7. Resuspend cell pellet in 100 μL of PBS.
8. Transfer cell suspension to a 1.5 mL Eppendorf tube.
9. Store specimens at $-70\ °C$ until DNA extraction.

Biopsy Specimen Procedure

1. Biopsy specimens are obtained under colposcopy observation. Place in PBS at $-70\ °C$ until DNA extraction.

15.16B DNA Extraction
Prepared Reagents and Equipment

1. RNase (20 mg/mL)
   RNase A (from bovine pancreas, Boehringer)
   Double-distilled water
   a. Dissolve 100 mg RNase in 5 ml double-distilled water.
   b. Incubate in 100 °C water bath for 5 minutes to inactivate DNases.
   c. Aliquot and store at −20 °C.
   d. Thaw on ice before use.
2. Extraction buffer (see Procedure 15.14.5)
3. Proteinase K solution (5 mg/mL) (see Procedure 15.14.6)
4. Phenol (see Procedure 15.14.8)
5. Chloroform-isoamyl alcohol (see Procedure 15.14.9)
6. TE buffer (see Procedure 15.14.10)
7. Anhydrous ethanol
8. 5M NaCl
9. 15 mL Corex tubes
10. Water bath
11. UV spectrophotometer
12. Scissors and tweezers
13. Floor centrifuge

Procedure

1. **Cell scrapes** suspended in PBS must be centrifuged, and the pellet resuspended in 2.25 mL extraction buffer.
   Biopsies are finely sliced with scissors and placed in 2.25 mL extraction buffer.
2. Add 250 µL proteinase K (5 mg/mL) (pre-incubated 1 hour at 37 °C.
3. Incubate at 37 °C until digestion is completed.
4. Add 25 µL RNase (20 mg/mL) (pre-incubated 5 minutes at 100 °C) and mix by inversion.
5. Incubate at 37 °C for 2 hours.
6. Add 2.5 mL phenol.
7. Mix slowly by inversion for 5 minutes.
8. Centrifuge at 6,000 rpm for 5 minutes.
9. Remove upper, aqueous layer containing DNA and place in a clean 15 mL Corex tube.
10. Discard organic phase.
11. Add 5 mL chloroform-isoamyl alcohol (24:1) to the tube containing DNA.
12. Mix slowly by inversion for 5 minutes.
13. Centrifuge at 6,000 rpm for 5 minutes.
14. Remove upper, aqueous layer containing DNA and place in a clean 15 mL Corex tube. Discard lower organic phase.
15. Add 5 mL chloroform-isoamyl alcohol (24:1) to the tube containing DNA.
16. Mix slowly by inversion for 5 minutes.
17. Centrifuge at 6,000 rpm for 5 minutes.

18. Remove the upper, aqueous layer containing DNA and place in a clean 15 mL Corex tube.
19. Add 50 μL 5M NaCl and 5 mL anhydrous ethanol to the tube containing DNA.
20. Precipitate DNA at -20 °C overnight.
21. Centrifuge precipitated DNA at 9,000 rpm for 45 minutes.
22. Discard ethanol.
23. Dissolve DNA pellet in 1 mL TE buffer.
24. Determine concentration of DNA by spectrophotometry.[34,60]
25. Precipitate DNA by adding 10 μL 5M NaCl and 2 mL anhydrous ethanol and leaving tubes at -20 °C overnight.
26. Centrifuge precipitated DNA at 9,000 rpm for 45 minutes.
27. Dissolve DNA pellet in TE buffer according to the spectrophotometric readings, ie, to obtain a solution of 1 μg/μL.
28. DNA is stored at -20 °C.

15.16C Restriction Enzyme Digestion

Background

The fragmentation of DNA molecules is done by restriction enzymes. All restriction enzymes always recognize the same specific DNA sequences. The fragmentation of viral DNA will permit to distinguish between types and subtypes of papillomaviruses because different HPV types do not harbor the same location for a given sequence. In other words, the size and number of DNA fragments obtained after digestion with a specific restriction enzyme differ for each HPV type.

Prepared Reagents

1. Migration buffer (0.1% bromophenol–50% glycerol–0.1% SDS)
   Bromophenol blue
   Glycerol
   10% SDS (see Procedure 15.13D.1)
   Double-distilled water
   a. Prepare solution of 50% glycerol by mixing 5 mL glycerol and 5 mL double-distilled water.
   b. Place 10 mg bromophenol blue in a 10 mL volumetric flask.
   c. Add 100 μL 10% SDS and increase total volume of 50% glycerol (step a) to 10 mL.
   d. Store at 4 °C.

Other Reagents and Equipment

Pst I restriction enzyme and its corresponding buffer (normally obtained from manufacturers or distributors)
1.5 mL Eppendorf tubes
37 °C water bath
Double-distilled water
Microcentrifuge

Restriction Enzyme Protocol

Prepare a total reaction of 30 μL as follows:

1. Add 10 μL DNA (corresponding to 10 μg DNA), 3 μL Pst I buffer, 4 μL Pst I enzyme (10 units/μL), and 13 μL double-distilled water to a 1.5 mL Eppendorf tube.
2. Vortex and microcentrifuge a few seconds.
3. Incubate at 37 °C in a water bath for 2 hours.
4. Stop reaction by adding 1.5 μL migration buffer. NOTE: Do not forget to include negative and positive DNA controls.

15.16D Gel Electrophoresis and Observation of DNA Fragments

Background

Gel electrophoresis is a powerful tool for the characterization of DNA molecules. Only small amounts of DNA are needed. Agarose gel electrophoresis allows rapid separation of restriction fragments on the basis of their molecular size and conformation.

Horizontal gels are more convenient than vertical gels. Horizontal gels are easier to handle and they are more stable at agarose concentrations lower than 0.8%.

DNA in agarose gels can be visualized by staining the gels with the fluorescent dye ethidium bromide and then using an ultraviolet transilluminator. The sensitivity of this staining technique depends on the amount of DNA present in the gel. The minimum amount of DNA that can be detected by ethidium bromide staining is about 2 ng in a 0.5-cm–wide band.

Reagents and Equipment

1. TBE buffer (Tris-borate-EDTA)
   Tris-base
   Boric acid
   0.5M EDTA (see Procedure 15.14.1)
   Double-distilled water
   a. Mix 10.8 g Tris-base, 5.5 g boric acid, and 4 mL 0.5M EDTA in a 1,000 mL volumetric flask.
   b. Increase total volume to 1,000 mL with double-distilled water.
   c. Mix well, and sterilize by autoclaving.
2. 0.7% Agarose gel
   Agarose
   TBE buffer
   500 mL Erlenmeyer flask
   Electrophoresis gel mold
   Comb for electrophoresis wells
   a. Mix 0.7 g agarose with 100 mL TBE in a 500 mL Erlenmeyer flask.
   b. Heat in boiling water bath or microwave oven until agarose dissolves and becomes clear and homogeneous.

c. Cool to 60 °C.

d. Pour agarose solution into electrophoresis mold to obtain 0.5-cm–thick gel.

e. Position comb 0.1 cm above bottom of electrophoresis mold.

f. Let gel cool at room temperature for 30 minutes.

g. Carefully remove comb and mount gel in electrophoresis tank.

3. Ethidium bromide (10 mg/mL)

   Ethidium bromide

   Double-distilled water

   a. Add 1 g of ethidium bromide to 100 mL double-distilled water. NOTE: Ethidium bromide is a strong mutagen. Wear a mask and gloves when working with it.

   b. Stir on a magnetic stirrer for several hours. Store in a dark bottle at 4 °C.

4. Ethidium bromide (1 μg/mL) (Working solution)

   Ethidium bromide solution (10 mg/mL)

   Double-distilled water

   a. Mix 25 μL ethidium bromide solution (10 mg/mL) with 250 mL double-distilled water.

Other Materials and Equipment

Electrophoresis tank and power supply
UV transilluminator
Kodak 22A Wratten filter
Polaroid camera
Polaroid film type 665 or 667
200 μL disposable micropipette
DNA-sized marker such as Lambda-Hind III

Procedure

1. Fill electrophoresis tank with TBE buffer to cover gel to a depth of 0.1 cm.

2. Slowly load molecular-sized marker in the first slot, and negative and positive DNA controls and digested DNA samples into other wells of the submerged gel using a disposable micropipette.

3. Allow all samples to migrate at 1-5V/cm.[34,60]

4. Run gel until bromophenol blue has migrated an appropriate distance.

5. Turn off power supply.

6. Remove gel from electrophoresis tank.

7. Place gel in a glass plate.

8. Stain gel with working solution of ethidium bromide for 15–30 minutes.

9. Rinse gel briefly in double-distilled water.

10. Examine gel with UV transilluminator.

11. Photograph gel on Polaroid film type 665 or 667.[60]

15.16E Southern Blot Transfer of Electrophoresed DNA Fragments

Background

Before transferring electrophoresed DNA fragments from agarose gel to a nylon membrane, the DNA must be denatured in situ by soaking the gel in alkali. Then single-stranded DNA molecules contained in the gel are transferred to a membrane in such a way that they retain their original pattern, ie, the relative position of DNA fragments remains unchanged during the transfer.

The transfer is obtained by placing the membrane against the gel and by blotting a solvent through it. In other words, the DNA fragments are transferred out of the gel by the capillary action of the solvent passing through the gel. This capillary action is produced by movement of the solvent, which is absorbed by a stack of paper towels deposited on top of the nylon membrane.[34,60]

Prepared Reagents

1. 0.25N HCl
   Commercial 1N HCl
   Double-distilled water
   a. Add 62.5 mL 1N HCl to a 250 mL volumetric flask.
   b. Increase total volume to 250 mL with double-distilled water.

2. Denaturation solution (0.4N NaOH–0.6M NaCl)
   Commercial 1N sodium hydroxide solution
   5M NaCl
   Double-distilled water
   a. Mix 400 mL 1M NaOH and 120 mL 5M NaCl.
   b. Increase total volume to 1,000 mL with double-distilled water.

3. Neutralization buffer
   5M NaCl
   1M Tris-HCl (pH 7.5) (see Procedure 15.14.3)
   Double-distilled water
   a. Mix 300 mL 5M NaCl and 500 mL 1M Tris-HCl (pH 7.5).
   b. Increase total volume to 1,000 mL with double-distilled water. Sterilize by autoclaving.

4. 10× SSC
   20× SSC (see Procedure 15.12A.9)
   Double-distilled water
   Mix 500 mL 20× SSC and 500 mL double-distilled water.

5. 0.4N NaOH
   1M commercial sodium hydroxide (NaOH)
   Double-distilled water
   Mix 400 mL 1M NaOH and 600 mL double-distilled water.

6. 0.2M Tris-HCl (pH 7.5) 2× SSC
   1M Tris-HCl (pH 7.5) (see Procedure 15.14.3)
   20× SSC (see Procedure 15.12A.9)
   Double-distilled water

a. Mix 200 mL 1M Tris-HCl and 100 mL 20× SSC.
b. Increase total volume to 1,000 mL with double-distilled water. Sterilize by autoclaving.

Other Materials and Equipment

GeneScreen Plus membrane cut to the dimensions of the gel
2 pieces of 3MM paper cut to the dimensions of the gel
Paper towels cut a little smaller than the 3MM paper
Glass plates
A glass plate with a support (larger than the dimension of the gel) in the center—this plate will be used for transfer of DNA fragments to the nylon membrane (see Figure 15.5)
2 pieces of 1M paper fitting in the glass dish
1 kg weight

Procedure

1. Place gel in glass plate.
2. Depurinate gel by soaking it in 0.25N HCl for 15 minutes with constant agitation at room temperature.
3. Briefly rinse the gel in double-distilled water.
4. Soak gel in denaturation solution for 30 minutes with constant agitation at room temperature.
5. Repeat step 3.
6. Neutralize gel by soaking it in neutralization solution for 30 minutes with constant agitation at room temperature.
7. Repeat step 6.
8. During step 7, wet pre-cut nylon membrane in double-distilled water for 2 minutes. Then immerse nylon membrane in 10× SSC for 30 minutes at room temperature.
9. Fill reservoir of transfer plate with 10× SSC and place each element (ie, 2 sheets Whatman 1M paper, gel, nylon membrane, 2 sheets Whatman 3MM paper, stack of paper towels, glass plate, and weight) in transfer plate as depicted in Figure 15.5.
10. Allow transfer to proceed for 18 hours. Replace paper towels if necessary.
11. When transfer is completed, immerse nylon membrane in 0.4N NaOH for 60 seconds to ensure complete denaturation of immobilized DNA.
12. Neutralize nylon membrane in an excess of 0.2M Tris-HCl (pH 7.5)-2× SSC for 5 minutes.
13. Allow membrane to air-dry on filter paper, with transferred DNA face up. NOTE: In order to check the efficacy of the transfer, it is recommended to stain the gel with ethidium bromide for 30 minutes and to examine by UV transillumination.

Preparation of Viral Probes

(see Procedure 15.12B and 15.13C)

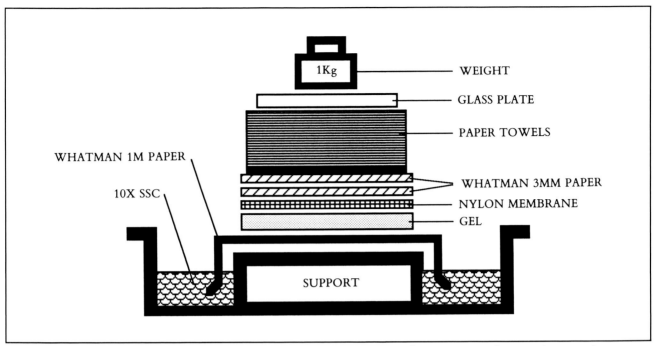

Figure 15.5 Schematic presentation of the Southern transfer of DNA from agarose gel to a nylon membrane.

DNA-DNA Hybridization, Washing Conditions, Autoradiography, and Dehybridization

(see Procedure 15.13D–G)

Autoradiogram Interpretation

Following hybridization of the filter with a given HPV type, the autoradiogram shows black bands, which correspond to restriction enzyme digestion patterns of the corresponding specific HPV type (see Figure 6.15). Types and subtypes of HPV are distinguished according to their characteristic restriction enzyme digestion patterns. About 0.1 HPV genome equivalents per cell can be detected by Southern blot hybridization. This is one of the most convenient methods for identification of specific HPV types.[6,54]

Polymerase Chain Reaction (PCR)

The polymerase chain reaction is a simple technique for amplifying nucleic acids invented by Mullis[44] in 1984 and developed by Saiki and coworkers in 1985.[59] It facilitates the detection of very small numbers of viruses or single-copy genes in fresh or fixed clinical specimens.

The method is based on the repetition of three steps:

1. Denaturation: The double-stranded DNA sample (template DNA) is denatured by incubation at high temperature.

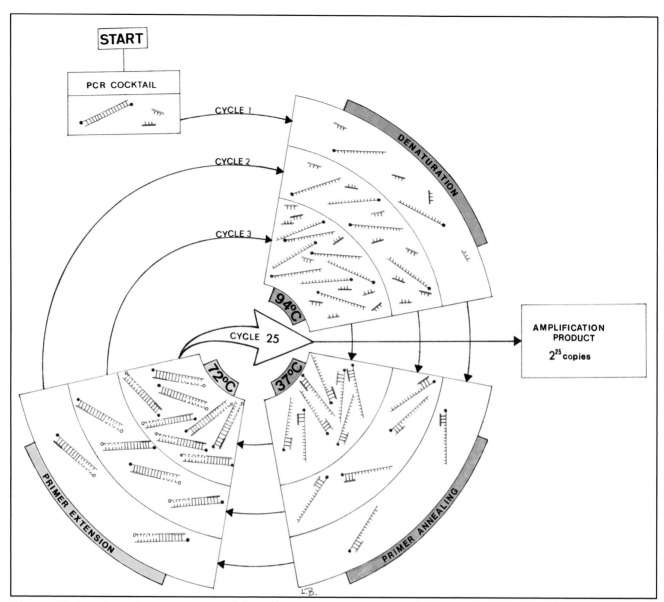

Figure 15.6 Schematic presentation of the polymerase chain reaction. Denaturation (94°C); annealing of primers (37°C); and primer extension (72°C) are illustrated with corresponding amplification of DNA molecules.

2. Annealing of extension primers: A pair of synthetic oligonucleotides (extension primers) complementary to template DNA are annealed when temperature is lowered. Each primer recognizes only one sequence of template DNA located on opposite strands at the extremities of the region to be amplified.

3. Primer extension: DNA synthesis proceeds in the 5′ to 3′ direction in the presence of DNA polymerase and deoxyribonucleotide triphosphates (dATP, dTTP, dCTP, dGTP).

These newly synthesized DNA molecules, then, as well as the original DNA molecule itself become template DNA for a second round of amplification (Figure 15.6).

Each set of these 3 steps is a cycle. The number of DNA molecules increases exponentially to 2^n, where n is the number of cycles.

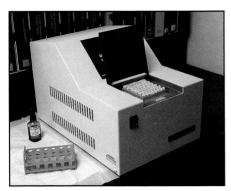

Figure 15.7 Illustration of the Thermal cycler (Perkin-Elmer/Cetus) designed for amplification of DNA.

DNA molecules double after each cycle. Repeated rounds allow amplification more than a million times.

Originally, the PCR technique used the Klenow fragment of DNA polymerase I of *E coli* (Saiki et al).[59] Because of the thermolability of this enzyme, it was necessary to add fresh enzyme after each denaturation step. The whole process was cumbersome. But recently, Cetus[58] considerably simplified the technique by eliminating the need to add fresh DNA polymerase at each cycle. They use a thermostable enzyme, Taq Polymerase, which is extracted from *Thermus aquaticus,* a thermophilic bacterium. Taq Polymerase proved to be an ideal enzyme for the PCR technique because it retains its activity after repeated exposure to high temperature. More recently, a purer preparation of Taq Polymerase, the AmpliTaq DNA polymerase, was genetically engineered by expression of modified form of the Taq DNA polymerase gene in *E coli.*

Taking advantage of the AmpliTaq DNA Polymerase, the Perkin Elmer Cetus group also introduced an automated instrument able to eliminate the manual transfer of the samples between incubation water baths adjusted at different temperatures, as required by the PCR technique (94 °C for denaturation → 37 °C for annealing of primers → 72 °C for primer extension). The DNA Thermal Cycler (see Figure 15.7) allows the user to program a specific thermal cycle profile that is optimized for his own samples. In the presence of template DNA, primers, dNTPs, Taq polymerase, and an optimized buffer, this instrument is able to perform repeated amplification cycles (up to 99).

The analysis of the samples is done using one or more of these following techniques:

1. DNA Dot/Blot hybridized with a radiolabelled oligonucleotide homologous to the amplified DNA segment. The result is the same as described in Procedure 15.15.
2. Electrophoresis of the sample followed by ethidium bromide staining of agarose or polyacrylamide gel. A band with a molecular weight corresponding to the projected amplified segment confirms the presence of the amplified segment. DNA amplification products of two or more different DNA templates can be designed to harbor different molecular weights in such a way that it is possible to distinguish each segment from one another by looking at the gel.
3. To further confirm the specificity of the band and to eliminate all false negatives (generated by a low amplification of sample), the Southern blot technique followed by radioactive probing and autoradiography should be used. Positive results are detected by the presence of a band corresponding to the molecular weight of the predetermined amplified DNA segment.

Detection of human papillomaviruses in genital lesions has been performed in many laboratories within the last two years.[8,9,11,15,20,29,35,41,42,52,66–68,74,75,78,82] Four main approaches have been designed by the users.

Table 15.3
Consensus Primers for Amplification of a Region Within the HPV L1 Open Reading Frame[35]

MY11: 5′ GCMCAGGGWCATAAYAATGG 3′ for positive strand synthesis
MY09: 5′ CGTCCMARRGGAWACTGATC 3′ for negative strand synthesis

NOTE: The letters C, G, A, and T are the four nucleotides. The letters M, R, W and Y are degenerate bases which could be replaced as follows: M $-> (A + C)$; R $->$ $(A + G)$; W $-> (A + T)$; Y $-> (C + T)$.

1. Low–recognition range primers.[11] A set of primers able to anneal with 2 different HPV types were designed. For instance, a single pair of primers which anneal to HPV-6 and also to HPV-11; another set of primers complementary to HPV-16 and also to HPV-33. DNA amplification products for HPV-6/11 and HPV-16/33 have different molecular weights (eg, 120 bp for HPV-6/11 and 200 bp for HPV-16/33). These two different DNA segments can be recognized in a Nusieve agarose gel stained with ethidium bromide, provided the amplification product is sufficient. This protocol permits differentiation between low-risk (6/11) papillomaviruses and high-risk (16/33) papillomaviruses, but does not permit distinction between DNA pairs (ie, between HPV-16 and HPV-33 or HPV-6 and HPV-11). To further recognize specific HPV type, the reaction products will have to be detected by dot/blot or Southern blot hybridized with specific radiolabelled oligonucleotides complementary to each HPV type.
2. High–recognition range primers[20,35] also called consensus primers (see Table 15.3).[35] These primers are designed to anneal to many different HPVs. For instance, a single pair of primers may anneal to HPV-6, HPV-11, HPV-16, HPV-18, HPV-33, and other types. Amplification of all these HPV types may occur. Recognition of specific types is possible using dot/blot or Southern blot hybridization with radiolabelled oligonucleotides specific for each type. A rapid screening alternative is also possible using hybridization with a consensus probe made of a mixture of two oligonucleotides (see Table 15.5) complementary to all the HPV types mentioned above.
3. Specific primers complementary to each of the HPV types can be designed: a set of primers capable to anneal to HPV-16 alone; another set to anneal to HPV-18 alone, etc (Young et al).[82] The molecular weight of the amplification product is different for each HPV type because the distance between annealed primers on different strands of template DNA is different. This approach permits confirmation of amplification of a specific HPV type by looking at the ethidium bromide-stained gel. Further characterization of specific HPV types can be obtained using dot/blot or Southern blot followed by hybridization with specific radiolabelled oligonucleotides and autoradiography.
4. This fourth approach is the same as the third approach except that a mixture of different specific primers is included in the

Table 15.4
Location of the Consensus Primers in HPV Genomes[35]

	Amplification		
	Location		
HPV Type	Primer 1	Primer 2	Product (bp)
6	6722–6741	7151–7170	448
11	6707–6726	7146–7165	458
16	6582–6601	7014–7033	451
18	6558–6577	6993–7012	454
33	6549–6568	6978–6997	448

same PCR reaction cocktail, allowing identification of more than one HPV type in the same DNA template preparation (Young et al)[82] by looking at the stained gel. Hybridization with appropriate probes is also possible.

Primers, Probes, and Controls

The analysis of sample specimens by the PCR technique requires the following:

1. Purified synthesized oligonucleotide primers
2. Purified synthesized oligonucleotide probes
3. Good control HPV DNA
4. Sample DNA preparation
5. Reagents for PCR reaction preparation
6. Application of PCR
7. Use of a technique for analysis of the amplification product

Synthesized Oligonucleotide Primers

Before starting the PCR reaction, it is necessary to select appropriate oligonucleotide primers that are complementary to the DNA template to be amplified. The primers must then be synthesized and purified.

Manos et al[35] designed a consensus primer pair (see Table 15.3) able to amplify a region within the HPV-L1 open reading frame, a region which is going to be retained if viral DNA integration has occurred in the infected cells. This point is particularly important because integration of viral DNA occurs frequently in cancer cells of the uterine cervix. These primers are degenerate in several positions (positions at which two possible nucleotides are inserted during synthesis of the oligonucleotide) which renders them complementary to genital HPVs (types 6, 11, 16, 18, and 33), and by inference to other HPV types. The location of these concensus primers in the HPV genome types and the length (in base pairs) of the corresponding amplified fragment is presented in Table 15.4.

Table 15.5
Consensus Probe: A Mixture of Two Oligonucleotides[35]

MY1019:	5′ CTGTGGTAGATACCACWCGCAGTAC 3′
MY18:	5′ CTGTTGTTGATACTACACGCAGTAC 3′

NOTE: This mixture of probes is complementary to HPV types 6, 11, 16, 18, and 33.

Table 15.6
Location of the Consensus Probes in HPV Genomes[35]

HPV Type	Location
6 (MY1019)	6771–6795
11 (MY1019)	6766–6790
16 (MY18)	6631–6655
18 (MY1019)	6607–6631
33 (MY1019)	6598–6612

Synthesized Oligonucleotide Probes

Synthesized oligonucleotide probes complementary to the amplified DNA segment must be prepared and obtained the same way as described in step 1. Manos et al[35] have selected two types of probes: consensus probes (Table 15.5) for identification of a large spectrum of HPV DNA types and specific probes (Table 15.7) corresponding to internal sequences that are specific to each HPV. The location of the consensus and specific probes on the amplified DNA template are reported respectively in Tables 15.6 and 15.8.

Selection of Good Control HPV DNA

At least three different controls must be included in each protocol: a positive control, a negative control, and one or more reagent controls.

a. The positive control is generally a sample that amplifies weakly but consistently. Frequently, positive controls are either recombinant plasmids containing HPV DNA or cell lines containing HPVs such as CaSki or SiHa cell lines for HPV-16, and HeLa cell line for HPV-18.
b. A good negative control is a proven negative sample previously characterized by PCR and/or other standard techniques such as Southern blot. The K562 cell line was used as a negative control by Manos et al (1989).[35]
c. All reagents (water, buffer, etc) should be included as controls with each amplification. The reagent controls should contain all of the necessary components of PCR reaction but without the addition of template DNA.

15.17 Polymerase Chain Reaction Procedure

15.17A Preparation of Sample DNA

Different approaches were developed by PCR users to prepare sample DNA for amplification.

a. Standard preparation of DNA extracted from fresh biopsy specimens or from cell scrapes obtained from the uterine cervix by the sodium dodecyl sulphate-proteinase K lysis technique (see DNA extraction protocol, in Procedure 15.16B). A similar technique was used by Young et al.[82]

Table 15.7
Probes for Detection of Specific HPV[35]

HPV6	5′ CATCCGTAACTACATCTTCCA 3′	(MY12)
HPV11	5′ TCTGTGTCTAAATCTGCTACA 3′	(MY13)
HPV16	5′ CATACACCTCCAGCACCTAA 3′	(MY14)
HPV18	5′ GGATGCTGCACCGGCTGA 3′	(WD74)
HPV33	5′ CACACAAGTAACTAGTGACAG 3′	(MY16)

b. DNA extraction from paraffin blocks[27] using a detergent (SDS) and a proteolytic enzyme (Proteinase K) as described in Procedure 15.14.

c. The use of a paraffin section without DNA extraction.[66,67] No detergent lysis and no digestion of proteins.

Reagents and Equipment

Toluene
95% ethanol
Eppendorf tubes
Microcentrifuge
Vortex

a. Place a single 5-10 μm paraffin section in a 500 μL Eppendorf tube.
b. Add 400 μL toluene and vortex a few seconds.
c. Centrifuge for 5 minutes.
d. Remove toluene.
e. Add 400 μL 95% ethanol and vortex a few seconds.
f. Centrifuge for 5 minutes.
g. Remove ethanol.
h. Desiccate the tissue pellet. NOTE: The tissue fragment is now ready for amplification by adding 100 μL of the PCR mixture, and allowing 40 cycles of amplification.

15.17B Rapid Preparation of Cell Scrapes
Reagents and Equipment

PBS (see Procedure 15.12A.1)
Sterile double-distilled water
50 mL conical tubes
Eppendorf tubes
Centrifuge
Ayres' spatula

a. Collect cell samples with spatula or swab.
b. Place spatula or swab in 50 mL conical tube containing 10 mL PBS.
c. Vortex tube to remove material from spatula and swab.
d. Remove and discard spatula and swab.
e. Centrifuge at 2,000 g for 10 minutes.

f. Remove and discard supernatant from each tube.
g. Resuspend pellet in 500 μL sterile double-distilled water.
h. Transfer the cell suspension in a 1.5 ml Eppendorf tube.
i. Denature cells by boiling for 10 minutes in water bath. NOTE: At this step, the sample is ready for PCR amplification. A 50 μL aliquot of this preparation is used for the PCR reaction. It is also possible to store frozen the denatured cell specimens at −20 °C until use. Another rapid preparation of cell scrapes and paraffin sections is also reported by Manos et al.[35]

15.17C Preparation of PCR Reagents

Reagents and Equipment

1. A pair of primers (20 bp) homologous to each of the DNA segment to be amplified. The primers are diluted in double-distilled water to make a 10 μm solution of each primer. Keep frozen at −20 °C.

NOTE: A commercial kit can be used in lieu of prepared reagents 2 through 6. The GeneAmp DNA Amplification Reagent Kit (Perkin Elmer-Cetus) contains all the reagents necessary for the PCR reaction: AmpliTaq polymerase, dNTPs, 10× reaction buffer, a control template (a 500 bp lambda DNA sequence) with corresponding primer 1 and 2 to test the kit reagents. Store at −20 °C.

2. 125mM $MgCl_2$
   1M Magnesium chloride solution
   Double-distilled water
   Mix 12.5 mL 1M $MgCl_2$ and 87.5 mL double-distilled water. Sterilize by autoclaving.
3. 1M KCl
   Potassium chloride (KCl)
   Sterile double-distilled water
   a. Add 74.55 g KCl in a volumetric beaker.
   b. Increase total volume to 1,000 mL with double-distilled water. Sterilize by autoclaving.
4. 1M Tris-HCl (pH 8.4)
   Tris base (Tris[hydroxy-methyl] aminomethane) (Trizma base, Sigma)
   Tris-HCl (Trizma hydrochloride, Sigma)
   Double-distilled water.
   a. Add 98 g Tris base and 30 g Tris-HCl to a volumetric beaker.
   b. Increase total volume to 1,000 mL with double-distilled water. Sterilize by autoclaving.
5. Gelatin (10 mg/mL)
   Gelatin
   Double-distilled water
   Dissolve 1 g gelatin in 100 mL double-distilled water. Sterilize by autoclaving.
6. PCR buffer
   125 mM $MgCl_2$
   1M KCl

Table 15.8
Location of Specific Probes in HPV Genomes[35]

Type	Location
6 (MY12)	6813–6833
11 (MY13)	6800–6820
16 (MY14)	6924–6943
18 (WD74)	6905–6922
33 (MY16)	6638–6658

1M Tris-HCl (pH 8.4)
Gelatin (10 mg/mL)
Sterile double-distilled water
   a. Mix 2 mL 125mM $MgCl_2$, 1 mL 1M Tris-HCl, 5 mL 1M KCl, and 2 mL 10 mg/mL gelatin.
   b. Aliquot and store at −20 °C.
7. dNTP mixture (these dNTP solutions are supplied by Pharmacia)
   dATP (100mM solution)
   dTTP (100mM solution)
   dGTP (100mM solution)
   dCTP (100mM solution)
   a. Mix 100 µL of each nucleotide with 1,600 µL of sterile double-distilled water.
   b. Aliquot and store at −20 °C.
8. Taq polymerase (Perkin Elmer Cetus)
   Before use dilute Taq polymerase 1:10 by mixing 1 µL of enzyme with 9 µL of double-distilled water.
9. Light liquid paraffin
10. Sterile double-distilled water
11. Positive displacement pipettes
12. Sterile 0.5 mL Eppendorf tubes
13. Microcentrifuge
14. Vortex
15. An automated instrument to perform the PCR technique (Perkin Elmer Cetus DNA Thermal Cycler, Figure 15.7).

15.17D PCR Technique

Special recommendations must be followed before starting the PCR protocol because many users of the PCR technique had to face the very serious problem of false-positive results. Kwok and Higuchi[31] suggest using the same principles applied to sterile handling of cell cultures to avoid cross-contamination. A list of precautions, reported in Table 15.9, will help to minimize the carryover of DNA from one tube to another and prevent false-positive results.

For those who wish to prepare their own reagents, follow the following steps:

1. Remove clinical and control specimens as well as all reagents from freezer and thaw in an ice water bath.
2. Dilute sample DNA to a concentration of 100 ng in 50 µL of sterile double-distilled water. For scraped cells denatured by boiling in water, use 50 µL.
3. Mix the following to obtain a 100 µL reaction in a 0.5 mL polypropylene microcentrifuge tube: 50 µL of DNA sample or denatured cell scrapes; 9 µL of PCR buffer; 4 µL of dNTP mixture; 5 µL of primer no 1; 5 µL of primer no 2; 23 µL of double-distilled water.
4. Inactivate proteases by heating to 95 °C in the PCR block heater for 10 minutes.

Table 15.9
Precautions to Prevent False-Positive Results

A. Physical separation of pre- and post-PCR reactions
Separate rooms should be used:
Room 1: used for preparation of DNA template
Room 2: used for preparation and storage of reagents
Room 3: used for setting up amplification reactions
Never bring in room 1 and 2: amplified DNA as well as reagents and supplies used in an area where PCR analyses were performed.

B. Alliquot reagents
All reagents used in PCR must be prepared, aliquotted, and stored in an area that is free of PCR-amplified product.

C. Positive displacement pipettes
Positive displacement pipettes are recommended in order to eliminate cross-contamination of samples by pipetting.

D. Meticulous laboratory techniques
Precautions must be taken not only in setting up the PCR reactions but also in all other technical procedures such as: sample collection, sample handling, and DNA extraction. Other precautions have also to be taken into account:
change gloves frequently
uncap tubes carefully to prevent aerosols
minimize sample handling

5. Add 4 μL of diluted (1:10) Taq polymerase to each tube.
6. Vortex briefly and microcentrifuge for 10 seconds.
7. Overlay the mix with 75 μL of light liquid paraffin.
8. The whole mixture is now ready for amplification in the DNA Thermal Cycler. (Read the Instruction manual for operating the Perkin Elmer-Cetus DNA Thermal Cycler carefully.) NOTE: DO NOT FORGET to turn on the Thermal Cycler 30 minutes before use.
9. Set the PCR machine for the following program. NOTE: Before starting the amplification reaction, always verify the complete program you wish to run in order to be sure you are using the appropriate amplification procedure.
Denaturation at 94 °C for 1 minute
Annealing at 55 °C for 2 minutes
Extension at 72 °C for 2 minutes
For a total number of 29 cycles
Add to this the following final cycle program:
Denaturation at 94 °C for 1 minute
Annealing at 55 °C for 2 minutes
Extension at 72 °C for 10 minutes
10. Place a drop of liquid paraffin in each well of the heat block to allow the tubes to fit closely providing the most satisfactory heat transfer to the reaction mixtures.
11. Place the tubes in the wells of the heat block.
12. Run the program. NOTE: It takes around three hours to complete 25 cycles. If you wish, you can run the cycles overnight because the soak program permits to keep the amplification mixtures at 4 °C until you are ready to analyze them by ethidium bromide stained gels, dot/blots, or Southern blots.

Analysis of the Amplification Product

Different techniques can be used for analysis of the amplification product: (1) the ethidium bromide-stained gels; (2) the dot/blot technique followed by hybridization with probes and autoradiography; or (3) the Southern blot technique followed by hybridization with probes and autoradiography.

1. Ethidium bromide gels. The product samples can be run directly on Nusieve agarose gel. A DNA-sized marker is included in each gel (Lambda-Hind III or 0X174-Hae III). Then the gel is stained with ethidium bromide and examined under ultraviolet illumination. The presence of a band corresponding to the size of the projected amplified sequence confirms that the sequence was effectively amplified. The absence of a band does not mean that no amplification has taken place. In such a case, it is necessary to use one of the two other techniques for analysis.

2. Dot/blot technique, hybridization, and autoradiography
   Description of these techniques are reported elsewhere in this chapter. Observe the following modification of oligonucleotide labelling. Oligonucleotide probes are very small pieces of nucleic acid which can be labelled at the 5′ termini with the T4 Polynucleotide Kinase and $[\gamma^{32}P]$-ATP (Amersham, 3,000 Ci/mmol) after dephosphorylation by bacterial alkaline phosphatase under recommended assay conditions. Target oligonucleotides are 5′ end labelled using the BRL 5′ DNA Terminus labelling System kit (Gibco-BRL) following the manufacturer's recommendations. Radiolabelled probe is separated from free nucleotides by Sephadex G-50 chromatography.[60] Use it without denaturation. If not used immediately, store at $-20\ °C$.

Prehybridization and Hybridization Conditions

1. Use the same prehybridization buffer described in Procedure 15.13D.
2. Add radiolabelled probe (5×10^6 cpm/mL hybridization solution).
3. Hybridize overnight at room temperature.
4. Wash membrane at room temperature with a solution of $5\times$ SSC–0.1% SDS for 5 minutes.
5. Repeat step 4.
6. Wash membrane at 37 °C with a solution of $5\times$ SSC–0.1% SDS for 30 minutes.
7. Repeat step 6.
8. Partially dry the blot, if you wish to dehybridize.
9. Autoradiograph (see Procedure 15.13G).

3. Southern blot technique, hybridization, and autoradiography
   Follow the same technique as reported in Procedure 15.16ff, taking into consideration the following modifications:
   1. Run the PCR product on agarose gel at 90 volts for 2 hours.
   2. Stain with ethidium bromide for 15 minutes.
   3. Observe stained gel on an ultraviolet transilluminator.
   4. Photograph gel.[60]
   5. Denature and transfer DNA fragments (see Procedure 15.16E).

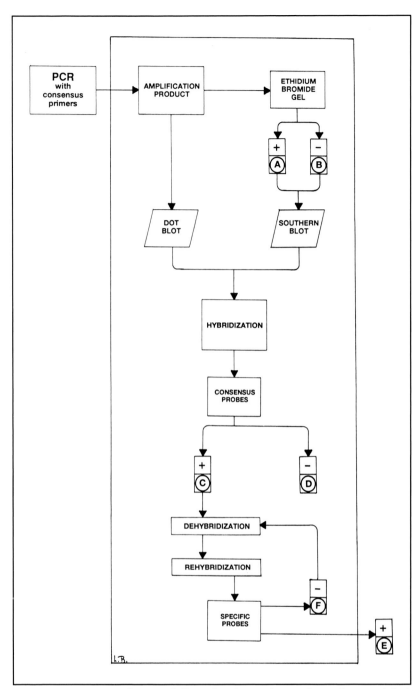

Figure 15.8 Procedure to follow for the analysis of samples amplified with consensus primers.

6. Prehybridize, hybridize, wash, and autoradiograph the membrane (see Procedure 15.13D–G).

Interpretation of Results

Figure 15.8 illustrates the procedure to follow for the analysis of samples amplified with consensus primers. The following is a key to 15.8:

A: The presence of a band in the ethidium bromide-stained gel, corresponding to the projected size of the synthesized DNA fragment indicates that the selected DNA segment has been amplified. Identification of a specific HPV type is obtained by Southern blot and hybridization with specific probes.

B: The absence of a band suggests that no amplification has taken place. However a low copy number of amplified DNA segment (ie, less than 100 fg of viral DNA) is not visible in the stained gel. For complete confirmation it is necessary to use the Southern blot and hybridization technique.

C: A positive result after hybridization with a consensus probe indicates that the sample contains a HPV-DNA of unknown type or at least of the type complementary to the consensus primers. In order to specify the HPV type involved, it is necessary to dehybridize and hybridize again with type-specific oligonucleotide probes.

D: A negative result after hybridization with a consensus probe indicates that the sample contains no HPV-DNA homologous to the consensus probe.

E: A sample positive to a specific probe is proved to contain the corresponding HPV type. Dehybridization and hybridization with other HPV type-specific oligonucleotide probes is also suggested to eliminate the possibility that the sample contains more than one HPV type.

F: A sample negative to a specific probe does not contain the corresponding HPV type but it is not necessarily negative for other HPV types. Repeat sequential dehybridization and rehybridization with other specific oligonucleotide probes to precisely type the involved HPV.

The same procedure can be used for analysis of samples amplified with specific primers except that the ethidium bromide gel shows the presence of bands with a molecular weight specific for each HPV type in order to differentiate between two or more different HPV types in the same specimen.

References

1. Bancroft JD, Stevens A (Eds): Theory and practice of histological techniques. 2nd ed. Churchill Livingstone, Edinburgh, 1982.

2. Beckmann AM, Myerson D, Daling JR, Kiviat NB, Fenoglio CM, McDougall JK: Detection and localization of human papillomavirus DNA in human genital condylomas by in situ hybridization with biotinylated probes. *J Med Virol* 16:265–273, 1985.

3. Brahic M, Haase AT: Detection of viral sequences of low reiteration frequency by in situ hybridization. *Proc Natl Acad Sci* 75:6125–6129, 1978.

4. Brigati DJ, Myerson D, Leary JJ, Spalholz B, Travis SZ, Fong CKY, Hsiung GD, Ward DC: Detection of viral genomes in cultured cells and paraffin-embedded tissue sections using biotin-labeled hybridization probes. *Virology* 126:32–50, 1983.

5. Brigati DJ, Budgeon LR, Unger ER, et al: Immunocytochemistry is automated. The development of a robotic workstation based upon the capillary action principle. *J Histotechnol* 11:165–183, 1988.

6. Caussy D, Orr W, Daya AD, Roth P, Reeves W, Rawls W: Evaluation of methods detecting human papillomavirus deoxyribonucleotide sequences in clinical specimens. *J Clin Microbiol* 26:236–243, 1988.

7. Chaiet L, Wolf FJ: The properties of sterptavidin, a biotin binding protein produced by streptomyces. *Arch Biochem Biophys* 106:1–5, 1964.

8. Claas ECJ, Melchers WJG, Vanderlinden HC, Lindeman J, Quint WGV: Human papillomavirus detection in paraffin-embedded cervical carcinomas and metastases of the carcinomas by the polymerase chain reaction. *Am J Pathol* 135:697–702, 1989.

9. Cornelissen MT, van den Tweel JG, Struyk AP, Jebbink MF, Briet M, van der Noordaa J, ter Schegget JT: Localization of human papillomavirus type 16 DNA using the polymerase chain reaction in the cervix uteri of women with cervical intraepithelial neoplasia. *J Gen Virol* 70:2555–2562, 1989.

10. Czegledy J, Gergely L, Endrodi I: Detection of human papillomavirus deoxyribonucleic acid by filter in situ hybridization during pregnancy. *J Med Virol* 28:250–254, 1989.

11. Dallas PB, Flanagan JL, Nightingale BN, Morris BJ: Polymerase chain reaction for fast, nonradioactive detection of high- and low-risk papillomavirus types in routine cervical specimens and in biopsies. *J Med Virol* 27:105–111, 1989.

12. de Villiers, E-M, Schneider A, Miklaw H, Papendick U, Wagner D, Wesch H, Wahrendorf J, zur Hausen H: Human papillomavirus infections in women with and without abnormal cervical cytology. *Lancet* 703–706, 1987.

13. Del Mistro A, Braunstein JD, Halwer M, Koss LG: Identification of human papillomavirus types in male urethral condylomata acuminata by in situ hybridization. *Human Pathol* 18:936–940, 1987.

14. Demeter T, Kulski JK, Rakoczy P, Sterrett GF, Pixley EC: Detection of human papillomavirus DNA in cell scrapes and formalin-fixed, paraffin-embedded tissue for the uterine cervix by filter in situ hybridization. *J Med Virol* 26:397–409, 1988.

15. Erlich HA (Ed): PCR technology: Principles and application. Stockton Press. New York. 1989.

16. Fu YS, Braun L, Shah KV, Lawrence WD, Robboy SJ: Histologic, nuclear DNA, and human papillomavirus studies of cervical condylomas. *Cancer* 52:1705–1711, 1983.

17. Gall JG, Pardue ML: Formation and detection of RNA-DNA hybrid molecules in cytological preparations. *Proc Natl Acad Sci* 63:378–383, 1969.

18. Garuti G, Boselli F, Genazzani AR, Silvestri S, Ratti G: Detection and typing of human papillomavirus in histologic specimens by in situ hybridization with biotinylated DNA probes. *Am J Clin Pathol* 92:604–612, 1989.

19. Gissmann L, Durst M, Oltersdorf T, von Knebel Doeberitz M: Human papillomavirus and cervical cancer. In Steinberg BM, Brandsma JL, Taichman LB (Eds). Cancer Cells: Papillomaviruses, Cold Spring Harbor Laboratory, Cold Spring Harbor, NY. 1987:275–280.

20. Gregoire L, Arella M, Campione-Piccardo J, Lancaster WD: Amplification of human papillomavirus DNA sequences by using conserved primers. *J Clin Microbiol* 64:969–976, 1990.

21. Gupta JW, Saito K, Saito A, Fu YS, Shah KV: Human papillomaviruses and the pathogenesis of cervical neoplasia. A study by in situ hybridization. *Cancer* 64:2104–2110, 1989.

22. Gupta JW, Gupta PK, Rosenshein N, Shah KV: Detection of human papillomavirus in cervical smear. A comparison of in situ hybridization, immunohistochemistry and cytopathology. *Acta Cytol* 31:387–396, 1987.

23. Gupta J, Gendelman HE, Naghashfar Z, Gupta P, Rosenshein N, Sawada E, Woodruff JD, Shah K: Specific identification of human papillomavirus type in cervical smears and paraffin sections by in situ hybridization with radioactive probes: a preliminary communication. *Int J Gynecol Pathol* 4:211–218, 1985.

24. Haase AT, Stowring I, Harris JD, Traynor B, Ventura P, Peluso R, Brahic M: Visna DNA synthesis and the tempo of infection in vitro. *Virology* 119:399–410, 1982.

25. Hallam N, Gibson P, Green J, Charnock M: Detection and typing of human papillomavirus infection of the uterine cervix by dot blot hybridisation: comparison of scrapes and biopsies. *J Med Virol* 27:317–321, 1989.

26. Hrding U, Sebbelow A, Daugaard S, Bock JE, Norrild B: Filter in situ hybridization: an evaluation of the FISH technique for HPV detection in cervical swabs. *J Virol Methods* 24:123–130, 1989.

27. Impraim CC, Saiki RK, Erlich HA, Teplitz RL: Analysis of DNA extracted from formalin-fixed, paraffin-embedded tissues by enzymatic amplification and hybridization with sequence-specific oligonucleotides. *Biochem Biophys Res Comm* 142:710–716, 1987.

28. John H, Birnsteil ML, Jones KW: RNA-DNA hybrids at cytological levels. *Nature* 223:582–587, 1969.

29. Kiyabu MT, Shibata D, Arnheim N, Martin WJ, Fitzgibbons PL: Detection of human papillomavirus in formalin-fixed, invasive squamous carcinomas using the polymerase chain reaction. *Am J Surg Pathol* 13:221–224, 1989.

30. Kulski JK, Demeter T, Rakiczy P, Sterett GF, Pixley EC: Human papillomavirus coinfections of the vulva and uterine cervix. *J Med Virol* 27:244–251, 1989.

31. Kwok S, Higuchi R: Avoiding false positives with PCR. *Nature* 339:237–238, 1989.

32. Langer-Safer PR, Levine M, Ward DC: Immunological method for mapping genes on Drosophila polytene chromosomes. *Proc Natl Acad Sci* 79:4381–4385, 1982.

33. Lewis FA, Griffiths S, Dunnicliff R, Wells M, Dudding N, Bird CC: Sensitive in situ hybridization technique using biotin-streptavidin-polyalkaline phosphatase complex. *J Clin Pathol* 40:163–166, 1987.

34. Maniatis T, Fritsch EF, Sambrook J: Molecular cloning. A laboratory manual. Cold Spring Harbor Laboratory, Cold Spring Harbor, NY, 1982.

35. Manos MM, Ting Y, Wright DK, Lewis AJ, Broker TR, Wolinski SM: The use of polymerase chain reaction amplification for the detection of genital human papillomaviruses. In Furth M, Greaves M

(Eds); Cancer Cells: Molecular Diagnostics of Human Cancer 1989:209–214; Cold Spring Harbor Laboratory, Cold Spring Harbor, NY.

36. Manuelidis L, Langer-Safer PR, Ward DC: High resolution mapping of satellite DNA using biotin-labeled DNA probes. *J Cell Biol* 95:619–625, 1982.

37. McConaughty BL, Laird CD, McCarthy BJ: Nucleic acid reassociation in formamide. *Biochem* 8:3289–3295, 1969.

38. McDonnell PJ, McDonnell JM, Kessis T, Green WR, Shah KV: Detection of human papillomavirus type 6/11 DNA in conjunctival papillomas by in situ hybridization with radioactive probes. *Human Pathol* 18:1115–1119, 1987.

39. McManus FA: Histological demonstration of mucin after periodic acid. *Nature* 158:202, 1946.

40. McNicol PJ, Guijon FB, Paraskevas M, Brunham RC: Comparison of filter in situ deoxyribonucleic acid hybridization with cytologic, colposcopic, and histopathologic examination for detection of human papillomavirus infection in women with cervical intraepithelial neoplasia. *Am J Obstet Gynecol* 160:265–270, 1989.

41. Melchers WJ, Schift R, Stolz E, Lindeman J, Quint WG: Human papillomavirus detection in urine samples from male patients by the polymerase chain reaction. *J Clin Microbiol* 27:1711–1714, 1989.

42. Melchers W, van der Brule A, Walboomers J, de Bruin M, Burger M, Herbrink P, Meijet C, Lindeman J, Quint W: Increased detection rate of human papillomavirus in cervical scrapes by the polymerase chain reaction as compared to modified FISH and Southern-blot analysis. *J Med Virol* 27:329–335, 1989.

43. Mullink H, Walboomers JM, Raap AK, Meyer CJ: Two colour DNA in situ hybridization for the detection of two viral genomes using non-radioactive probes. *Histochemistry* 91:195–198, 1989.

44. Mullis KB: The unusual origin of the polymerase chain reaction. *Scientific American* 262:56–65, 1990.

45. Myerson D, Hackman RC, Meyers JD: Diagnosis of cytomegaloviral pneumonia by in situ hybridization. *J Infect Dis* 150:272–277, 1984.

46. Myerson D, Hackman RC, Nelson JA, Ward DC, McDougall JK: Widespread presence of histologically occult cytomegalovirus. *Human Pathol* 15:430–439, 1984.

47. Nagai N, Nuovo G, Friedman D, Crum CP: Detection of papillomavirus nucleic acid in genital precancers with the in situ hybridization technique. *Int J Gynecol Pathol* 6:366–379, 1987.

48. Nuovo GJ, Richart RM: Methods in Laboratory Investigation. A comparison of biotin- and ^{35}S-based in situ hybridization methodologies for detection of human papillomavirus DNA. *Laboratory Invest* 61:471–476, 1989.

49. Nuovo GJ, Richart RM: A comparison of slot blot, Southern blot, and in situ hybridization analyses for human papillomavirus DNA in genital tract lesions. *Obstet Gynecol* 74:673–678, 1989.

50. Nuovo GJ, Richart RM: Buffered formalin is the superior fixative for the detection of HPV DNA by in situ hybridization analysis. *Am J Pathol* 134:837–842, 1989.

51. Ostrow RS, Manias DA, Clark BA, Okagaki T, Twiggs LB, Faras AJ:

Detection of human papillomavirus DNA in invasive carcinomas of the cervix by in situ hybridization. *Cancer Res* 47:649–653, 1987.

52. Pao CC, Lin C-Y, Maa J-S, Lai C-H, Wu S-Y, Soong Y-K: Detection of human papillomaviruses in cervicovaginal cells using polymerase chain reaction. *J Infect Dis* 161:113–115, 1990.

53. Pardue ML: In situ hybridization. In Hames BD, Higgins SJ (Eds); Nucleic acid hybridization, A practical approach. IRL Press, Oxford, 1985:179–202.

54. Piper MA, Unger ER: Nucleic acid probes: A primer for pathologists. ASCP Press, Chicago. 1989.

55. Reid R, Fu YS, Herschman BR, Crum CP, Braun L, Shah KV, Agronov SJ, Stanhope CR: Genital warts and cervical cancer. VI. The relationship between aneuploid and polyploid cervical lesions. *Am J Obstet Gynecol* 150:189–199, 1984.

56. Richart RM, Nuovo GJ: Human papillomavirus DNA in situ hybridization may be used for the quality control of genital tract biopsies. *Obstet Gynecol* 75:223–226, 1990.

57. Rigby PW, Diekmann M, Rhodes C, Berg P: Labelling deoxyribonucleic acid to a high specific activity in vitro by nick translation with DNA polymerase I. *J Mol Biol* 113:237–251, 1977.

58. Saiki RK, Gelfand DH, Stoffell S, Scharf SJ, Higuchi R, Horn GT: Primer-directed enzymatic amplification of DNA with a thermostable DNA polymerase. *Science* 239:487–491, 1988.

59. Saiki RK, Scharf S, Faloona F, Mussis KB, Horn GT, Erlich HA, Arnheim N: Enzymatic amplification of B-globin genomic sequences and restriction site analysis for diagnosis of sickle cell anemia. *Science* 230:1350–1354, 1985.

60. Sambrook J, Fritsch EF, Maniatis T: Molecular cloning. A Laboratory manual. 2nd Ed. Cold Spring Harbor Laboratory, Cold Spring Harbor, NY, 1989.

61. Schmid CW, Jelish WR: The Alu family of dispersed repetitive sequences. *Science* 216:1065–1070, 1982.

62. Schneider A, Kraous H, Schuhmann R, Gissmann: Papillomavirus infection of the lower genital tract: Detection of viral DNA in gynecological swabs. *Int J Cancer* 35:443–448, 1985.

63. Schneider A, Sterzik K, Buck G, de Villiers E-M: Colposcopy is superior to cytology for the detection of early genital human papillomavirus infection. *Obstet Gynecol* 71:236–241, 1988.

64. Seligman AM, Hanker VS, Wasserkrug H, Dmochowski H, Katzoff L: Histochemical demonstration of some oxidized macromolecules with thiocarbohydrazide (TCH) or thiosemicarbazide (TSC) and osmium tetroxide. *J Histochem Cytochem* 13:629–639, 1965.

65. Shevchuck MM, Richart RM: DNA content of condyloma acuminatum. *Cancer* 49:489–492, 1982.

66. Shibata DK, Arnheim N, Martin WJ: Detection of human papilloma virus in paraffin-embedded tissue using the polymerase chain reaction. *J Exp Med* 167:225–230, 1988.

67. Shibata D, Fu YS, Gupta JW, Shah KV, Arnheim N, Martin WJ: Detection of papillomavirus in normal and dysplastic tissue by the polymerase chain reaction. *Laboratory Invest* 59:555–559, 1988.

68. Shibata D, Cosgrove M, Arnheim N, Martin WJ, Martin SE: Detection of human papillomavirus DNA in fine-needle aspirations of metastatic squamous-cell carcinoma of the uterine cervix using the polymerase chain reaction. *Diagn Cytopathol* 5:40–43, 1989.

69. Singer RH, Ward DC: Actin gene expression visualized in chicken muscle tissue culture using in situ hybridization with biotinated nucleotide analogs. *Proc Natl Acad Sci* 79:7331–7335, 1982.

70. Southern EM: Detection of specific sequences among DNA fragments separated by gel electrophoresis. *J Mol Biol* 98:503–517, 1975.

71. Sternberger LA: The unlabeled antibody peroxidase-antiperoxidase (PAP) method. In Immunocytochemistry, 2nd ed., John Wiley & Sons, NY, 1979:104–169.

72. Stoler MH, Broker TR: In situ hybridization detection of human papillomavirus DNAs and messenger RNAs in genital condyloma and a cervical carcinoma. *Human Pathol* 17:1250–1258, 1986.

73. Thiéry JP: Mise en évidence des polysaccharides sur coupes fines en microscopie électronique. *J Microscopie* 6:987–1018, 1967.

74. Tidi JA, Parry GCN, Ward P, Coleman DV, Peto J, Malcolm ADB, Farrell PJ: High rate of human papillomavirus type 16 infection in cytologically normal cervices. *Lancet* (8635):434, 1989.

75. Tidy JA, Mason WP, Farrell PJ: A new and sensitive method of screening for human papillomavirus infection. *Obstet Gynecol* 74:410–414, 1989.

76. Unger, ER, Budgeon LR, Myerson D, Brigati DJ: Viral diagnosis by in situ hybridization; Description of a rapid simplified colorimetric method. *Am J Surg Pathol* 10:1–8, 1986.

77. Unger ER, Brigati DJ, Chenggis ML, Budgeon LR, Koebler D, Cuono C, Kennedy T: Automation of in situ hybridization: Application of the capillary action robotic workstation. *J Histotechnol* 11:253–258, 1988.

78. van den Brule AJ, Claas EC, du Maine M, Melchers WJ, Helmerhorst T, Quint WG, Lindeman J, Meijer CJ, Walboomers JM: Use of anticontamination primers in the polymerase chain reaction for the detection of human papilloma virus genotypes in cervical scrapes and biopsies. *J Med Virol* 29:20–27, 1989.

79. Wagner D, Ikenberg H, Boehm N, Gissmann L: Identification of human papillomavirus in cervical swabs by deoxyribonucleic acid in situ hybridization. *Obstet Gynecol* 64:767–772, 1984.

80. Winkler B, Crum CP, Fujii T, Ferenczy A, Boon M, Braun L, Lancaster WD, Richart RM: Koilocytotic lesions of the cervix. The relationship of mitotic abnormalities to the presence of papillomavirus antigens and nuclear DNA content. *Cancer* 53:1081–1087, 1984.

81. Wu TC, Mounts P: Sensitive detection of nucleic acids and protein of human papillomavirus type 6 in respiratory and genital tract papillomata. *J Virol Methods* 25:31–47, 1989.

82. Young LS, Bevan IS, Johnsoon MA, Blomfield IL, Bromidge T, Maitland NJ, Woodman CB: The polymerase chain reaction: a new epidemiological tool for investigating cervical human papillomavirus infection. *Brit Med J* 298:14–18.

83. Yun K, Molenaar AJ, Wilkins RJ: Detection of human papillomavirus DNA in cervical lesions by in situ DNA hybridization. *Pathology* 21:1–4, 1989.

Rare Lesions of the Cervix

Rare cervical lesions include leimyoblastomas, leiomyosarcomas, rhabdomyosarcomas, angiosarcomas, fibrosarcomas, carcinosarcomas, malignant fibrous histiocytomas, malignant lymphomas, and melanomas. Histologically, these tumors are similar to those encountered in other sites. Cytologic recognition is difficult, mostly because of lack of experience, since only a few cases of each of these conditions have been reported. In general, cells from sarcomas tend to remain isolated on the smear and display bizarre shapes. Often the nuclei contain very prominent macronucleoli. Signs of differentiation may sometimes suggest the diagnosis: the presence of melanin pigment in malignant cells points towards a malignant melanoma. In most cases, however, while the diagnosis of malignancy is obvious, the type of neoplasm may not be accurately determined from the smear.

Further Reading

Abell MR, Ramirez JA: Sarcomas and carcinosarcomas of the uterine cervix. *Cancer* 31:1176–1192, 1973.

Bokun R, Perkovic M, Babotin J, Milasinovic D, Mojsovic D: Cytology and histopathology of metastatic malignant melanoma involving a polyp of the uterine cervix. *Acta Cytol* 29:612–615, 1985.

Brand E, Berek JS, Nieberg RK, Hacker NF: Rhabdomyosarcoma of the uterine cervix. Sarcoma botryoides. *Cancer* 60:1552–1560, 1987.

Chiu Yu H, Ketabibi M: Detection of malignant melanoma of the uterine cervix from Papanicolaou smears. *Acta Cytol* 31:73–76, 1987.

Harris NL, Scully RE: Malignant lymphoma and granulocytic sarcoma of the uterus and vagina. *Cancer* 53:2530–2545, 1984.

Izumi S, Hasegawa T, Tsutrsui F, Kurihara S: Carcinosarcoma of the uterus. *Acta Cytol* 29:602–606, 1985.

Massoni EA, Hajdu Sl: Cytology of primary and metastatic uterine sarcomas. *Acta Cytol* 28:93–100, 1984.

Retikas DG: Hodgkin's sarcoma of the cervix. *Gynecol* 80:1104–1107, 1960.

Taki I, Aozasa K, Kurobawa K: Malignant lymphoma of the uterine cervix. *Acta Cytol* 29:607–611, 1985.

Zaloudek CN, Norris HJ: Adenofibroma and adenosarcoma of the uterus. *Cancer* 48:354–366, 1981.

▣ Index

Numbers in **boldface** refer to pages on which illustrations appear.

C

C-myc oncogene, **133,** 166
C4–1, cell line, 123
Candida, **19,** 21, 39, **45,** 52, **60,** 249
Capillary loop, 195–196
Capsid antigen, of papillomavirus, **110,** 122, 126
Carcinogenesis
  animal, oncogene involvement in, **133**
  cervical, 22, 197
  genital, 166
  role of papillomavirus in, 119
Carcinoma, 53, 133–134, 165–169, 218, 327
  adenosquamous, 180–181
  cervical, 75–76, **90,** 119, 126, 128, 147–148, 166, 179, 183
  early invasive, squamous, **172–175**
  HPV isolation from, 123, 125, 131–132
Carcinoma in situ, (CIS), 17–18, **20,** 22, 149, 195, 217
CaSki, line of cervical cancer, 130, 314
Cell image analysis, **218–219**
Cell spread, 11, 13, 66–67, 110, 151
Centrocytes, in lymphocytic cervicitis, **61**
Cervical lesion(s), 18, 22, 119, 243, 252
  cryosurgery as treatment for, 198
  herpetic, **47–48**
  HPV in, 123, **126**
  intraepithelial, 147, 201
  squamous, association with adenocarcinoma, 179
Cervical neoplasia, 179
  association with HPV, 129, 195
  intraepithelial, grade 1 (CIN 1), **20,** 22, 148, 193
Cervical stenosis, 199, 201
Cervicitis, **20,** 52, 56, **61–62,** 169
Cervix, 1–**2,** 194, **198**
  cancer of, 75–76, 165–166
  infections in, 122, 125
  in pregnancy, 55, **66,** 202
  squamous lining of, 80, 56
Chemotherapy, **20,** 54, **65**
Chlamydia, **19,** 38
  endocervical cultures for, 194
  trachomatis, 38, **44,** 52, **60, 133**
Choriocarcinoma, 55
Chromatin, 2, 12, **79,** 168
CIN, 18, 148–149, 193, 195
CLASSVEE system, operating instructions, 227–235
Clinical menarche, 26
Cloning, molecular, of recombinant papillomavirus DNAs, 122
"Clue" cell(s), 38, **42**
Cocci, in "mixed" flora, 37, **41**
"Color index" (C.I.), of stains, 247
Colposcopy, 22, 193–194, 200, 202, 261
  diagnosing HPV infection, 82, 91
  HPV-type tests, 132
  investigation of abnormal Pap tests by, 197
Columnar epithelium, 2–**3, 10–11,** 74, **182,** 194, 252
Computerized reporting, 213–214, 227–235
Concretions, psammomalike, on smears, 7, **14**
Condyloma, 18, 85, 125
  acuminatum, 74, 89–**90,** 122–123, 166
  genital, detection and localization of HPV DNA in, 285
  sexual transmission of, 91

Condylomata, 120–121, 126, 128–129, **133, 195–196**
Conization, 190, 200–**201**
Consensus primers/probes, **312–314, 320**
Contraception/contraceptives, **20,** 27, 56, **133,** 147
Controls, 271, 295, 313–314
"Cornflakes", on smears, 251, **253**
Corynebacterium vaginalis, 38
Cryosurgery, 55, 91, 198–**199**
Curschmann's spirals, 251, **255**
Cyanophilic cytoplasm, **11,** 26, 149, 168
Cytology, 18, 38, 83, 200, 217, 219, 224
  biochemical/morphologic, 259
  exfoliative, 122, 132
  screening, for cervical intraepithelial lesions, 147
Cytolysis, **33,** 37, **41**
Cytomegalovirus, **19,** 40, 285
Cytometry, flow, 217–**218,** 219
Cytoplasm, **11, 13,** 181, **187,** 249, 264, 274
  of benign cells, changes due to chemotherapy, 54, **65**
  of cervical carcinomas, 167–168
  concentric striations, of invasive squamous carcinoma, **174**
  ground glass, in glassy cell carcinoma, 180
  hematoxylin stain of, **70**
  in LGSIL, 148
  mucin-containing, in AIS, 180
  of repair cells, 150
  orangeophilic, of dyskeratocytes, **76, 100**
  staining of, in HPV infection, **102**
Cytotrophoblast, 55, **67**

D

Decidualization, of cervix, during pregnancy, **66**
Dempster-Shafer evidential reasoning (UMS), 223
Denaturation, of DNA, 284, 300, 307, 309, **310–311**
Desmosomes, 2, **9,** 274
Diabetic nullipara, 226
Diathermy, for eradication of HPV lesions, 91
Diplococci, 38
DMBA (dimethylbenzenthracene) and malignancy of warts, **133**
DNA, 88–**90,** 132–**133,** 283, 302–303, 309–311, 314
  extraction, 296–**297,** 299, 303
  ploidy, 218, 225–226
  replication of, 130, 284
  sequence, 122, 125, 127–129, 261
Döderlein bacilli, **33,** 37
Dot blot, **89,** 132, 296–**297,** 299–**301,** 319
Dyskaryosis, 22
Dyskeratosis, 73–74, 79–80, **95**
Dyskeratotic cell(s), **100–101, 103, 108**
  in LGSIL, **93–94, 96, 99**
  in HGSIL with HPV infection, 85, **104–105**
Dysplasia, 17–18, 22, 54, 64, 76, 79, 148–149

E

E coli DNA polymerase I, 122, 288, 311
Electrodiathermy, 198–199
Electron microscopy (EM), 73–**78, 80–87,** 120, **126–127,** 274
Embedding media, 260–262, 274, 276–**277**
Endocervical
  canal, 1, **8,** 196, 199, 243

Immunoassays, enzyme-linked, diagnosis by, 38
Immunocytochemistry (IC), 90, 285
Immunocytology, 259
Immunofluorescence, techniques, disadvantages of, 267
Immunoglobulin, 266
Immunohistochemistry, 129, 132–**133**, 266–267, 270
Immunoperoxidase microscopy, 84, **268**
Immunoprecipitation analysis, 132
In situ hybridization (ISH), **111**, 129, 283–286, 289–292
"Indian files", **58,** 149, **152**
Intercellular bridges in keratinizing carcinomas, 166
Intermediate squamous cell, **11,** 26–27, **31–33, 66,** 249, 251, **253**
International Committee on Taxonomy of Viruses, 123
Intraepithelial lesion, 18, 52, **81–82, 85–87, 133–134,** 198
Intraepithelial neoplasia, 54, 125, 166
Involucrin, and keratinocyte pattern of synthesis, 125
IUD (Intrauterine device), 39, 56, 68, **197**

K
K562 cell line, 314
Karyolysis in HSV, 40
Karyopyknotic index, 29
Karyorrhectic nucleus, 52, 54, **65**
Karyorrhexis, 40, **76, 78, 99**
KB, cell line, HPV-18 in, 123
Keratin, 52, **101, 109,** 166, 249
Keratinization, 73, 79–80
    in carcinomas, 167–168
    in cells, **92–94, 174**
    in squamous epithelium, 52, **58–59**
    under PV stimuli, 129
Keratinocyte, 89, 125, 130–132
Keratoacanthoma, **90,** 125
Kinetics, reassociation, and papillomavirus nomenclature, 124
Koch's postulates, etiologic agent of cervical cancer, 166
Koilocyte, 76–78, 80–81, **99–100,** 122
Koilocytosis, 74–76, 82, **95,** 149
"Koilocytotic atypia", 75–76

L
Lactobacilli, 28, 37–38, **41**
Laryngeal papilloma, 120–123, 125, **133**
Laser therapy, 53, 91, 194, 200–201
Leiomyoblastoma/Leiomyosarcoma, 327
Leptothrix, 39, **43**
Lesion, 55, 84, 88–**90,** 128, 166, 194–196, 217
Leukocyte, 27, 38, 53, 168, 220
Leukoplakia, oral, **133**
LGSIL, **20,** 81–82, **92–97, 99,** 107, 148–149, **151**
Lymphocyte, 7, **14,** 52
    and inducing antigens, 267
    differentiation from small cell carcinoma, 168, **175**
Lymphocytic cervicitis, **14, 61**
Lymphogranuloma venereum, 38
Lymphoma, 52, 54, 327

M
Macrocytosis, 53–54, **63–65**
Macronuclei in clear cell carcinoma, 181
Macronucleolus, 53, **63,** 168, 181, **187**

Macrophage, 7, **14,** 52, **61**
Malignancy, 17, 54, **90,** 123, 166, 169, 193
Melanoma, **90,** 125, 327
Menstrual cycle, 26–27, **30–32**
Metaplasia, immature, differentiated from HGSIL, 150
Metaplastic cell, 51–52, **60,** 252
Microcomputer systems, 214–215
Microconvolution, 195, 197
Microinvasion, 196, **198, 201**–202
Microinvasive carcinoma, 167–168, **170–172**
Microscopy, (See also Electron microscopy), 84, 259–260
microTICAS system, 224
Microvillosities in koilocytes, **77–78**
Mitochondria, **79,** 274
Mitosis, 2, 53, 166
Mixed association
    anisokaryosis in, **106**
    cellular (HPV and HGSIL), 87–88
    HGSIL and HPV infection, **103–105, 108–109**
Miyagawanella, 38
Molecular hybridization, 83, 90, 121–122, 284
Monoclonal antibodies, diagnosis by, 38
Morphology in prediction of disease outcome, 18
Mosaicism, **196–197**
Mucoepidermoid tumor, 180
Mucosa, **90,** 119, 219
Mucus, 3, 51, 55, 252
    inspissated, 7, 251, **255**
    reaction to stains, 264, 266
Multinucleation, 7, **13, 63, 67**
Myc oncogene, and HPV, 128
Mycelia, 39, 45
MYCIN certainty factors (UMS), 223

N
Naboth's eggs, 3
Nabothian cysts, in normal transformation zone, 194
"Navicular" cell, 28
"Nearocarcinoma", 75
Neisseria gonorrhoeae, 38, **133**
Neoplasia, **133,** 165–166, 179, 327
Neural network, 223, 226–227
"Nick translation", 288, 292
Nuclear/cytoplasmic ratio (N/C ratio), 150, 244
Nucleic acids, 121, 283, 309
Nucleoli, 168, **172–173, 184–185**
Nucleus, 77–79, **85, 127,** 129, 169, 194
    "naked", 37
    of repair cells, 150
    reaction to stains, 249, 264, 266, 290
    sarcoma, 327

O
Oligonucleotide, **310,** 312
Oncogene, 130, **133**
Open reading frames (ORF), 127–128, 166
Organelles, **78,** 260, 274
Ovarian function and cytohormonal smear, 27

P
Palmar myrmecia, HPV isolation from, 125
Papanicolaou, **13,** 17, **19,** 193